Krav Maga

Krav Maga

Use Your Body as a Weapon

Boaz Aviram

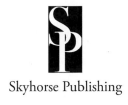

Skyhorse Publishing

Skyhorse Publishing books may be purchased in bulk at special discounts for sales promotion, corporate gifts, fund-raising, or educational purposes. Special editions can also be created to specifications. For details, contact the Special Sales Department, Skyhorse Publishing, 307 West 36th Street, 11th Floor, New York, NY 10018 or info@skyhorsepublishing.com.

Skyhorse® and Skyhorse Publishing® are registered trademarks of Skyhorse Publishing, Inc.®, a Delaware corporation.

Visit our website at www.skyhorsepublishing.com.

10 9 8 7 6 5 4 3

Library of Congress Cataloging-in-Publication Data is available on file.

Cover design by Richard Rossiter

ISBN: 978-1-62873-612-0
E-book ISBN: 978-1-62914-017-9

Printed in China

ACKNOWLEDGMENTS

I am deeply grateful to all those who contributed to this book.

I especially wish to thank:

Sgt. Major Eli Avikzar, RIP, Immi's successor in the Israeli Defense Forces and my Krav Maga instructor.

Sgt. Major Immi Lichtenfeld, RIP, the first Israeli Defense Forces head of Krav Maga and its creator. He was my friend and training advisor.

Sgt. Pablo Dreispiel (Eli Avikzar's deputy chief). He was my first Krav Maga instructor in the Israeli Defense Forces.

Lt. Col. Giora Cohen and Lt. Col. David Gerstein. They supported me when I was the head of Krav Maga in the IDF.

Raanan Pshigoda and Col. David Ben Asher. They supported me in my Krav Maga career.

My son Brandon Taelor Aviram. He took the pictures for this book.

My friend Steven Hartov. He encouraged me and guided me with my project of writing this book.

My student Tomasz Jeziorski. He modeled in the pictures.

My neighbor Ruben Serrano. He participated in the defense vs. multiple opponent pictures.

My father Col. Harry Aviram and my mother Shoshana Aviram.

CONTENTS

FOREWORD

Throughout history, law enforcement has been successful in curbing crime, but never in completely destroying it. In modern democracies, though adult citizens have the right to pursue life, liberty, and happiness, any day could still turn into a life or death confrontation in an instant.

Just as individuals have the right to vote, they should also have the right to control their fate. Many times false perceptions lead to bad habits. As a result of living in a civil environment, our survival skills are being suppressed.

While we rely on trained professionals in many aspects of our lives, we should also be able to resort to the basics if everything else fails. This book shows readers how to use their bodies in a physical confrontation.

In a real-life survival fight, one cannot afford to simply exchange blows to see who can take more than the other. A methodical way to react to danger and to eliminate it is achieved through intensive Krav Maga training. For a skilled Krav Maga fighter, it should not take more than a few seconds to end the fight and survive. The starting point of Krav Maga is the realization that if you finish your opponent, you finish the fight. In modern society, the preference would be to avoid such extremes, but if you want to live, you need to consider this option at all times. A thorough analysis may reveal that in certain scenarios this is your only option.

Krav Maga was the official self-defense and hand-to-hand combat system of the Israeli Defense Forces (IDF) from its inception. The name comes from the Hebrew words *Krav* for fight and *Maga* for contact. The first IDF Krav Maga chief instructor was Imrich Lichtenfeld (Immi Sde-Or). Second was Eli Avikzar, and I was third.

The Krav Maga approach to fighting is a result of comprehensive analysis of all the dangerous elements that are involved in a confrontation scenario. To master control over your body for the purpose of self-defense, you need to identify the situation, identify the most immediate threat, and instantly overcome it using your body. Learning the principles of Krav Maga will give you the tools required to prevail.

The most important contribution this book can make is to give you the security and calm in life that is the basis for excelling in any other field—as Immi used to say: "So may one walk in Peace."

The book is for anyone who feels the need to hone his self-defense skills, or just get a thorough understanding of the split-second process. Students, instructors, civilians, military, and law enforcement personnel would all benefit from it. It is recommended for judiciary system officials as well, for a clearer understanding of the mechanism behind successful self-defense processes, to help better serve communities, and constituents.

While I did not intend for this book to be used by those in the fields of sports or entertainment I realized it would be a great source to well-known professional boxing trainers and mixed martial arts fighters. Superior fighting knowledge might end a fight sooner than expected. To have full control in a street fight, you must be able to see all the combat options and prioritize what takes the minimum amount of time. The same applies to fighting sports, except some of them have fewer dangers, and therefore allow additional tactics. Learning Krav Maga could help athletes make sense of what they are doing and how to do it better. An audience might see less pain, less sweat, and more knockouts. I believe that once you can easily perceive the basic elements of your activities, you can then excel in them.

Krav Maga was designed to provide training methods with optimal self-defense capabilities while maintaining strict safety during training. The key to this system is the correct hierarchy of prioritization! However, the Krav Maga known outside the military is not the IDF Krav Maga, but another form of martial arts marketed to civilians.

Modern martial arts generally have rules that make it very difficult for fighters to kill each other in an instant. They provide social activity, entertainment for spectators, and a controlled release of violence. When the student is engulfed in this environment, he becomes part of it and it becomes part of him.

While martial arts, boxing, and wrestling provide some help in overcoming fear, they very seldom give students an ability to control their opponents in hand-to-hand combat scenarios. Martial arts and fighting sports have rules that were designed to reduce injury. Some non-competitive martial arts geared toward combat have proven hard to learn due to a lack of communication that may have persisted over generations.

The Israeli underground forces had to train their members in hand-to-hand combat. Carrying weapons was restricted under British rule and access to weapons was limited anyway. Daily risk was confronted with the stick fighting method, based on sword-dueling techniques. As members of underground organizations gathered, they used sports fighting skills as part of their training. As the IDF was established, the need for a systematic uniform training system arose. Immi was chosen to implement the system because of his superior skills.

By observing animals we can see how they use their bodies for hunting and survival. Cubs hone their hunting and survival skills through wrestling their parents. The human race, over the years, has concentrated its resources on devising weapons. In the old world, it was essential to learn how to use each handheld weapon for hunting and fighting. In the new world, however, as technology gave advantage, most military battles were won with large, high-tech weapons.

Throughout the historical development of fighting weapons, there were certain scenarios where hand-to-hand combat was needed to bridge gaps in a fight for personal survival. Wars were not won through hand-to-hand combat, but while many lives were saved because of it, the confidence of those trained increased.

Soldiers could see that there were scenarios that would limit the use of a particular weapon, due, perhaps, to a malfunction or to other obstacles in the environment. This would require resorting to hand-to-hand fighting. Just being prepared would reduce their anxiety and increase their confidence.

Let's face it, whether armed soldier or policeman, there could be a moment that your weapon does not work. In that moment you are reduced to a civilian who has to fight with his bare hands to save his life. The least a military organization can do for its members when sending soldiers on a life and death mission is to teach them life-protecting skills.

Historians can look at piles of bones and ancient wall drawings and conclude that in each era, humans were fighting according to their anatomy. If they walked low to the ground, they tended to fight that way with more ease. Often they needed to support their bodies with more than their legs.

It might have been more comfortable for them to grab and wrestle their opponents. When able to stand erect, they used their hands to strike and legs to kick. In the later stages of development, they could pick a log of wood and strike their prey as well as their opponents. They could use their environment by smashing their opponent's head on rocky ground. They used their intelligence to devise weapons. Techniques used for hunting were tried on enemies.

Krav Maga is a systematic approach of prioritizing the most critical components of hand-to-hand combat scenarios. The objective of controlling an opponent in the split second he is in range is key to the process. By learning pressure points and effective manipulation techniques, trained individuals gain the advantage they need to succeed in hand-to-hand combat. Techniques include striking, kicking, pressuring, tearing, blocking, deflecting, and using leverage on the body as needed.

The reaction time principle must be considered at all times to ensure no early arrivals for our opponent, and no late departures for us. In Krav Maga, students learn principles through techniques for each possible range of fighting from three body positions: standing, lying, and sitting.

While the objective of self-defense is not to get hurt, the top priority in training is learning to identify scenarios where one needs to kill before being killed. By learning to assess the possible outcome and intensity of various dangers, students learn to develop sound judgment and awareness which can instantly be applied without hesitation.

Krav Maga students cover self-defense and hand-to-hand combat principles in an intense learning environment. The instruction method is crucial to ensure that at the end of the short program (three days to two weeks), each of the trainees has the ability to fight with his bare hands and win.

Additional two-week training is required to qualify as an instructor. At the end of the Krav Maga instructor's course, the student is required to participate in a series of full-contact fights where he is graded on his ability to execute his learning skills, and develop confidence in his ability.

In addition, Krav Maga instructor candidates are assigned to teach a few classes and are evaluated and corrected on their ability to meet the teaching objectives. This time is also used to facilitate repetition, rehearsing the material learned.

Krav Maga techniques are taught in steps where complex motion, principles, correct sequential execution, and best tactical solutions are demonstrated first, then broken down and simplified, and then put back together and allied with sparring drills.

Students need to fully understand all aspects of their training, and should practice each step about ten times in a prescribed order. The correct order is designed to instill a chain reaction with body parts moving in the correct sequence that will save the student's life in threatening scenarios. Instructor corrections instill effective techniques and give the students tools to assess and correct their techniques.

Once the training methods and process have been set to provide maximum reality and minimum injury, students need to be exposed to reality and learn to overcome the obstacle. The sparring drills are designed to test, reinforce, and correct the way students apply principles in a hand-to-hand combat scenario. This is the most essential section of the training process.

LESSONS FROM HISTORY

Before gunpowder and automatic weapons were developed, hand-to-hand combat was a key fighting method for armies. Weapons served as an extension of the hand, facilitating a small movement and extending soldiers' reach.

Assume that you were a handgun instructor and your assignment was to train a person to fight a pistol duel. The most realistic approach would be to have a competition and see who would live and who would die, but that defeats the purpose. If you have advanced body armor for the students, you could have them shoot each other and determine who shot first. You must consider that protective gear would have limiting effects on speed of reaction and field of vision. If you did not have body armor, you might use air pistols with protective goggles.

The advantage of using a pistol is the split-second result you get when pointing it at your opponent and pulling the trigger. Self-defense is a more involved process, and even if you happen to have a pistol in your possession, there are scenarios where it would be useless.

It is obvious that various guns have different weight, accuracy, and range. Lighter guns are faster to draw. It would be best if you could mimic the exact scenario while training in order to succeed in combat. Instead we practice with shooting targets. In combat shooting, the time it takes to hit the target is what's measured.

The accuracy can be seen on the target. We compare the speed of drawing from one student to the other, and determine which one was faster. If we see

that each one is consistent with his results, we assume that the student with the faster draw and accuracy would kill the one without.

But for the question of how to teach people to improve their accuracy and speed, the answer would be training with the right technique. The proper technique is one that conserves movement. If you do less, you are quicker. In instinctive pistol shooting, it takes a few hours of training for the shooter to learn to draw and shoot thrice in less than 1.2 seconds.

Repetition creates habits. If we start repeating something before we learn the right technique, we're not only wasting our time but also creating a bad habit. That takes up further time. A better idea is to get it right the first time before repeating it again and again. Gunfighting is not a game. It is a life or death experience.

Imagine you have to teach someone good swordsmanship, or hand-to-hand fighting. Hopefully, you would teach them techniques that show you value their life as much as you do your own. The likelihood of them using these techniques in real life is small, but you would still want to feel your instruction is worth it and watch them succeed.

While reading the following overview of the history of weapons in combat, I would like you to think of the training methods that were used.

Non-gunpowder weapons varied throughout history. Egyptian carvings dating back to 1200 BC show sport fencing with protective gear and judges. The Greek and Roman civilizations favored short swords and light spears. The collapse of the Roman Empire around 476 AD brought heavy weapons from barbarian invaders. Guns eventually replaced the bow and arrow. In the 14th century, lighter swords were brought back since gunpowder made heavy armor obsolete.

In the 15th century, dueling to death was popular in Europe. In the 18th and 19th centuries, the legal system made dueling more of a contest than a fight.

In the 16th century, with the development of print, there was a great increase in fencing treatises—sword-fighting books written by teachers, and paid for by noblemen. In some cities, carrying swords was forbidden for obvious reasons.

Since modern societies don't allow swords, there is not much use in learning swordsmanship for hand-to-hand fighting. Stick fighting however has techniques taken from fencing, and could be extended to objects other than swords, such as rifles.

The need for local farms to protect their properties and lives, for authorities to enforce the law, and unfortunately for criminals to succeed in their crime all led to a stronger development of the martial arts. Militaries, too, realized that there are always gaps in fighting methods, and despite having weapons, a soldier might sometimes need to resort to using his bare arms to fight.

In almost every part of the world hand-to-hand combat has existed in one form or another. If we look into the historical context of hand-to-hand combat, we can identify various patterns. The first pattern we see is that there were elements of combat-tested techniques modified in civilian sports. This may have been the result of teachers looking for simple, injury-proof training methods for young children, or of governments enforcing penalties, or of the commercializing of these arts, which watered down their lethal elements.

There are two methods of delivering a blow. First is a boxing-like movement, and the second is the traditional karate strike. While equal in force, the boxing-style strike has a greater range and is easier to execute. The boxing-style strike uses gravity and shift of weight to support the strike, while the traditional karate-style strike uses a sudden tightening of your body's muscles to deliver a short blow. The longer range of the boxing blow facilitates greater acceleration to a higher speed and is more efficient in creating a knockout effect. The traditional karate-style strike is more suitable for breaking boards of wood, but the composition of wood fibers is quite different from the human body's protective tissues. The traditional straight karate strike takes longer to execute and requires slight preparation. Since even a split second is of the essence and the force used is more efficient with the boxing style, it has won popularity in the martial arts field.

From the split second you decide to move your body and deliver the strike, all you need is to aim at the opponent's chin. You then need to accelerate your arm to maximum speed, and maintain that speed as your fist lodges in your opponent's face. The opponent's skull will then shake the brain and nerves to a concussion.

The ancient Olympics had fighting sports. Sparta is believed to have had boxing around 500 BC. Spartans used boxing to strengthen their fighters' resilience. Boxing matches were not held since Spartans feared that it would lead to internal competitions, which could reduce the morale of the losers. Sparta did not want low morale on the battlefield.

For many years the question of Bodhidharma's existence has been a matter of controversy among historians. A legend prevails that the evolution of karate began around 5 BC when Bodhidharma arrived to the Shaolin temple in China from India, and taught Zen Buddhism. He introduced a set of exercises designed to strengthen the mind and body. This marked the roots of Shaolin-style temple boxing. This type of Chinese boxing, also called kung fu, concentrates on full-body energy blows and improving acrobatic level. Indian breathing techniques are incorporated, providing control of the muscles of the whole body while striking. This promotes self-resistance that helps achieve balance and force when striking and kicking. Krav Maga shows that it is not the most efficient approach. It is certainly forceful, but cannot be mastered quickly enough, and also does not promote a natural and fast reach to the opponent's pressure points, nor does it adhere to the principle of reaction time.

In fact, Shaolin kung fu considered boxing-style strikes and what are known today as karate-style strikes as well. But the method of force used for the impact involved total muscle tension orchestrated by blowing out air rather than the gravity acceleration principle used in Krav Maga. For some reason, lunging with the attack was not perfected to a simple lunge, but instead to a more complicated jump or rollover. It appears they were not able to apply the concept of timing to the most efficient way of lunging forward. Perhaps they saw the need to make the body resilient, not knowing why people get hit even after training. Not being able to prioritize training with reaction time, but rather making the body more resilient, would probably not work in case of a very sharp object. Instead, they tackled many problems and aspects of fighting without prioritizing.

Karate, originally known as Kenpo in China, crossed to Okinawa, and changed its name. Karate became a competition sport in the beginning of the 20th century.

Breaking boards, ice blocks, glass bottles, and acrobatic performance with weapons were used to exhibit self-defense. Semi-contact and full-contact sparring competitions were held too. In China, fights in local villages were held as a form of display to attract challengers, prospective students, and potential instructors. In the west, sport competitions provided publicity and reputations for atheletes as well.

The development of Chinese boxing to karate in Okinawa, to Kyokushin, which is full-contact karate, shows the transformation of self-practiced hand techniques into full-contact sports karate. Many Korean martial arts have elements of Japanese martial arts, and it is believed that their founders took seminars in Japan at some point of their training.

In comparing karate and Krav Maga, we notice various differences. In traditional karate, the advance forward has the rear foot sliding forward from a low dip stance into a forward dip. When comparing straight punches in boxing and in Krav Maga, there are two major differences. First, take into account the limitations of reaction time. The punch is lunged into the opponent's face as the gap is closed, before the front foot has landed. Second, training in Krav Maga separates the retraction of the hand and stresses that the body should never come to a centered position to help with a quick linear motion backwards. Instead, Krav Maga recommends staying in this newly angled stance until students recognize what needs to be done next to end the fight. Fortunately, this also helps finish the punch and ensure the full body weight has shifted to the desired direction before rushing to the next punch. If the speed is kept at its maximum at the time of the blow, this ensures a knockout!

Closing the distance to reach an opponent, karate fighters are taught to lunge their rear leg for a kick as their upper bodies remain static. They are taught to contract their abdomen and hip muscles as they send their hands and legs for a blow.

The way the foot or hand makes contact with the opponent's pressure point depends on how it fits the targeted part of the body. For example, the shin or open hand for the groin, the ball of the foot or open hand to the chin, the heel or palm to the sternum, the knife side of the foot, or extended fingers for the throat.

Krav Maga fighters close the gap by pushing their toes and shifting their weight forward. They are trained to pivot their torso for greater reach. Lunging forward, they kick with their front foot and land on their rear foot. The momentum of the kick is being generated with gravity as they throw the ball of the foot in their opponent's groin or torso in an upward motion (depending on the availability).

The speed is kept at its peak by swinging the leg to ninety degrees. The contact point of the foot should preferably be the heel or ball of the foot. The ankle should be kept in a neutral position upon contact, so the ligaments are not in an overstretched position. This is a safety feature that will minimize trauma upon contact with the opponent's bones.

When executing hand strikes, karate fighters utilize the same advance motion they use for kicking. All the muscles in the body are tightened during the strike, and the hand is swung from under the armpit forward, as the torso is kept static. The strike ends with a release of breath followed by a scream, in an attempt to deliver all the "energy" to the opponent's body.

In the Krav Maga hand strike, the only tightened muscles are those of the forearm and fist. The body lunges forward, initiated by the push of the rear foot's toes. The weight is shifted forward by pivoting towards the direction of the strike. As the body springs to close the gap from a walking stance to a forward lunge, the front hand is extended with a complete torso twist, creating an arm-and a shoulder-length range.

The body reaches its maximum twist where one shoulder is behind the other, towards the direction of the opponent. The hand is retracted back, in front of the body, while the body continues in a forward motion, nearing a complete stop a split second after the hand has been completely retracted. This sequential motion facilitates maximum body weight to support momentum during contact.

The retraction of the hand allows maximum speed and range during the contact. A complete stop is caused by an initial slowdown before the contact. The motion of the legs allows for maximum speed and ease in reaching the target, with the least muscle energy consumption. It can be executed easily with full force during physical exertion or calm.

English boxing is rooted in the 18th century and French boxing in the early 19th century. Ba Gua Zhan (Chinese Fighting System) was popular in the 19th century. Taiji is an offshoot of Ba Gua Zhan used for exercise and meditation. We can see the same pattern in America where Tai-Bo was derived from Muay-Thai (Thai boxing). When used for exercise, arms and legs mimic combat techniques to induce rapid heartbeat. However, most physical fitness instructors do not see the need to understand what the correct fighting techniques should be.

Greco-Roman wrestling was first known in the 18th century. The term was created for athletic activity in connection with ancient Greek and Roman fighting competitions. "Wrestling" became a western word used to define any kind of unarmed fight.

Japanese records tracing back to 24 BC suggest that one of the emperors ordered two men to wrestle in his presence, so we can date wrestling's origins to a time long before it became part of Greco-Roman culture. According to the story they fought mainly through kicking. One survived and even as his opponent broke his ribs and fell to the ground, the winner kept kicking him to death.

Documentation shows the founding of an old jujitsu school during the middle of the 16th century. In the middle of the 17th century, cultural exchanges between China and Japan by means of immigration caused a debate as to the source of striking and kicking techniques. For many years, Japanese jujitsu was perfected, lacking blows and kicks.

Jujitsu consists of throwing, striking, choking, joint breaking, and the use of small weapons. For soldiers in a tight space, short daggers facilitated the development of a related grappling system.

If I had to comment on the reason Japanese jujitsu did not have many blows and kicks, I would think it was to find a more socially acceptable form of wrestling in Japan.

In any form of civilian fighting, defense and offense were carried on until the opponent surrendered. The name jujitsu was used in Japan to describe any wrestling confrontation. It was first introduced to Europe at the end of the 19th century.

In Japan, families living on farms trained their guards to protect their lives and property. Agricultural tools were often used as weapons. The first hand-to-hand combat documented in Japanese history was named Daito-Ryu. It was followed by consequent systems such as jujitsu, aikijitsu, judo and aikido.

For many years Japan was divided into kingdoms and clans while the Samurai served as the knights of the ruler. The Samurai had followed their code of honor called the Bushido.

Bujutsu (loosely translated as "science of war" or "martial art") is the general Japanese term for fighting systems taught to the Samurai, using the body and the weapons which were available at the time. They learned to use the sword, the shield, and the bow as major weapons. After the Samurai class disbanded, some used this system in crime. Schools in various weapon-fighting systems opened to teach bow-shooting, sword-fighting, or jujitsu.

When learning self-defense techniques in jujitsu, the general approach is to stop the threat and bring the opponent to the ground. This approach is time consuming, and could also open up an opportunity for other attackers to overpower a defender.

Additionally, the jujitsu approach is to block a weapon, a strike, or a kick with a pliers-like grip using two hands, continued by a throw to the ground. Using two hands for every block is not the most efficient and convenient move since it does not facilitate a simultaneous counterattack. Therefore, it is definitely not the answer for a continuous or repeated attack.

In a battlefield full of swarming enemy soldiers and their swords, it would not be a good idea to waste time trying to throw an opponent to the ground and then choking him. The same thought applies to the street, where you may have to fight multiple opponents. You do not want to stay more than two seconds in the same place. This makes you wonder if today's jujitsu could be a result of a system watered down by civilians, where a few generations of instructors had concentrated on safe throws and breaking falls. To answer their students questions on how to apply it back to self-defense, they tried to reconstruct the training system but to no avail.

A few of the descendants of Samurai families and other instructors opened schools for the martial arts. They realized that most of their students were young adults with local families. The jujitsu training methods developed in the Japanese dojos were sufficient entertainment for students. When students visited other jujitsu schools they knew what to expect.

The Samurai era was over, and no one was carrying swords. While sword-fighting techniques were often applied to fighting with bare hands, they did not provide optimum balance. Since past swordsmanship training methods were limited to agreed-upon attack and defense drills designed to limit training injuries, as these training methods were being applied to hand-to-hand fighting jujitsu, they did not see the necessity of new training methods.

Jigoro Kano, born to a wealthy family, studied jujitsu when he was young and developed his own techniques. He was dedicated to reforming jujitsu, integrating it with mental and physical education. In 1882, at age 23, he called his system judo. He formed the Kodokan, Japan's judo institution, and integrated judo as the national sport approved by the ministry of education.

As a sport, the deadly techniques were extracted, and the soft techniques were perfected. According to Jigoro Kano, "you force your opponent to make his body rigid and lose his balance, and when he is helpless, you attack."

The rules in judo were designed to allow getting a grip of only your opponent's clothes. Judo practitioners were given the chance to perfect their ability by throwing each other to the ground in a safe environment. Gripping just the sleeve and the lapel, you twist your opponent's torso shifting his weight onto one leg, out of balance, and it becomes easier to trip or throw him down.

In judo, you are allowed to lift your opponent onto your hips or shoulders and throw him to the ground, or to tilt his weight to one leg and sweep him off the ground. This can be done by changing directions while pulling the opponent toward you. A clean throw, where the opponent falls clean on his back, wins a judo match.

To promote safety and avoid injuries in this sport, students would learn to break a fall before being thrown to the mat. Judo is now a modern Olympic sport.

In judo, athletes attempt to first shake their opponents off balance, always redirecting the opponent's resistance. This has to be decisive and the throw should take two seconds. Hesitation allows the opponent to gather counter-resistance, and the initiating athlete will then need to immediately look for another angle.

There are various judo ground holds which are designed to keep your opponent's shoulders on the ground. As your opponent tries to get out of the hold, you shift your weight and counter his force in a new direction. If he gets out of this hold, you grab him again in the nearest gripping position available.

If you hold your opponent on the ground for twenty-five seconds, you get a point as well. Arm-bars or chokeholds leading to your opponent's surrender can also be a winning strategy.

Throwing an opponent to the ground as opposed to striking or kicking them is common in other martial arts. When used in self-defense, you may buy time before finishing him on the ground, but try to end it as quickly as possible.

The Russian version of judo, Sambo, originates from the early 20th century. The originator spent six years training at the Kodokan. Upon returning to Russia, he taught the Red Army and the secret police judo. Judo was converted to Sambo in the 1930s. Russian Sambo is a mix of judo, wrestling, and jujitsu, where athletes wear the judo top with wrestling tights. The suit top is used to hold contact with the opponent, and the bare legs for grabbing in a wrestling style.

Brazilian jujitsu was created at the beginning of the twentieth century. In traditional judo, you first throw your opponent to the ground and then restrain him with a chokehold or an arm-bar. In Brazilian jujitsu, the training system explores other possibilities, although only within the realm of holding the opponent's judogi. Recently they added grappling training without the judo-gi as they geared their fighters to participate in mixed martial arts competitions. In Brazil, the word jujitsu was used for all martial arts. The Brazilian Jujitsu Association is actually a Brazilian Judo Association.

Brazilian jujitsu athletes have competed in mixed martial arts tournaments where light strikes are occasionally permissible. However, it appears that none of the participants had any great skill in punching and kicking, since neither resulted in a knockout. Not knowing how to fight in the kicking or punching range forces judo opponents to close the gap and "fight" from a closer range. However, if one of your opponents knows how to end the fight in a longer range, close-range fighters may never get a chance to employ their knowledge. Rules restricting soft pressure points in sports fighting promote tactical gaps that jeopardize athletes in self-defense scenarios.

In 1927 Morihei Ueshiba created his own training method, the aikido. He was a senior Daito-ryu student who decided to leave the system and create his own discipline, aiming to demonstrate the movement of the universe as a combination of martial arts and religious training.

Aikido techniques consist of manipulating the bones of the human body. Practitioners use evasive defense moves and counterattacks on the opponent's wrists or neck. A simple yet effective manipulation of the wrist can lead to a throw to the ground.

With techniques borrowed from sword-fighting, aikido engages the arm or leg of the attacker with a circular body and arm motion to redirect the attacker's force before he has a chance to resist. The opponent can be thrown to the ground with a wrist, neck, or leg manipulation. Once the opponent develops resistance, the aikido master suddenly throws the attacker into a new direction.

Aikido is not a competitive sport and not a true form of self-defense either. It is marketed by some associations and instructors as a form of self-defense, although its creator really intended for it to be an art for itself.

Once you have been gripped by a determined aikido professional, your chances of surviving are slim to none. However it is very hard for an aikido professional to catch a kick or a punch that is not projected. Their movement is very coordinated, but too slow for shadow boxing.

Aikido training takes a long time to complete. During the training, students develop extraordinary coordination and great skills to predict attacks. Aikido techniques are great once in reach. However, they often fail against a skilled attacker if he does not project his attack.

The aikido sword technique is precise and powerful, but based on a slow and controlled motion. A jab with a wooden stick or a slash with a fencing sword would leave the aikido professional helpless.

The training method emphasizes defensive moves. A school cannot train its students well in defense if it does not provide challenging attacks. Attack moves need to be perfect so that defense is strengthened.

Aikido techniques promote an evasive circular motion while the defender is positioned behind the attacker's back. A linear motion is faster than a circular motion.

An aikido fighter would try to counter a boxer's jab by grabbing his wrist and executing a full body pivot, but the boxer could retract his hand quickly and stop the whole motion right there. This allows the boxer to attack again, in the direction the aikido fighter is moving. If the aikido would try to counter a speedy retracting kick, he might find himself out of balance without sufficient time to recuperate.

For aikido to be a realistic form of martial art, hand strikes, preferably in the Krav Maga style, should be utilized during the defense training to facilitate maximum attack speed. Aikido practitioners who attempt to learn Krav Maga may realize that many of their techniques and principles have to go through major changes.

Since the human body weighs more than the hand, years of aikido training would not be sufficient to move it fast enough out of the way of a boxing jab or a wrist whip delivering a stick blow. A successful initial engagement would hardly ever facilitate a full move of the body behind a well-trained attacker.

While aikido techniques could prove deadly, they do not provide enough safety in self-defense and hand-to-hand combat scenarios, especially against a quick and unanticipated attack.

The constant break in motion with an average of at least three to four directional changes per technique surpasses the human reaction time. This puts the aikido practitioner in danger subject to a quick strike or a kick from his initial opponent and any others that may be in the area.

Aikido is a great art. Practitioners allow one another's bodies to be manipulated and thrown around in various directions using gravity and common sense.

If we try to adapt aikido into a complete self-defense method, we cannot ignore human reaction time, and therefore we cannot allow inefficient moves that take more than two seconds and give our opponent an opportunity to recuperate and plan another attack. We do not wish to leave the outcome to chance.

We may want to look at its source in order to understand why a great master would create an art that is so ineffective in self-defense. Since it comes from sword fighting, we can understand the safe training techniques, where only one student attacks, while the other defends, as opposed to both attacking and defending at the same time.

This gives students more control and safety. Obviously they do not try to really cut each others' necks off. They just pretend to attack in full force and speed, giving each other a head-start to practice their art safely.

In aikido, the sword-fighting motion is applied to the arms. Adapting to this, however, can be a problem, since you are no longer encountering a heavy sword but a quickly jabbing hand.

During your Krav Maga course, you will encounter mostly aikido leverages and locks used for teaching how to restrain a person and how to escape someone who tries to restrain you. However, the traditional circular body motion attributed to aikido has been modified to a pivot, while standing in one place. This makes for a faster execution of defense and counterattacks in shorter ranges, where an opponent closes the gap and tries to attack with kicks, punches, stabs, or clubs.

We can thus conclude that martial arts have added or deleted techniques from all its forms to improve their systems. The martial arts also enhance many athletic skills. In street fighting, however, a trained opponent may have the upper hand on some fighters, but not all.

Most arts have at least one area they specialize in. For example, boxing is good with punches, karate with kicks, and judo with grappling. If the opponent is not good with one of these, the fighter has a much higher chance of winning.

In Krav Maga, however, the whole approach is to design the system from the top down. It does not take a lot of force to control an opponent with a kick to the groin. Even with a protective cup, a devastating kick to that area would fold the person in half. Krav Maga, however, teaches its students how to specifically defend that one area, which makes kicking it increasingly difficult.

During a full-contact fight, Krav Maga students wear boxing gloves and attempt to knock each other out. An experienced instructor who teaches how to throw a knockout punch should teach his students to extend their fists into the opponent's face lightly.

When practicing defenses and counterattacks, Krav Maga students maintain maximum speed to provide reach and the surprise element. However, they do not fully extend their hands or legs upon impact with their training partners' bodies. This preferred training method helps preserve realistic speed, distance, and momentum of body mass, with a shock that's surprising enough to stop the opponent while also preventing deep-tissue damage.

In comparing prior martial arts to Krav Maga, we see that training methods and techniques were modified keeping the reaction time very specifically in mind.

One of the modifications was delivering the hardest punch possible in the quickest time to control opponents through their pressure points. Techniques that involve holding the opponent to the ground for a prolonged time were omitted.

Krav Maga is a new approach. Rather than repeating the errors of traditional systems, Krav Maga has explored new ways the human body can be used for self-defense.

The idea is not to get hurt in the process. Considering reaction time, you have a split second to identify the danger, and another split second to react. The process of danger elimination starts by first sensing it and then by commanding your body to counter it. The entire process averages two to four seconds at the most.

In Krav Maga, the student should learn mechanics of knockout strikes in one hour. Basic kicks are taught in the next hour. Blocking off hand strikes and kicks are taught in another hour. Close scenarios of grappling and ground fighting are taught in three more hours. Knife and stick attack and defensive techniques are taught in five more hours. You can learn all other kicks and hand strikes ever devised in two hours. You can spend a few hours on advanced training, learning various combinations for attack or defense. You can spend a few hours on full-contact fighting, and the whole process can be completed in twenty-one hours.

Students are advised to kick under the belt, not just because the groin is one of the most vulnerable pressure points, but also because its position allows your kick to reach maximum distance and speed. Aiming higher or lower would require more time, as those spots wouldn't be the absolute closest and easiest to reach target.

Using the element of surprise moving into full speed from standing still, for kicking and punching, shift your weight forward and slightly down instead of relying on major muscle groups to do the work. You are falling forward due to gravity, and following that by lunging your leg muscles forward. Your weight shifts to the appropriate direction and will support the mass required for a knockout strike, or a devastating kick.

The Krav Maga approach to ground fighting is very different. The student learns to prevail in any possible situation by attacking available pressure points with very little manipulation of his body weight to counter the opponent.

If you find yourself on the ground while your opponent is standing, as he is getting close to you your first choice would be to kick upward.

If your opponent sits on top of your stomach, trying to punch or choke you, you would first block the punch, or remove his wrist from your throat, and then bring your heels close to your seat and push your hips up, throwing his body off yours. This would force him to fly off your body, and he would not be able to attack you again. As he is lifted off the ground with your hips, punch him in the groin. If his head is near yours, push it to the side or poke one of his pressure points, like his neck or face.

If you got caught in a neck hold from the back, you would need to lift his elbow up and get out of it before reaching for one of his pressure points.

If he is kneeling beside you, leaning over your head while trying to punch you or choke you, move his thumbs off your throat, or block his punch. As you maintain a grip on his arm which is closer to you, you flip his body with your legs, smashing his head on the ground. If the ground is too soft to smash his head, kick him in the groin as well. Then, immediately get up.

The few techniques taught in Krav Maga seem to work, as opposed to all judo techniques and some wrestling techniques. What they do not counter is those wrestling scenarios where your leg is already twisted behind your back and you try to get out of it as you are locked up. This situation is comparable to letting someone tie you up with a rope and then stand behind you, leaving you completely defenseless.

Since the human response time is two split seconds, any attempt to harm you that takes longer should be successfully foiled if you are trained to be most efficient.

The advantage of Krav Maga is that it is the most efficient self-defense training system. Other martial arts have components that would not apply in the context of hand-to-hand combat. Perhaps most people who originally developed martial arts lacked the generations' accumulated common sense. Perhaps they were reluctant to pass on their true experience in order to keep their position.

If you see a tiger and a monkey fight in different styles, you would understand that they have different styles because they have different anatomies. Krav Maga is definitely not a form of mixed martial arts. It is a new and improved way to approach a previous method.

Theoretically, any technique could be used successfully if executed in the right timing. Attacks should occur when the opponent is caught by surprise and does not have enough time to devise a counterattack. In plain words, it means catching and blocking the opponent's attack before it is too late. Efficient movements give you the edge.

In Krav Maga, understanding the concept of reaction time is crucial. Krav Maga takes into consideration that depending on the scenario, certain techniques are less time consuming than others, and would be quicker to use. In addition Krav Maga prefers techniques that are easily executable for a weaker person.

Should students learn another martial art after learning Krav Maga? There could indeed be many benefits, such as an enjoyment and deep understanding of another aspect of the art or the human body, but I believe that mastering Krav Maga provides all the necessary self-defense and combat skills.

Would a fight to survive adhere to the judo rules or aikido training routines? If we train in boxing, then in karate, then in aikido, and then in judo and jujitsu, we would indeed have a greater set of capabilities. However, that also could be the downfall of our survival attempts.

Not being able to separate or combine techniques and determine when or why to use them would leave us to our intuition. I would rather see more planning done during downtime with less reliance on intuition in combat. Krav Maga training should encompass all the essentials of successful techniques to survive.

As you learn Krav Maga you learn how to optimize the use of your body by analyzing the danger, understanding reaction times, knowing the principles of delivering kicks and blows, deflecting a strike or a kick, and escaping grappling. You learn how to use your arms to fight and how to handle an armed opponent with your bare hands.

While there are many training systems that were dealing with the same issues before Krav Maga, they lacked the experience and understanding both instructors and students now have.

Krav Maga was kept as a military secret for the first twenty years. When Immi was close to his retirement, he opened a school in Tel Aviv. He gradually made Krav Maga Israeli martial arts, similar to the Japanese dojo.

The dojo, in western terms, was basically a gym geared with equipment for training in the martial arts. Initially, students did not have belts, but they eventually decided to add the belt grading system. In 1976, during an interview, Immi said that when a martial art becomes a sport, like judo for example, lethal moves have to be restricted. This destroys the basic principle of Krav Maga. "You automatically end the fight when you put an end to your opponent." While judo was the first martial art to have belts for grading, karate, others, and civilian Krav Maga followed with the belt ranking and with the restriction of their lethal elements.

Initially, the Krav Maga training gear was sweatpants or military pants, and later martial arts suits, or pants and T-shirts. Immi felt that civilians should not learn exactly what is taught in the IDF. Military training priorities were modified to fit civilians.

As Immi started teaching as a retirement hobby, his students followed with a more intensive business form. The one-week military curriculum needed to be spread over four to five years like the rest of the martial arts in order to fit to the existing business model of the dojo system.

Long-term memberships made monthly tuition more affordable. In urban locations, most students were schoolchildren that needed an after-school activity. Simpler training systems are more profitable. One of the problems with fast teaching was immediate business competition. There was no commercial advantage to sending kids home after two weeks of training for a fee comparable to that of the local karate school.

Extensive fitness additions to the classes gave a good workout and attracted those who wanted more than just to learn self-defense. Part of the reason for the simplification was to make it easy for everyone to teach and to learn.

Some civilian instructors attempted to change the grading system to differentiate them from others. Realizing the potential of Krav Maga as an intensive form of learning, they reverted to a new form of recognition that resembled the military style. In the military, fashion played a role in rank designations. A coat-of-arms-style badge, a bar, stars, or olive leafs in the IDF were symbols of rankings.

The benefits of civilian Krav Maga include the inclusion of small children, who could not participate in the original IDF Krav Maga. The IDF was suitable for adult men and women only.

Small children can benefit from activities suitable for their age in a protected environment, but it takes considerable time for them to fully understand and control their bodies. Therefore, small children need a modified approach. By the same token, an adult participating in a class geared towards kids would not get maximum benefit from it.

Finally, since the program is designed to keep students in training for a period of four to five years, it becomes obvious that there were secrets being kept for many years. Twenty-one hours of a core military curriculum tended to get lost and at times never found in the five hundred hours stretched over five years.

The first civilian curriculum was comprised of a technical list of material for belt levels, where the student started with hand strikes, basic kicks, releases from one or two holds, and an increase in the load of knowledge through an advancement in belts. It was advised that students should spend three months on lower belts, and pass their test with increments of six to nine months in the higher belts.

Various positions and angles were added, and the knife and stick training was pushed to the higher belts. To add a challenge, one needed to perform double and triple spinning kicks at the black belt level—acrobatics that were long before extracted out of the IDF program.

For many years there were no books or written instructions on how to teach the art in civilian schools. However, instructors needed to pass a course at the Wingate Institute for Physical Education. Various schools offered various levels of instruction, and knowledge was kept hidden.

While Krav Maga was the name used in the Israeli Defense Forces and in the Civilian Krav Maga Association for hand-to-hand combat training, its training methods were different. Immi was reluctant to share a superior hand-to-hand combat system with youth and civilians.

Unlike state education institutions, where students join at the beginning of the year, they could join whenever they wanted at martial arts schools. Much of the time students learned principles by practice without understanding them completely.

The required lecture was at times skipped by the student or omitted by the instructor. Instructors could test students two grades lower, and higher belts were needed for testing higher-level instructors. Although civilian associations attempted to keep good quality control, the product became closer to its package, the belt.

Selective teaching, disrespectful students, and ego games caused the creations of separate associations. In any martial art, first degree to third degree black belts are given according to skills or fighting abilities, and beyond that rest on favoritism.

At some point the association did not offer new challenges, and after Immi died, instructors figured out that they could promote themselves faster if they opened their own schools.

Many organizations teach civilian Krav Maga; the name Krav Maga is being used for a variety of different training systems.

Where the civilian school environment is a place to play, the IDF environment is designed for more pure learning. An impartial instructor does not allow for anything other than a strict intensive learning process of hand-to-hand fighting skills.

During a full-contact practice, the instructor stops the match when there is an obvious advantage for one of the soldiers, corrects the one who didn't do so well, and explains why one combatant gained the upper hand.

The full-contact fight is performed in front of the group, one pair at a time, and is interrupted many times. This facilitates group learning as each mistake is corrected. There is no time or opportunity to settle accounts.

In the making of Krav Maga, a scientific approach was applied. The training method was defined as the need to train soldiers in a hand-to-hand combat system in a short amount of time. Hand-to-hand combat is a possible interaction between two humans. The interaction involves reaction time, pressure points, blows and kicks, strangulations, knives, clubs, and other weapons. The reaction time was the crucial point for training.

Referring to the first example in this chapter, the most efficient move proved to have the upper hand. The first question asked was, how does a person hurt, restrict movement, or kill another person? The next question was what techniques have the most time efficient

motion? The assumption is that the person who will execute the technique fastest will have the advantage to go in for the kill.

Once students get comfortable in confronting deadly risks, they gain confidence and avoid overuse of force. From there you look at ways to control an opponent without killing him as long as you feel comfortable that you are not risking your own life. You then use the same tactics in defenses, and release from holds.

Observing various martial artists, Olympic athletes, and circus acrobats can stretch the limits of expectation in what kind of motion one could encounter if attacked by an unknown opponent.

However you need to recognize that techniques should be extracted from their core. Devising new safety rules for training and assuring each specific and important drill is kept close to a realistic scenario is crucial to maintain the quality of the training. The training should include scenarios that could be executed by most skilled athletes.

Safe and realistic training methods allow students to gain confidence in executing techniques that will work in real life. At the same time the methods allow partners to apply a maximum force attack without being bogged down by their training partner, who may have no control over his counterattack.

The motion of getting close to the opponent is one of the most important parts of the technique. Students learn that if they are at an attacking range without needing to move, they lose their surprise advantage if they do not attack immediately as their opponent enters the range.

The moves of the kicks and punches are illustrated with comparison laws of physics and mechanics. For example the front kick's motion resembles a seesaw motion, and the side kick resembles corkscrew motion, while a roundhouse kick's motion is generally a combination of both.

In Krav Maga, one of the keys is human biomechanics. The force of the strikes or kicks is measured by the trained instructor's judgment. Concentrating on training steps that lead to maximum efficiency and correct sequential execution leads to maximum speed and shift of mass in the direction of attack. This leads to the maximum force possible by humans. With this technique, an average person trained to punch in Krav Maga can generate a force of at least one and a half times his body weight into the strike with sufficient speed for a knockout. Since the mass is given, the training should stress proper technique to utilize the mass in maximum speed. Shaolin monks might have been able to pick up fight techniques from observing animals, but I don't think that's what Darwin would've recommended.

Some boxers learn to throw an effective knockout punch in their subconscious. In Krav Maga, the instructor's job in the first hour of training is to program the student to perform the correct technique with each training step.

Immi, in his ideology for peace, believed that if everyone would feel safe and have respect for their neighbors' force, there would be less violence in the world. However, the question of whether or not to keep some knowledge to ourselves was a central one. In other words, instructors should understand each student's personality to make sure the knowledge will not be used for the wrong purposes.

Another concern was whether or not we want to hold the information from certain nations. In recent years it became clear that the most dangerous weapon is the human mind. Unfortunately, in Western societies, this subtle understanding did not create enough fear and determination for all citizens to learn hand-to-hand combat.

In 2001 a few average-size non-athlete terrorists overcame airplanes full of people and used the planes as weapons, emphatically demonstrating the need for teaching good people how to fight the bad people in the world.

The same approach should be taken to gun safety. If you want to own guns, you need to teach your kids about gun safety. Kids can find ways to get their hands on almost everything to satisfy their curiosity. I think that if you want safety you need to learn the potential of threats to safety.

This book is about understanding how the human body can become a weapon. Krav Maga was originated by Immi Sde-Or, in 1940. It was in the IDF, where Immi, the former boxer, wrestler, student of jujitsu, gymnastics acrobat, and soldier in the British legions trained in Fairbairn Fighting Methods honed his teaching skills, further adapting the system to the IDF needs. It was further developed under Eli Avikzar, from the 1960s to the 1980s.

My addition to the training methods emanated from careful application of earlier founders' principles. As a fan of the system, I found myself comparing everything I'd previously learned in judo, jujitsu, karate, and aikido. I replaced every older technique I knew with a better, improved Krav Maga twist.

I needed to understand the complete process of a knockout punch in order to replace and renew the karate punch, which I've used to break boards of wood in the past.

I then set up steps and an explanation system to teach hand strikes in one hour. One hour was the IDF standard for teaching this technique. However, the steps and the explanation were too broad, and did not facilitate a satisfactory achievement of goals.

In writing this book I believe I've analyzed the theory of hand-to-hand combat to the core. Since I've found some prior additions to the system dubiously presented, I have satisfied my curiosity in tying loose ends.

Although there are many people in the world that somehow were involved in the history of Krav Maga, they did not happen to develop it. In addition, some caused a decline in Krav Maga's reputation by misinforming others or because they misunderstood the system.

From my research of the martial arts, the possibility that few people have come to the same conclusions around the same time in history did not appear. No other Martial Arts have the precise core elements suitable for self-defense as pure Krav Maga does!

On occasions, I've asked a few senior civilian Krav Maga instructors how they would teach the knockout punch mechanism. Most answered that they do not teach, but just let students practice with punching bags and let them improve on their own. If I had to ask myself why I came to learn Krav Maga, I would look for a better answer.

I teach how to execute a knockout punch in the first hour of training my students. While there are pressure points that do not require the application of such a great force, we need to be able to close the gap in a split-second motion and attack. No one assures us that the opponent's throat or groin would be an easy target, and there could be slight changes in a split second.

It is important that even in a self-defense scenario, a defender should be able to deliver a blow with great power. This should serve as a great motivation for the student to practice effective defenses against challenging attacks.

In addition, I've found many instructors are confused about which techniques to choose, or what to teach first. And of course students inherit that confusion from their instructors. I attempt to organize and prioritize Krav Maga concepts to help control this.

I am sure that there are quite a few great Krav Maga instructors out there, and people who contributed in one way or another to promote this field, but for the purpose of this book, I have picked only the source, the original Krav Maga head instructors from the IDF Fighting Fit Academy.

Krav Maga originated with Immi Sde-Or (Imrich Lichtenfeld, 1910–1998).

Immi was born in Budapest and raised in Bratislava, the capital of Slovakia. His father Samuel was a famous detective in Bratislava. Prior to that, Samuel had been a circus acrobat. Beginning in 1907, Samuel ran the Hercules Gym where he taught jujitsu and wrestling.

At age 18, in 1928, Immi won the Slovakia Youth Wrestling Championship. A year later in 1929, he won the Slovakia National Wrestling Championship. In the same year he won the National Boxing Championship, as well as the international Gymnastics Championship.

In the late 1930s when Hitler's youth gangs started to single Jewish young men out on the street, Immi said when you encountered them it was a hit or run. Immi got more satisfaction in hitting. Confronting several opponents at a time, he quickly realized that the sport had very little to do with street fighting, and began to reevaluate and redirect his knowledge.

In 1940 he boarded a ship to the Holy Land. Saving a drowning fellow in the freezing water, he got a severe ear infection, and had to be operated on in Alexandria. The British were stopping Jewish immigrants from entering Palestine, so in Alexandria Immi volunteered in one of the British brigades hoping for a permit to enter. After two years of service, he was allowed to live in Israel.

In 1942, Immi taught his skills to underground organizations that were established to defend the Jews' interests in Israel under the British rule of Palestine. He taught swimming and hand-to-hand fighting. In 1948, he became the chief hand-to-hand instructor in the IDF.

The system was constantly changing due to the need for a quick system that anyone could use within a small budget in limited training time. Male and female soldiers alike had to learn to use a comprehensive system that would protect their lives in times of need.

Israel was lucky to have Immi. At the time, they needed to train citizens in guerilla fighting to give ordinary people the confidence to defend themselves, or to risk their lives in a small guerilla mission. He modified the techniques and training systems to fit the military environment. With his prior background, he had a pretty good idea of all the ways to prevail in a hand-to-hand combat scenario. Under the time constraint of the Israeli Defense Forces, and with the need to tailor a system suitable for any male or female soldier, coupled with the opportunity to intensively train a mass amount of soldiers, a lot of experience was gained.

When you're constantly seeing the whole picture, you can draw conclusions and make improvements to your training methods. Teaching hand-to-hand combat with at least 20,000 hours of intensive instruction, striving to bring each soldier to the same level of combat experience in the very little training time allotted, he distilled the training system.

In 1968, twenty years later, Immi retired from the IDF. A few years earlier he had opened civilian schools, first in Tel Aviv, and later in Natanya, Israel. After Immi retired, his favorite student Eli Avikzar became the chief of the IDF Krav Maga.

Eli Avikzar was born in Casablanca, Morocco, in June 1947. In a hostile Arab environment, he got his first taste of street fighting. At age 16, in 1963, he immigrated to Israel.

In 1964 he began training with Immi in his civilian school. In 1965 Eli added judo and jujitsu to his training in other schools. Immi thought that it would be good for students of Krav Maga to augment their training by obtaining black belts of other sports and broaden their horizons. The idea behind it was to encourage the development of a well-rounded education in fields related to your art.

Some Krav Maga students came in with no prior experience, while others already had a background in one or many martial arts. Some techniques from other martial arts were added in earlier years to Krav Maga, thus demonstrating the various differences in approaches and the superior effectiveness of Krav Maga.

In 1968, Eli was appointed as the IDF head of Krav Maga. In 1971, Eli received his judo black belt and the first civilian Krav Maga black belt. In 1977 he received his black belt in aikido from the European Association in Germany.

Eli, with his additional background in aikido and judo, had brought another view to the table, and was able to look at Krav Maga with fresh perspective. As Immi and Eli recounted, in those days they were developing counter-techniques to all the other martial arts.

Continuing with the IDF tradition of developing and perfecting reality-based training methods, Eli Avikzar devised additional tactics and training techniques.

In 1978, Immi established the civilian Krav Maga Association and appointed Eli Avikzar in charge of rank and training curriculum.

The Krav Maga Association made connections in Europe and the United States to demonstrate and teach the system to the Jewish communities and the local police forces. However, at some point, the quality of Krav Maga training declined.

Eli retired from the IDF in 1981. In addition to his military career, he had a civilian school for Krav Maga, which he inherited from Immi. I replaced Eli as the Krav Maga chief instructor in the IDF.

I would like to recount the events that led me to become one of the chief Krav Maga instructors at the IDF Fighting Fitness Academy.

At about 10 years old, I moved to the suburbs of Tel Aviv, and as the new kid on the block, I found myself confronting local kids who were looking for a new victim for bullying. One time, for example, I happened to club a kid to the floor using a leg of a wooden chair that was thrown out in the yard. Running into the next high rise building and using a fire hose, I stopped other bullies using water pressure.

At elementary school, I was dropped and held to the ground with a judo technique. I was very independent, but I guess the leaders of the class did not take kindly to me. I thought then that I should be more proficient about fighting, and learn an art, so I started with judo and then moved on to jujitsu for a few years with a former Dutch-military jujitsu instructor and a gymnast that immigrated to Israel.

The jujitsu training was similar to judo, only knife training was added and the sport had more chokes, head holds, and street holds than judo. In judo you were only allowed to contact the opponent's clothes.

Jujitsu training included practicing breaking free of various holds and chokes, and defenses against limited strikes. The blocking method vs. hand strikes and kicks appeared to be the same. You crossed your outer forearm to create a pliers-like grip, and applied it in any direction.

When we were sparring, it was judo. We practiced releasing from various holds and grabs, and added a jab or kick to the groin, and followed that with a judo-style throw to the mat.

To handle a knife-holding attacker, we either took hold of the knife with the pliers-like grip, which would lead to a throw, or manipulated the opponent's wrist by throwing him to the ground. Once the opponent fell, we followed with a kick or a stomp to the head or rib. Many times, the wrist manipulation caused the knife to drop to the ground, and the pain in our partner's wrist would cause him to surrender and tap the mat twice. That was a signal that he was in great pain, and we should stop inflicting pressure on his wrist.

If you're attacked on a sidewalk, however, and your opponent taps the ground twice, I hope you don't release him. You instead need to punch him in the face, kick him in the groin and check that your technique works before you walk away. It is advisable that you take the knife away from him. You do not want him getting up from a coma, or one of his friends using the same knife against you again.

Jujitsu kicks and hand strikes practice on that level were a smack to the face with an open hand, a hammer punch from the top down, and an abrupt foot jab to the groin, with no explanation of the technique.

Around the eighth grade, I tested my jujitsu training to stop a kid attempting to hit me in the face. I kicked him in the groin once and he bent forward and stayed in that position for five minutes. In high school, I remember an occasion where a student started to verbally harass me in front of the class. I grabbed him by the throat. He was shocked and never dared to bother me again.

When I got to the brown belt level it turned out I had to learn karate or boxing.

The karate style available then was called Shotokan. The martial arts became my hobby, and I used to train three to four times a week in various schools, occasionally training with visiting judo instructors from the Kodokan, Japan's largest judo academy. At one point I learned that you could stop any judo practitioner who is trying to flip you with a simple one-handed push to his hip. I saw my opponent doing it, I did it back, and it always worked.

As a teenager, my street and school fighting was limited to a few occasions. One night, I fought a gang member near a movie theatre by kicking his rib, and as he fell forward to the ground, I marked about five fist strikes to my next opponent's face leaving him shocked but standing still. That night I ran home through back alleys, hoping not to be found by the rest of the gang members.

I immediately realized that my karate training methods gave me bad habits. By practicing how to strike with full force but stopping one inch away from the target, never having contact with the opponent's face, in real life the bad training habit became reality. Once your body already advanced forward, you would not have the time to think.

In 1975, various Israeli karate instructors formed a team and participated in the Japan Masutatsu Oyama's World Full Contact Karate Tournament where our karate instructor knocked out the American contender. Consequently our karate school changed styles from Shotokan to Kyokushin Kai.

Training involved breaking at least two one-inch boards and full-contact fighting. The idea behind breaking wooden boards was that if you could break the wood, you could break another person's bones. While the sparring rules allowed full-contact kicks to any part of the body, except the groin, throat, and knee, hand strikes to the face were disallowed. The system therefore was not equipped with effective blocking techniques to counter boxers and kick-boxers.

To learn pressure points we would go over a routine of standing in front of our training partner and marking all kinds of attacks to various pressure points with full concentration. We would take deep, yoga-style breaths and follow it with screaming to make the punch more powerful. This made our muscles tighten, which would give us a false psychological perception of power.

Since not all pressure points have the same accessibility, and since each pressure point requires a different degree of application of force, a thorough explanation should have been substituted for this training method.

The tactical method of fighting was to wear out the opponent through roundhouse kicks to the opponent's calves or thighs, and then trying to knock the opponent out by punching his solar plexus or kicking his face. I used to come home late at night after biweekly training sessions, grab a heavy-duty garbage bag, fill it with ice, and leave it on my shins as I watched TV. Many times I went to sleep with it. Reflecting back on these tactics, had anyone explained to us that the pain resulting from the low kick to the calf causes distraction that buys us time for the follow-up punch, we could have ended our sparring much faster and more decisively.

For a black belt in Kyokushin, I was required to pass the 100-man Kumite. This entailed fighting 100 opponents one after the other, taking about two to three minutes a person, so if you did not knock them out, you would end up with more exertion time, thus leading to hyperventilation and possibly bursting lungs. Many people dropped out from exhaustion toward the end. It was a three- to four-hour job.

During the years of training we had European high rank guests that came to train with us, and on occasions teach a seminar. At one point I remember facing a 4th Dan aikido that wanted to defend himself using aikido as I attacked him with karate.

I was 17, and already had prior confrontations with various martial artists, but never before had to fight an aikido black belt. The thought was not a pleasant one.

Those familiar with aikido throws know that if the aikido man does not let go of his grip as you are tossed in the air, you end up landing on your head, and badly injured. Letting the wrist leave the grip lets the training partner land on the ground in a safe way. Luckily, he was not even able to grab my punches or kicks for a throw.

During the first year of basic commando training, and between border incursions, my infantry troop was sent to participate in a series of social seminars on a resort in the Mediterranean.

It just happened to be the same time as other groups were there, including soldiers recruited from disadvantaged families. These soldiers grew up in a rough environment, and were on the border of a life of crime. The IDF drafted those in the hope that they might become good soldiers and good citizens.

Since I had to take care of a few errands, I had arrived to the resort early. I learned later that my troop had already arranged for me to settle their accounts.

Before I had a chance to ask for directions to the dorm, I found myself surrounded by a group of the bad soldiers. One got closer, and started to accuse me of stealing his sneakers. He chest-bumped me, and his friend slapped me in the face. At that point I immediately hit the one that was leaning on me with an inverted roundhouse to the temple, and as he fell down, I leaned on his shoulder, and kicked the one behind him with my military boot impacting his sternum bone with the heel.

The second soldier fell as well, but after ten seconds he jumped up, grabbed a long and narrow metal cylinder and charged at me. One of my troop mates was coming with his M-16 assault rifle, and I shouted at him to throw his weapon to me.

He did and I was going to use it to block the cylinder. I did not need to, since the attacker fell back to the floor getting a second jolt in his nervous system from the kick I gave him a few seconds earlier. To disperse the rest of the group, I got into a fighting stance, rolling up my sleeves, and looked at them with an intimidating glare. They took off.

In the evening we were standing in attention, clean-shaven with shined boots ready to leave the base. We were heading out for a drink at the local bar in town. Unfortunately I was standing in the back line. That was when I got stabbed in the back.

I felt a tickle in my rib, turned my head and saw one of the sergeants standing behind me with a red face, as a silhouette of a short soldier was retracting a knife in a straight stab motion.

I touched my back, and felt blood. I did not move, fearing that I might create more damage to my kidney. This was a planned revenge. I was sent to the hospital for a week. Luckily the cut was just in the lower back muscle, between the kidney and the spine.

After I ended my basic commando training, I had my mind set on becoming a Krav Maga instructor at the IDF Fighting Fitness Academy.

I was transferred to the Fighting Fitness Academy, which is where I met Eli Avikzar. He led me to his assistant Pablo, and offered me a spot in helping teach Krav Maga.

Pablo was excited about sparring with a black belt in Kyokushin. He gave me a few quick explanations about Krav Maga, showed me a few moves, and off we went. After a few minutes I realized I was using his techniques against him. Krav Maga was that simple.

A few days later, I decided to pay a visit to my old Kyokushin School after one year of absence. Suddenly, I was noticed by the instructor. "You did not come to training! You must fight!" In the martial arts world, students are expected to continue their training even after they get a black belt. I arrived there, and no one cared if I was in basic training at the IDF.

Beating was a common tactic used around the world to encourage class attendance. I was quickly standing in front of the new champions lined up for me.

My first and last opponent was taller and heavier, and had bursting muscles.

In my last year of infantry training, I lost all my muscle build. Lack of sleep, long jogs with full gear, and a lack of protein all took their toll.

I was given bandages to put on my knuckles when I realized these were the new rules in that dojo. Face punching was legal, and I was glad to be back in business. He started to dance as I stood still. He threw about seven roundhouse kicks: low to the legs, high to the face. I brushed them all off, standing still in one spot. He stopped and held his hands high, protecting his face.

I threw one left punch with my hand while closing the gap. My fist and forearm passed through the tight space between his forearms, reached his face, passed it, and retracted. In a split second, less than a minute after the fight started, I saw his body following his head, and his feet lifted up as he fell down.

Someone went to bring cold water to revive him. I was not allowed to fight there anymore. My former karate instructor reported to Eli Avikzar the next day trying to learn Krav Maga. I have never returned to my karate school since.

The year was 1980. After taking three hours of Krav Maga, I came to realize that seven years of training in almost all other major martial arts were a waste of time. The difference was a result of a genius.

I was assisting in training Krav Maga at the IDF Fighting Fitness Academy, and later joined a Krav Maga instructor's course as a student where I was assisting the instructor as well. I developed a professional friendship with Eli Avikzar, the head of Krav Maga, and he entrusted me with all Krav Maga activities in the IDF Fighting Fitness Academy. After a few months, I used to meet him daily in the coffee shop and give him all the news that happened in the Academy. A few months later Eli Avikzar retired and I became officially in charge.

There were short two-week Special Forces training courses, special unit officer's courses, and at some point one-week self-defense for female recruits.

The highlight of the training was the Krav Maga instructor course, which served soldiers and officers in various units. Of course, the purpose was to create instructors who could go back to their units and spread hand-to-hand combat training techniques to their comrades.

I felt I was very lucky to be there.

I never in my dreams thought I would end up in the Fighting Fitness Academy. I had the best trainers in the world, and the best arena to train. I had witnessed the power of the system by supervising hundreds of full-contact fighting sessions in courses I had designed.

In each course were a few females, and a few black belts in various martial arts, and at the end of the course it seems that females used the techniques as well as males, and the newly trained soldiers had an advantage over those who had prior extensive experience in martial arts.

As I was told by Eli, it took time to unlearn. Years of practice in other martial arts embedded unrealistic instincts into many of the academy's students.

In the IDF curriculum, you teach hand strikes in one hour, and the lesson needed to be complete. Students need to learn the correct technique to execute knockout punches. They need to know how to use the quickest motion to reach the target, and how to accelerate to a sufficient speed that creates a momentum sufficient enough to cause a concussion.

In karate, when you break boards, your aspiration is to develop a knockout punch. Many civilian Krav Maga instructors follow the same philosophy as boxing trainers. Train on a heavy bag until you have a good punch. I disagree since bad technique combined with repetition creates bad habits that are hard to get rid of.

After hours and between teachings, I had opportunities to train with an Russian Sambo ex-champion and then-current Israeli Boxing Champion. I remember asking the boxer to try to punch me in the face. He could not touch me, since I blocked them all. I wanted to test the techniques with an authentic boxing champion to make sure we did not miss anything.

Since I was teaching in the IDF, Eli introduced me to Immi and for the next five years I would meet Immi almost every weekend. Immi was in his seventies and felt it was his obligation to take me under his wing as I was teaching in the IDF.

We used to meet Saturday mornings for espresso. Many times, a few of his black belt students used to stop at the Café Ugatti in Netanya, greet him and be invited to sit with him as well. He used to go over and over the importance of basic principles. Immi always paid for dinner. If any of his students reached for his wallet, Immi used to execute a wrist lock on the poor student and say: "I am the oldest, therefore I pay."

As I was assuming responsibility at the IDF for all Krav Maga activities, Immi and Eli recommended that I also join civilian activities and get tested for a belt to secure a position in helping the Krav Maga Association activities.

During that time I used to teach for Eli at his civilian gym. It kept me busy, but I felt I did not learn anything new, and that the civilian black belts did not know more than a third of what I already knew.

In 1983 I retired from the IDF. I then started to teach Krav Maga for security personnel of the Aviation

Authority until 1986. In my free time I attended a Krav Maga coaches course at Wingate University and added another diploma to my collection.

The coach certification program was designed for athletic trainers who were teaching national teams but had never earned a bachelor's in physical education. This was an equivalent program that concentrated on the professional enrichment of trainers while leaving their learning in the field they were teaching to their professional associations.

Occasionally I was sent by the Krav Maga Association to train the Jewish communities of Frankfurt and Antwerp in Krav Maga. I've led an intensive women's Krav Maga seminar designed to prevent rape at the request of the Tel Aviv Municipality.

Prior to immigrating to the US, I received a Krav Maga top expert recognition from retired colonel David Ben Asher in the IDF, who once served as head of the Fighting Fitness Academy. At the same time I received a letter of excellence from Immi.

My first two weeks in the US were in Philadelphia, Pennsylvania.

I trained Alan Feldman for two weeks. Instead of wasting time on the civilian curriculum, I gave him the training I thought he needed to be able to handle himself in Krav Maga, and signed his diploma as his instructor. Immi's signature appeared above the title as the president of the Krav Maga Association.

On one of my trips back to Israel I learned that Eli had quit his role as head of the Krav Maga Association Rank Committee in 1987. He had left the association and opened his own school named Krav Magen.

Sports martial arts were the starting point for Immi, and Krav Maga was the starting point for Eli. For me, Krav Maga was the ending point of my training. I've recognized its benefits as superior to any martial art I've encountered before. For Immi and Eli, teaching Krav Maga as a form of civilian martial art was the last stage of their career. When I finally realized that Krav Maga had turned into another civilian martial art, I refused to be part of any civilian association.

The average Israeli travels the world, and quite a few Israelis have studied various martial arts from all over. In Israel, you can find almost any kind of martial arts school. The first foreigner in Japan to attain the fifth black belt degree in Nin-Jitsu is an Israeli. Israel is also a place of great cultural exchange. In addition to the Jewish, Christian, Arab, and other populations, many scholars of the world come to visit Israel. Krav Maga was unknown to civilian life until 1960, and it took twenty years for Krav Maga to reach civilians in Israel.

After Immi's death, quite a few Israeli martial artists started to claim they were teaching Krav Maga. Some of them attempted to learn through observing training in civilian schools. Some Israeli instructors that claim they teach Krav Maga have no clue what Krav Maga is. Many are still bogged down by years of other martial arts knowledge, not knowing what to teach and what not to teach. Those who want to become certified Krav Maga instructors need to take intensive courses.

The name might have been the same, but civilian Krav Maga was not Krav Maga. It was becoming a form of mixed martial arts. New instructors felt comfortable with changing styles, adding styles, and forgetting about their application to reality. I believe their approach mainly resulted from limited experience, or experience that was too broad and did not give them the ability to prioritize.

Currently, there are both legitimate and illegitimate users of the name Krav Maga. The legitimate ones are those that completed the Israeli Defense Forces Krav Maga instructor course. The second group of legitimate users is those who learned the civilian Krav Maga from either Immi or Eli, or their students. This system was never intended to teach everything about military Krav Maga. The civilian Krav Maga proved to be just another activity class, but Immi had intended to keep IDF Krav Maga within the military and not in civilian life. Over time, they realized that it did not have the benefits of the IDF Krav Maga. Illegitimate users use the name like it is a generic brand name that everyone has a right to use. They ignore the fact that it is really a name for a specific system started by Immi Lichtenfeld and developed in the Israeli Defense Forces Fighting Fitness Academy, not in any dojo, and surely not in a judo, jujitsu, karate, or aikido dojo.

Krav Maga is a very complex training system. The whole picture involves how to define and get from the beginning of the training experience to the end, intensively. While every person is different and there are many different approaches, I hope this book will serve as a guide to direct students and instructors in achieving their goals.

Eli died in May 2004 leaving Avi Avisadon as his heir in the Israeli Krav Magen (KAMI). Avi was the most qualified follower student, since he was Eli's deputy in the IDF from 1977 to 1979, and later served for twenty years as the Naval Commandos Krav Maga instructor.

Shortly after, the original Krav Maga Association was dissolved. Instead there were a few new ones. Every association leader became the most authorized and certified authority. That path was clearly not for me. My level was at least at Grand Master.

During the last twenty-five years in the US, I've been invited to teach intensive seminars to the Italian

Krav Maga Association, police officers in Rome, the Krav Maga Association in Nice, France, and US local and federal law enforcement students. In 2002, I was invited to train the New Jersey state police troopers and SWAT team in instinctive and tactical shooting using pistols and machine guns. I've taught intensive seminars to various American organizations and universities. I also taught as a guest in some civilian instructors' classes.

Endless repetitions of basic hand-to-hand combat skills could turn Krav Maga into a form of fitness. However, while Krav Maga is meant to be executed with ease, increasing the degree of physical difficulty for core or cardio training should be balanced out by maintaining the techniques in their original patterns and contexts.

Adjusting techniques to fit a musical rhythm, meditation, relaxation, or increase of heart rate defeats the purpose of Krav Maga as a hand-to-hand combat system. The danger is that when the need for self-defense arises, the techniques can't be reverted to their original purpose.

Since the training environment does not resemble real life, it is up to the instructor to create the resemblance. It is highly important not to confuse the student's perception.

Students need to train in a fashion where the overall purpose is not to win a fight by flipping the opponent, but by being in a position where the opponent is under his training partner's control.

Many training methods attempt to simulate full-contact fighting by just limiting it to light contact. That defeats the purpose of training because students end up using sports techniques all the time.

A serious Krav Maga school should allow full-contact fighting, including hand strikes to the face, blows to the groin, or pokes to the eye. While promoting safety is important, the fact is that it decreases the student's street fighting capabilities.

When I see Krav Maga teaching, I expect to see the best way to use the human body in a survival-type confrontation, not a quest for entertainment or physical fitness.

Krav Maga lessons are about spending a few minutes clarifying what the purpose of various techniques is, and then spending a few minutes practicing the parts and the whole, testing it to see if it is a knockout punch or not, and immediately correcting any major errors all within the time frame of an hour.

I believe Krav Maga instructors should feel a responsibility to prepare students to defend their lives.

I believe the more law-abiding citizens that are trained in self-defense and hand-to-hand combat, the better off the world will be.

PREPARING FOR FACE-TO-FACE CONFRONTATION

I would like to start this chapter with some of the most crucial principles for protecting your life.

Danger analysis involves an assessment of the risk you are willing to take to confront a dangerous situation. It involves controlling your opponent in your territory. Think of an uncomfortable situation where you feel your basic human rights are being violated. Someone is attempting to forcefully take something you have a claim to and you are not willing to give it up. At times, you can sense danger. At times, you will instinctively react. However there are a few things you must understand. The following would eliminate any hesitation when time is of the essence.

If you have the time, ask yourself if you can avoid or mitigate the danger. You may choose to walk away, thus potentially being followed, giving the attacker a chance to attack you later in a more convenient time. The problem is that once you let a dangerous person in your personal space, you are not in control of your safety anymore. If he attacks you, most of the time you will not be able to defend yourself. If he attempts to punch or stab you, you will not have enough time to block it even with years of training.

Since you do not know what the attacker is all about, never assume what he wants. He could just want a dollar, or he could be a psychopath that wants to kill you. You must not let the attacker cross your personal range without you attacking him first. If you allow him

to get close to you without you reacting, you may never have a chance to live.

Your chances of survival drop to 50 percent if you let an attacker in your territory. Use your judgment, but think about your mother, your wife, and your kids before you think about sacrificing your safety and letting him attack you.

If you don't react on time, you have wasted all your training, and you may waste your life.

While using public transportation, a taxi, a limo, a train, or an airplane, your personal range becomes the entire vehicle, the entire train, or the entire aircraft. In a high speed, in the middle of nowhere, in the air, or at sea, when a vehicle is hijacked, all the passengers' lives are in danger. You must control your fate by controlling your territory.

Your reaction time is the time it takes your brain to recognize a dangerous motion and send a command to your body to move the danger away from you.

If you are on the defense, you will always be one step behind the person on the offensive.

Krav Maga considers the reaction time that is crucial in effectively blocking an attack. If your opponent was two steps away from you, his best option would have been to use his front leg to kick you. This would have been the fastest move his body would have been able to take. If he tried to do anything else, it would have taken him at least another split second longer to execute.

When you notice him starting to close the gap, counter his best option with a swift defense and simultaneous counter strike. Any hesitation on his part would make his attempt futile.

After deflecting a kick or punch, follow with an immediate strike to the face or to the groin. In Krav Maga, you execute both defense and attack at the same time, limiting the opponent's attempts to attack back.

While training, you start by testing various techniques of blocking and counterattacks, taking into account all possible scenarios. However, in real life, you cannot afford to waste time thinking about what technique you are going to use. You need a simplified principle.

The distance you should keep from your opponent should be greater than your outstretched arm. If you are at close range face-to-face, the distance for the attacker to slap your face is about the same for your hand to pop and protect your face. Considering the distance is the same, you both have the same time to attack. However, if that is the case, there is no time left for reaction, and if he attacks first, you lose.

The equation is that long distance attack equals a short defensive motion plus reaction time. Unfortunately, I've seen many students left unaware of this basic, and many times their instructors, knowingly or not, take advantage of it. The instructor may strike a student from close range to show the student they cannot block the attack. The students then may feel that they need to practice a few more years to improve their speed.

Although in sports sciences there are constant attempts to test runners for fast twitch muscles, when it comes to motion reaction in a self-defense situation, the variances in individual reaction times become less important if a defender can be aware of it and start his defense a split second earlier. The idea is to stand away at least a hand and a shoulder from your opponent so that you will be able to block, and if you are closer than that you will not.

On a higher level, you must remember that if you do not react as your attacker enters your space, you will never be able to block his attack. You must reach for his wrist when he starts to move into the attack; vigilance is key.

Even if the attacker did not punch you, but just moved quickly, you should deflect his wrist so that in case he does attack, his motion will be deflected out of your body.

In defense, you are deflecting his hand or leg, and in attacking you are simultaneously preventing him from attempting to strike again.

Many times you might see a person's arm flailing around your face in slow motion. That usually won't trigger your instinctive reaction, since its speed could not result in a devastating blow to your body. However, a swiftly moving object or body should trigger an instinctive defense from your body or hands.

Your body would move away from the object, or your hand or leg would deflect the object away from you. To move your body, you would need to identify the danger ahead, otherwise move the object away from you with your hand. This is due to the simple fact that your body weighs more than your hand.

If an attacker catches you in a hold, you will break out of the hold with the techniques you will learn in this book. As he holds you, take advantage of the fact that you are not being punched or kicked and hone in on his pressure points, while trying to get out of the chokehold.

If the opponent has his hands to your throat, your instinct is not to punch him, but to move his thumbs from your windpipe. Remember, it takes two split seconds to break a windpipe.

If you identify your attacker's intent ahead of time, you should strike him with your hand before he grabs you. Your advantage is that both of his hands are extended in his attempt to grab you, so you can extend one hand while pivoting your body behind it for greater reach. So if your hand is extended, you can reach his throat ahead of time before he grabs your body.

When attempting to hold the opponent's body you need at least two split seconds to harm the opponent. The move usually involves getting a good grip, and then manipulating it in a way that inflicts pain, cuts off oxygen supply, breaks the neck, or throws the person on the ground headfirst.

If in great pain, the opponent cannot strike back. However, since it takes two split seconds for the task, the defender has time to free himself before the pain is inflicted. He has one split second to realize that the opponent has grabbed him, and another split second to stop it.

After the imminent threat is relieved, a quick strike, kick, or finger jab neutralizes the opponent. Multiple attacks may be used if the first attack did not work. This will lead you to victory.

If you find yourself in an unplanned grappling scenario, take comfort in the fact that his hands aren't striking or grabbing you. You still have two split seconds to react.

Vision

To ensure you do not miss any attacks, you need to concentrate your vision on the center of the attacker. As you suddenly notice your opponent, look to the center of his body to assess the danger.

Your vision should shift along the perpendicular line at the center of the opponent's body. You would stay at eye level prior to lunging at him, to accurately measure the distance you need to cover as you plan. Keep your vision at eye level, but look to the center of his body. You will see his arms and legs in the corner of your eyes. This way, you avoid distraction.

If you look away for even a second, you could have missed a motion that is coming from the opposite direction. Even if the opponent is looking at the sky, the floor, to his left, or to his right, or over your shoulder, do not follow his line of vision, unless you are standing far away from him. If you do change the direction of your vision, you will not be able to see an attack coming.

The student learns to identify which part of the opponent's body would be approaching the defender's territory first. Territory pertains to a distance that is a few steps away from one's body. When an opponent crosses that distance, the defender cannot afford to wait any longer. He must execute a defense and attack back.

Motion

One should be able to strike in maximum range, at maximum speed and with minimum motion required and needed to obtain the target. Your body weight should help to support the momentum of the blow or kick. A balanced stance at the start and finish of the attack or defense makes you ready for the next move. Getting into a balanced position and then figuring out what to do from this stance could prove fatal; don't worry about balance before you begin to execute your attack or defense.

Once in motion, the balance needs to be continuously kept by coordinating and shifting the body. In a sports match, one can get comfortable in a planned stance before the referee gives the start signal. In reality, you never know what position you will find your body at when you're being attacked. If you had advance notice, you would be balanced so you can react with quick motion in any direction. You should not, however, waste time thinking about it. If you do, it might be too late. It prompts your opponent to suspect and pay greater attention to your moves, and then give you his best shot. You really do not want this to happen.

The punch should be fast enough that it should impact the opponent's chin before you land on the ground after you lunge in a springing motion. Once you decide to punch, you want to complete it and strike the opponent before giving him a chance to block it.

The body starts to lunge forward. The hand starts to move toward the target. As it gets close to the opponent's chin, your body pivots right behind, allowing the hand to extend further, and the body's mass to shift and support the force of the impact. Your rear shoulder is behind the shoulder of the punching hand to facilitate maximum range. Passing the chin by a few inches, you retract to maintain speed and are ready to see the results.

Your hand starts at zero and accelerates to maximum speed. To maintain maximum speed, your hand must not stop at contact. If it did stop, that means you slowed down a second before on the way to a complete stop. This means that you were not at full speed upon contact.

To facilitate maximum speed when striking, we must not immediately stop when we reach the target since it could change positions an inch forward or an inch backward. We therefore estimate where the target is, and want to ensure we strike at maximum speed an inch before and an inch after.

To maintain the speed when our body is completely stretched forward, and the hand is fully extended, we use a whip motion where the hand passes the target and returns to its initial position. The body must not attempt to shift its weight for a neutral position move before the hand completes the return. If it does, the first strike is a waste, since the weight has shifted to another direction before the strike was completed. From empirical experience an average person can be trained in one hour to be able to efficiently maximize a straight strike with speed without projecting his strike, to at least one and a half times his body weight. This is empirically sufficient to cause a knockout, impacting the opponent's chin with bare knuckles. When we strike, we want to do it right the first time. Why take chances?

As you strike, you find a window of opportunity. You do not worry about being off balance nor do you worry about being thrown on the floor. You spring forward, taking advantage of the speed and range of motion to strike, letting your front foot land.

As you retract, another reason why you wait a second before bringing your center of gravity back to the center of your body, is that you want to ensure your body weight was in motion during the strike. Since it is faster to move the hand than the body, the hand should be completely retracted before the body returns to a neutral position.

If you did not have enough speed and mass in your strike you must conclude that your body was trying to keep up with your hand and therefore must have started its retraction before the hand finished the punch. Unfortunately, this causes your body to pull in the opposite direction of the strike. This does not achieve the right amount of body weight concentration to support the punch, and also works against you by pulling your hand back before you hit the target. A maximum body weight shift in the direction of the hand strike delivers a more powerful punch.

Understand that while it is easy to use your hand to block an opponent, it takes more time to lift your foot for a kick. For kicking you will need to shift your weight to the base foot, which is the foot that is on the ground while you are using your other foot to kick. A better choice is to learn to twist your hips and shift your weight so your center of gravity is pulling your body for a landing on your base foot, readying your kicking leg for action. Understand that an attacker standing at a distance of about two steps can kick you faster than punch you, because to punch, he has to take two steps to reach you. As he executes the first step, he kicks and closes the gap of the second step.

If an attacker is within one step of you, it is faster for you to punch him, or vice versa, than for him to kick you, or the other way around. Since you learn to attack simultaneously, you need not concern yourself with what the attacker is going to do. You block and attack according to the range. If your attacker is taking the slower course, you block the unexecuted fist in the short range, or the unexecuted kick in the long range, and attack simultaneously. The opposite limb is not going to reach you before your opponent has shifted his weight in the short distance, or before the two-step gap has closed.

In grappling scenarios, you can use the opponent's pressure points while standing, sitting, and lying. At times when the attacker is pushing or pulling you, you may need to change direction. You need to go with the pull or push faster to surprise him and at the same time change direction to reposition your body out of harm's way. This leaves him with nothing to pull or push. If you are attacking him at the same time, you end the confrontation. If you do not, you may need to keep diverting the direction he is trying to take by stepping to a slightly different angle.

This principle is easily demonstrated in arm wrestling. While your opponent is applying full ninety-degree force to your hand, you can twist your wrist and do the same but at a different angle. It will take your opponent a split second to completely follow the change, and until then you have taken his arm down an inch. If you now lead to another angle, you have gained another inch. Do this four to five times, and you have won.

Safety in Training

Learning hands-on skills enables us to handle dangerous situations and expose students to a dangerous environment. But if the danger is not curbed, the purpose of learning is defeated with the student's injury. It would be ridiculous if a person who wishes to learn how to protect himself would get seriously hurt during the training.

It is not unheard of for a serious injury to be inflicted in training. This might occur because of unsafe training methods, or due to a self-destructive mindset, the belief that hard work and suffering build spirit and resilience. What good is it to train oneself to become resilient with strong spirit, if one's body becomes dysfunctional in the process?

During training the environment should be safe, and both the instructors and students need to be safety oriented and safety smart. The instructor should create a safe environment by spacing the students at sufficient distance from each other when the basic techniques have been learned, and teach them how to fall safely. In addition, he must teach students how to protect their training partners.

During practice, all training partners are in danger; however the one in the role of attacker is in more danger than the defender.

Krav Maga techniques make the attacker vulnerable as the defender is executing a simultaneous defense and counterattack in a force sufficient to stop follow-up attacks.

Since the attacker is required to attack the defender using all techniques, the defender knows what the attacker is going to do, and has the opportunity to block the attacker at an increasing pace. The defender should not take advantage of his training partner, controlling his counterattack.

Understand the risk involved in not knowing and not being able to control the training environment. You should take great caution to prevent harm to self, training partners, and bystanders.

Self-Defense Protection and the Law

The right to bear arms should be interpreted as the right to self-defense.

Attempts have been made to restrict individual human rights in favor of society through legislation. But the act of self-defense is an immediate response to imminent danger.

When I eat an animal's flesh, I contemplate this: This animal lived its short life to its full expectation, in its own context. There was a point where the animal sensed it was fighting for its life after it has been tricked and overpowered. And the next thing it is sitting on your table like nothing ever happened. It is all over for that animal. This animal could be you.

We need to identify possible last seconds of our lives even if they take us by surprise, and react with determination to overcome imminent danger. If we do not, it is all over for our families and us.

Survival is the need to exist and preserve your full potential. Clean and easy ways to kill in society have been developed. Inventions like the gun give the user some great advantages. The human mind can use almost any object as a weapon. Using a gun for self-defense does not always give optimal protection. You could be outsmarted and not have enough time to react before using your gun.

You could be a civilian in normal society that prevents law-abiding citizens from carrying weapons. Whether you are a man, a woman, an able youth, a soldier, an officer or a Secret Service agent, you may find large gaps in your personal protection. Feeling unsafe can cause your subconscious to worry, which wastes your energy.

The moment you feel you have the upper hand, you minimize the damage you inflict on your opponent, unless it jeopardizes your safety. In Krav Maga, you are trained to control the level of severity by controlling the depth of your strike.

To facilitate reasonable safety, we try to identify a threat as early as possible and avoid as many threats that we can in our daily routines.

Modern governments strive to provide their citizens with a safe living environment. Yet daily, people lose their lives in precarious situations that could have been easily controlled.

We learn not to talk to strangers when we are small. We learn to differentiate suspects according to the place and time of the day, their clothes, their behavior. We learn to notice if they are busy minding their own business or watching us as their prey.

We learn to limit our children's Internet communications, not to put them in a situation where they could be outsmarted and become victims. We learn to protect our computers from hackers who might steal information or our financial assets. We lock our doors and windows as well. But we know, where there is a will, there is a way.

We know that a reasonable time for emergency help to arrive is about ten minutes. We know that many times, the police arrive too late to do anything but write a report. The alarm does not protect our lives and property; it just gets the police and us aware that something is going on. It is up to us and the police to protect our assets and especially our lives. With today's crime patterns, ten minutes may not be enough for a burglar to break into our homes, load everything on his truck, and take off, but it is definitely enough time for him to kill everyone in the house and take off.

For civilians, law enforcement, and soldiers, chances are that at the end of the chain of safety, armor, and weapons that can make the job easier and impersonal from a great distance, attacker and defender might eventually meet face to face at any given time and in any given place.

If we keep all that in our mind, and once in a while think of possible scenarios, and review our safety plans, we can ensure that we are still in a state of reasonable safety.

You have learned the principles of self-defense. You have gained an understanding of reaction time, and you should be able to now assess your advantages and disadvantages in maintaining your safety. The most important things to avoid are situations where you could be totally surprised. Assessing the dangers in each environment ahead of time should easily become your second nature.

Generally when we see someone attacking, we conclude that he is guilty of creating violence. Hopefully lawmakers realize that you have a right to live, and if someone is trying to kill you, you might kill him. More important, they need to realize when you reach the break-even point of no return. You cannot really afford to wait until you are distracted with a slap. That might confuse you and buy your attacker time to kill you. Society should not expect you to bleed to death before you are allowed to kill in self-defense. By the same token it is illogical to be expected to wait until the opponent's blade is in your territory speeding to your heart. Reaction time should be the break-even point to determine if killing someone could have been avoided or not.

Self-Defense for Women

The major question in approaching teaching women self-defense is: Should you concentrate on the shorter range, letting the attacker grab the woman and assuming he will not kick her or punch her or slap her and give her a concussion before she can react?

If you concentrate on escaping close scenarios, you may build false confidence. You should teach pressure points and striking or manipulation techniques as well. Most importantly you should teach reaction times, the time it takes to start and complete possible attack attempts, and the time it takes to successfully initiate a reaction and foil these attacks. If a woman is only prepared to react when someone lays a hand on her, it might limit her combat options. What if an attacker is aware that many women learn self-defense and will try to surprise her in a countering way? What if you have multiple attackers? You should learn how to identify dangerous scenarios, analyze them and react to each potential threat as soon as possible.

In Krav Maga, you cover close scenarios completely, but you should also learn to respond to danger and eliminate it in its earlier stages, from a kicking or punching distance. Therefore, teaching women self-defense in any other form is obsolete. As a woman all you really need to learn is Krav Maga.

Pressure Points

Although the human body is full of pressure points, those selected for the purpose of self-defense and hand-to-hand combat should be accessible in the split-second window of opportunity a defender has, also bearing in mind the relative body positions of the attacker and defender.

For example, if the defender is standing erect, and the opponent has his arms high to the sides of the face, the defender would punch his chin. The main reason is that the punch fits well with regard to the height and angle of the chin.

From a closer distance, an elbow to the jaw or a strike to the temple or neck would be effective. Some pressure points are preferred over others, but we should consider their accessibility in deciding which to go for first.

In general, straight strikes have the greatest range. Once you are close, straight strikes can be too short, and therefore your motion would not have a long enough plane to accelerate and develop sufficient speed. You may need to use a circular motion in your strikes to gain sufficient force.

Everything, including pressure points, is relative. We need to learn to control the opponent in a way he can't harm us. This can be done with psychological deterrence, trickery, or physical distraction, or increasing the level of damage. The outcome of our efforts would cause our opponent delayed reaction, disorientation, incapacitation, or death.

We will look at the human body in a few perspectives. The first perspective is the aim. We should prioritize our aim to points that are easy to reach in an instant and will give us the desired results.

If you want to strike the head but you can't, strike another area. Our bodies could be positioned such that their head is hard to reach; they could be sitting on our stomachs while we're lying on the floor, for example. In this scenario, if we strike his head, it would not be in the first strike.

We should take into consideration the distance of the pressure point from our striking limb, and how accessible it is. We can strike, push, tear, or poke according to that distance.

We can also use leverage on joints to manipulate the opponent's body, throw him to the ground, or break his finger. A break of a finger will cause a short trauma and will stop the opponent, buying us time.

When striking, we need to make sure we have enough room for acceleration to develop sufficient force. We may poke or tear if we are closer. We may also use the opponent's body weight to deliver a blow to one of his own pressure points, like by throwing him on his head. We must however realize that a conscious person would try to mitigate his fall by landing on less vulnerable parts of his body, whether he was trained to do so or whether it was natural instinct.

Sixty percent of the human body contains water. The body is built from cells in the form of organ tissue, cartilage, bones, muscle tissue, and other types of tissue. The bone tissue is structured to protect vital organ tissues. The cartilage tissue connects bones to smooth out friction and absorb shocks. The organ tissue is the building core of organs.

Each organ has a slightly different tissue that has its own individual characteristics. For example, the brain tissue has a thinking capacity, where electric pulses are exchanged back and forth between the sensory and memory parts. The liver and kidneys have filtering characteristics, and are aided by enzymes that contribute to dissolving toxins.

Arteries supply blood with nutrients, and oxygen to organs. Tendons and ligaments connect bones to muscles. Nerves function as sensors. The brain has a few centers to analyze data from censors, and give commands to various organs of the body, for example, shivering when it is cold. Shivering is a muscular motion that generates immediate heat.

For our purposes, we divide the human self-defense system into two mechanisms. First, the inner mechanism, which causes a chain reaction designed to stop harm. This mechanism is activated after harm has already been inflicted to the body. Fear can cause hyperventilation and butterflies in the stomach, but a broken windpipe will cause fainting to conserve oxygen supply to the brain.

The fear factor also helps the body to function in emergency situations. The rapid heartbeat and the release of fats and hormones provide readiness for an increase in potential physical activity to help counter the danger.

Let us remember that a man with a broken windpipe still has about fifteen minutes to live. However, he would be unconscious and his revival would depend on someone coming to his help and puncturing a hole in his windpipe so he can breathe. There is a technique that might work at times, depending on the severity of the injury, where the windpipe is relocated to help restore breath.

The second is the outer mechanism. Upon sensing danger, it triggers an instinctive reaction and moves our bodies out of the range of danger, or blocks an attack depending on the opportunity.

In selecting pressure points, we need to consider the manner and outcome of their use.

We learn pressure points so we can know how much life we have left in each scenario, and how much life the opponent is left with. This will let us evaluate what to avoid and what to pursue.

Let us compare the brain and organ tissues to a sponge to understand what happens when they are hit. When you squeeze a sponge, the water in it shifts from one cell to another. Similarly, when this happens to the brain or vital organs, it causes a trauma or concussion. It activates the self-defense mechanism. Therefore, sensations of pain and loss of consciousness are designed to limit further injury.

Internal bleeding, lack of oxygen supply, and tearing of the spinal cord can cause death. Tearing of the spinal cord can cause paralysis. Striking major muscle groups like pecs, hamstrings, thighs and calves, causes a concentration of lactic acid. This is painful and temporarily limits the motion of the body in the respective area.

Striking areas with cartilage and ligaments can cause overstretching or tearing of the ligaments and the cartilage tissue. Overstretched or torn ligaments can fill up a joint with synovial fluid that swells it to prevent further damage and inflict severe pain and immobility. If torn, one cannot walk, until it has been repaired.

It takes enormous impact to crack the skull. One needs to use a golf club, or a baseball club, or have a motorcycle accident. However, a strike to the face uses the inner skull to impact the soft brain tissue. The motion needs to be fast. Using the skull to protect the inner tissue subjects it to harm by keeping it susceptible to a punch. There is no need to fracture the skull in order to cause concussion. A speedy impact will cause a shift of brain fluid, or cause internal bleeding and affect the inner tissue, cells and nerves, and veins, thus causing a trauma, or concussion.

I would like to note that all limbs have nerves that cause pain when the body senses an injury. Most times it is easier to attack the limb, cause the damage, and let the nerve send a message to the brain, letting it know that this limb is out of use and hence causing the body to restrict its own motion out of caution.

We will now get a clear picture of where the pressure points are from each angle of approach.

Hair (for gripping): We can pull someone's hair to throw them to the ground and smash their head on the ground. We can do this from the front and smash their face on our knee, on a bar counter, or all the way down to the floor.

Skull: The adult skull is normally made of twenty-two bones. Except for the mandible, all the skull bones are joined together by sutures, which are semi-rigid articulations formed by a bony ossification called Sharpey's fibers. The fibers permit a little flexibility.

Top of the head: The top of the head is where the frontal cranial bones join. Sharpey's fibers, which have a

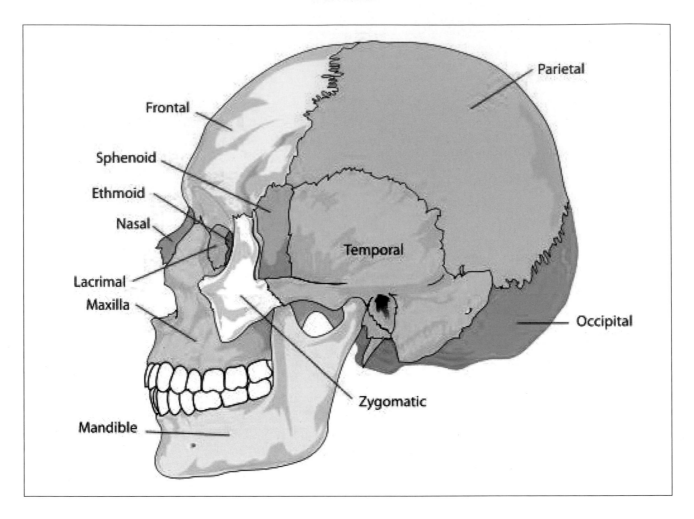

toothcomb structure, are much more enhanced. Forceful strikes or throwing a person on top of his head will cause trauma to the cranial cavity. You can also grab the top of the opponent's head and pull him down for a knee-strike to the face. There is very little resistance that one can generate in response to a pull on the top of the head.

Edge of the eyes: A strike to the cavity around the edge of the eye will cut skin on the bone and cause bleeding and blurry vision.

Eyes: Aiming to poke someone's eyes is not recommended since the opponent may move his head, and your fingers will instead hit a sturdy bone. However, a controlled scratch or a closer poke using both hands to hold the opponent's head still will cause pain and give you control from a close distance. It is one preferred method to get out of a grapple.

Place your open hands on the opponent's cheeks, and insert one thumb into the eye cavity. Keep pushing until he reacts by jumping backwards. Scuba divers who are used to high pressure may need three quarters of your thumb pushed in a slow motion before reacting. If you jab quickly, it will trigger a faster reaction,

mostly out of fear. Gouging out eyes is not an easy task as the opponent does not stand still.

Temples: Skull bones are weak at the temple. An artery and large nerve lie close to the skin. An accurate strike can cause a concussion. If the artery is severed, a massive hemorrhage compresses the brain, which can cause death.

I personally have used this technique in real life. I used a roundhouse punch with my middle knuckle protruding. My attacker was unconscious for at least few minutes. I did not stay around for him to wake up.

A roundhouse kick would cause severe damage. A strike using the edge of the palm would cause damage as well. However, we need to know that roundhouse kicks are optional only if the person is close to us but not attacking us. If we utilize the reaction time principle, we would never allow this, and in order to strike as he is moving closer, we would straight punch his face. If a person grabs us in a low bear hug, we can aim for his temple as well.

Ears: Striking the ears with cupped hands can rupture the eardrums, which causes severe pain. The attacker's instinct then is to leave you alone and cover his own ears. When caught in a bear hug, you can scream in the attacker's ear, causing more pain. You can also bite his ear causing him to let go of your body.

Nose: Any blow to the nose can break its thin bones, causing extreme pain, watering of the eyes, and breathing difficulties. This buys you time for the next more severe attack.

Nasal bridge: With a little force, you can push upwards from under the nose at a forty-five degree angle and move the attacker's body away from you if he grabs you in a bear hug. You can then smack your own thumb with your other hand's palm, which will create an accurate blow to the nasal bridge. You will encounter no resistance, and he will encounter great pain and disorientation.

Teeth: You can break your opponent's teeth in a kick or hand strike. This would give your opponent a headache and also buy you time. Your opponent may need a few seconds to assess the damage to his own body.

Chin: A punch to the chin can cause a concussion if you learn the hand strike techniques mentioned in this book. The lighter version will buy you time.

Mouth: Biting someone's lips or tongue will give him severe pain, causing temporary stunning. When you stop biting, your opponent will be busy dealing with the pain. The tongue is full of nerves and muscle.

Jaw: An uppercut elbow to the jaw can cause a concussion if the jaw is closed, since it delivers a strike to the back of the brain with the jaw as leverage. If, however, the jaw is open, it could get dislocated, and your opponent will accidentally bite his tongue. This will cause severe stunning and pain, and possibly a concussion as well.

Throat: A blow to the throat can crush the windpipe, which causes stunning and immediate fainting. Pushing your thumbs or fingers to your opponent's throat, or circling the rest of your fingers around it will break the windpipe as well. One should be careful of plucking, where your opponent may attempt to grab your windpipe from the side and tear it. After about fifteen minutes you would be dead from lack of oxygen to the brain. If you push one finger down to the cavity below the windpipe, you can easily take an aggressor down.

Side of the neck: A chop to the side of the neck can close the carotid artery and keep it from delivering blood and oxygen to the brain. This would cause

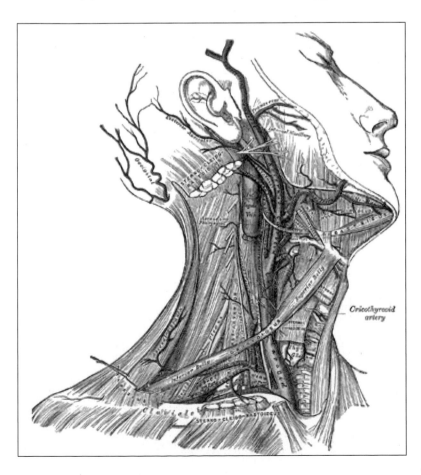

unconsciousness. At times a knife hand chop to the side of the neck can strike the vagus nerve and slow down the heart rate, leading to dizziness. Slashing your opponent's throat with a sharp object will tear his artery and make him severely bleed, perhaps to death. Your opponent could use your shirt or a rope to strangle you. You might not immediately feel it, and you have to realize you have to get out of it in less than three seconds before you faint.

Clavicle hollow: A downward hammer blow or a knife hand-strike can fracture the clavicle (collarbone). This will cause severe pain and lack of mobility in the arms. A knife stab in that cavity will cause a puncture in the carotid artery, which will cause severe bleeding and death.

Back of the head or neck: A powerful blow to the back of the head can cause concussion or a broken neck where the head is used to leverage the neck vertebrae. A broken neck means severed vertebrae, pressuring or cutting the spinal cord, or releasing cerebral fluid creating high pressure in the brain. This can cause immediate death. Holding the attacker's head with both hands in a spinning motion can break the neck or cause disk damage. Depending on the force, the opponent can be temporarily stunned, or he can die.

Armpit: A large nerve close to the skin in the armpit, when kicked, causes severe pain and paralysis. If your attacker is holding a knife with his front arm in front of his shoulder and above, you wait for him to extend it in a stabbing motion. You lean your upper body backward and then kick his armpit. This will cause the knife to fly out of his hand, and he will stop attacking you. To ensure you do not miss, it is suggested to use the outer side of your foot as contact as opposed to the ball of your foot.

Sternum: The heart is underneath the lower part of the sternum. A kick to the sternum with a heavy shoe can stun the opponent causing his heart to change its rhythm. The person will drop to the floor until his rhythm comes back to normal. You aim a kick for the chin if he attacks you with a knife, aiming for your abdomen, but it might land on his sternum which will stop his attack as well. Refer to the scissors kick technique for a low hold knife attack in the knife defense chapter.

Chest pectorals: Large muscles, when kicked, will cause severe pain due to accumulation of lactic acid, and cause a temporary stunning of the upper body.

Nipples: A large network of nerves passes near the skin at the nipples. Biting them can cause extreme pain and temporary stunning. This technique can usually be used in rape prevention, when the woman bites the attacker's nipple.

Celiac plexus: A dense cluster of nerve cells and supporting tissue is located behind the stomach in the region of the celiac artery, just below the diaphragm. Rich in ganglia and interconnected neurons, the celiac plexus is the largest autonomic nerve center in the abdominal cavity. Through branches, it controls many vital functions such as adrenal secretion and intestinal contraction. A blow to that area, if it penetrates it, may temporarily halt visceral functioning.

In Krav Maga, we rather teach our students to prefer the false ribs area to the sides, if they duck for a low punch, or if they knee to that height. The reason behind this is that it is hard to be accurate at that angle. An athlete could have large muscles protecting this area, while an overweight person can have fat used as

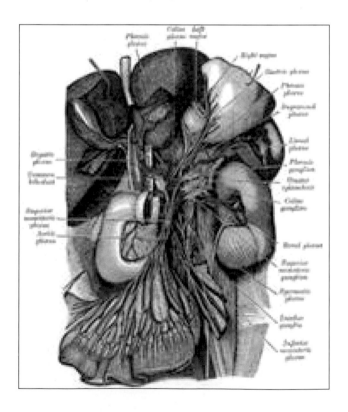

protection layer. However, if a window of opportunity allows us to hit that pressure point, we should know that the solar plexus is a center for nerves that controls the cardio-respiratory system. A blow to this location is painful and can stun the opponent, taking the breath out of his lungs. A more powerful blow shocks the nerve center and causes unconsciousness.

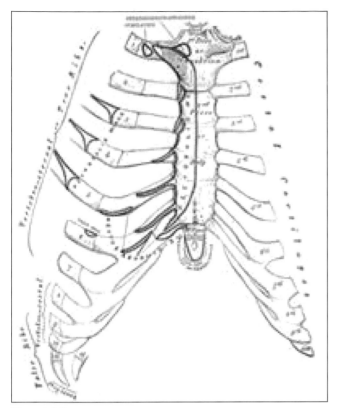

Front View

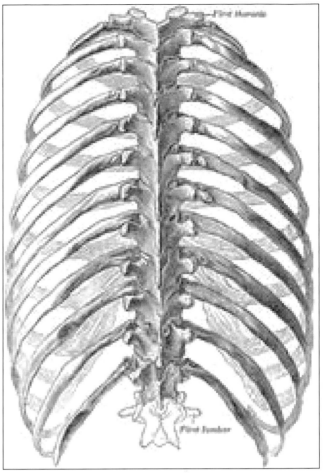

Back View

False and floating ribs: The last five ribs are called false ribs. Three out of the five false ribs are attached to each other with cartilage. The last ribs on the bottom are small in width, and only attached to the ribcage at the spine. They are the weakest in the ribcage. A blow to the floating rib will easily fracture it. If on the right side, the fractured rib can cause internal injury to the liver; fractured ribs on either side can possibly puncture or collapse a lung.

Kidneys: The kidneys are located underneath the floating ribs at the back of the human body. If the person is standing with his side or back to you, you can strike them with a roundhouse kick, or a knife hand chop (slapping motion). This causes shock and possibly an internal injury. Internal injuries can cause pain and infection, and if not treated, can later cause death. A stab in the kidney can cause death due to severe internal bleeding.

Stomach: A blow to the abdomen, when the opponent does not contract his muscles, can cause a shock.

This is a direct blow to the intestines, and while the abdominal muscles are not contracted, the intestines are not protected. A shift of internal fluid and an immediate intense pressure on the intestines causes a shock, and any food in the upper part may be vomited. It also can cause internal bleeding.

Liver: A blow or a kick to the liver, located on the front right side under the ribs, can cause laceration. It can drop your opponent to the floor immediately.

Waist and hips: We generally aim our kicks to the groin area but with the ball of the foot to take into account the possibility the opponent might move a bit in the last split second. This means we might end up kicking his waist or upper thigh. Kicking the pelvis bone unbalances the opponent's center of gravity. We want to make sure our ankle can take the impact, and as a rule of thumb we always kick with either the ball or the heel of the foot for a front kick or the heel for a side kick. This keeps the ankle joint in a neutral position, which can take a greater impact without injury.

The reason why we aim to the opponent's belt area is very simple. Our kick originates from the same area in our body. Kicking in a linear motion forward will give us the longest range and will keep the rest of our body out of reach from the opponent's kicks. We would only kick lower if our hands are tied up in a wrestling hold with the opponent, or against a committed knife stab.

Roundhouse kicks would not be our first choice, since a front or a side kick is much easier, and faster to execute, and simple. However, getting out of the way of a lunging opponent while keeping a kicking range would be a perfect scenario to put the roundhouse kick into use. If an attacker is lunging with a straight knife stab we would throw our hips and shoulders in the direction of the attacker's front hand. This will throw our center of gravity pulling our body out of the line of the blade and will at the same time drive the force of the roundhouse kick to the groin.

Testicles: One of the Krav Maga favorite pressure points. This would be the first choice for a kick. In close combat, and in any wrestling situation, this pressure point is almost always accessible. Testicles have many nerves. The pelvis bone could be used as a vice to squash them with a powerful kick. Squashing can be done with a hand. Tight jeans would only help a forceful strike.

The key is to strike underneath the body, between the thighs. A blow to the testicles can cause stunning, severe pain, trauma, shock, loss of consciousness, or even death from a related neurogenic shock.

A single blow to the testicles is the most effective way to immobilize a man. This area is richly supplied with nerves and a blow can stop him in his tracks for ten to twenty seconds.

Testicles were the centerpieces of an unusual legal case heard in Papua New Guinea in 1995, which saw two young women jailed for six years. The women, from the Highlands province of Chimbu, both managed to kill their husbands by crushing their testicles—a form of death not well known in Australia.

One woman knocked her husband unconscious with a swift kick to the groin. He later died, doctors reported, from "severe bruising of both testicles." The other woman grasped her husband's testicles and "pulled down hard" to get him to remove his foot from her neck. The post-mortem found that he suffered profound neurogenic shock resulting from "a smashed left testicle."

Neurogenic shock: A life-threatening medical condition in which there is insufficient blood flow throughout the body, caused by a sudden loss of signals from the sympathetic nervous system that maintains the normal muscle tone in the walls of blood vessels. These blood vessels relax and become dilated, resulting in pooling of the blood in the venous system and an overall decrease in blood pressure. A neurogenic shock can be a complication of an injury to the brain or spinal cord.

While Australian urologists agree that crushed testicles can cause inordinate pain, they doubt whether they can actually cause death. There would have to be other factors such as a ruptured bladder or septicemia involved as well.

In Krav Maga, we wait for a person to be bent in half and in trauma. We then continue with a downward hammer-fist to the back of his neck. While there is no concrete evidence confirming whether kicking or squeezing testicles can cause death, a hammer punch to the back of the neck surely will settle the argument. The person can die, and what can be left for the Australian pathologist is to determine if it was from the blow to the groin, or to the back of the head. Piece of cake!

Thighs: A kick to the thighs causes an accumulation of lactic acid in the large muscle, the quadriceps. This causes trauma and severe pain. It stops the attacker and buys you a little time. Side kicks can be effective for this purpose. If you must kick this area, a kick to the lower thigh, closer to the knee, would be your preferred spot.

Knee: Kicking the knee from the side causes the cruciate ligaments to stretch and even tear. At the same time, the cartilage tears as well. This causes immobility as the knee joint gets filled with synovial fluid to protect it from further injury.

The attacker is immobilized with great pain, and cannot do anything but hold his knee. The cruciate ligaments stabilize the femur bone in the upper leg, with the tibia bone in the lower leg below the knee. The kneecap is hard to break with a kick.

Coccyx bone: The coccyx is the last bone of the spine. It is a preferred place to kick when an opponent turns his back on you to prepare for a roundhouse kick, or just to escape.

A kick to the coccyx will cause him to fall on to his face. A hard kick causes trauma as well and also a broken bone, which can take six months to heal. If closing the gap as the opponent turns his back, you can also knee that bone.

Hamstring: A kick to the hamstring can cause muscle spasms and slow down the opponent's mobility.

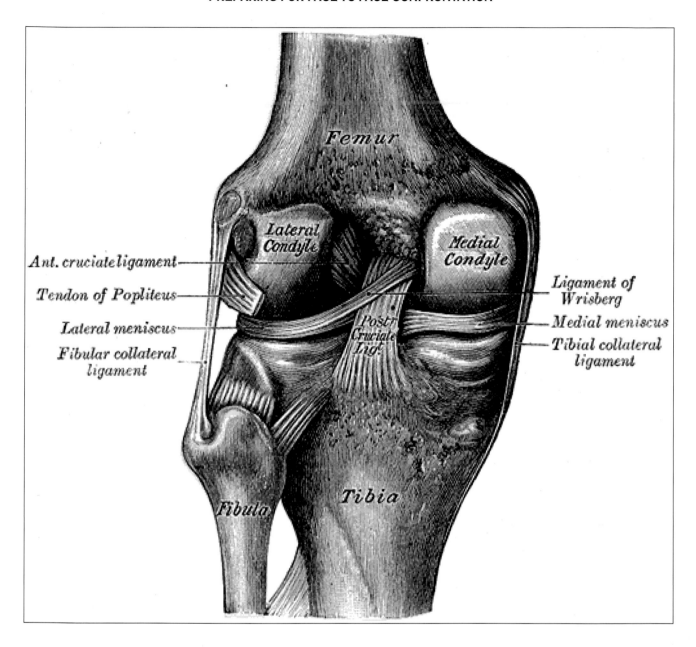

Calf: A roundhouse upward kick to the calf tosses both the opponent's legs in the air, and he falls down. However, it would not be the preferable mode of attack. You have to come around him at the right angle, otherwise you waste a valuable second or two. Another result is a muscle spasm.

Shin: When the opponent grabs you from behind, kick him in the shin with your heel and scrape it with your shoe. This causes great pain, and he will lessen his grip on your body.

Top of the foot: The top of the foot has small bones that can easily be fractured with a stomp. When an opponent grabs you from behind or from the front you can stomp on his foot. This causes fracture and severe pain, and limits the attacker's mobility as well.

Achilles tendon: It is located in the back of the heel. Make sure you protect yours. When you spring forward to kick your opponent, make sure you land properly on the base foot. Make sure your landing leg is right in the center of your gravity. Land the ball of the foot first and heel second, and make sure your foot does not get caught and you twist your ankle. This will keep your mobility intact. Remember that you need to land your base foot in about a forty-five-degree angle so your kicking leg will be comfortably able to reach maximum kicking range, without having your body center of gravity shift over your base foot risking your tendons.

The Achilles tendon is named for Achilles, an armored Greek soldier who was most vulnerable at his heels. A smart opponent would try to cut his tendon, taking advantage of the heavy armor that would slow him down.

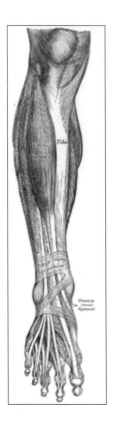

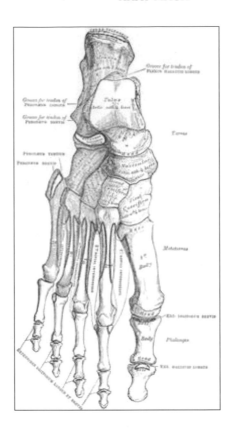

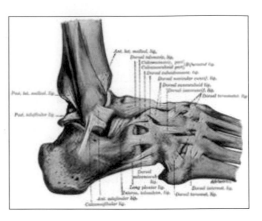

All joints: We use most of them to control the opponent by causing him severe pain and immobilizing him. Shoulders, elbows, wrists, fingers, knees, ankles, toes, the neck area, and weak parts of the spine are all vulnerable points in the body. We use the shoulder joint and elbow joint to manipulate the opponent's body.

We mostly use the opponent's wrist to hold him in place, or to throw his body to the ground or on to a second attacker to buy time. We also use pressure on the joints to escape from holds.

Wrestlers often inflict unbearable pain on the knees by attempting to overstretch the ligaments and tear the cartilage. We can escape a wrestler's attempt by either pulling our leg out of his hands quickly, or moving toward him with a punch before he completes his attempt. It is very uncommon to use knees as pressure points in this manner, and it is not as quick as using other pressure points available. A man with no shoes could have his toes targeted as well.

Specific Warm-Up

Years ago, when I was training in various martial arts and visiting various schools, I noticed a range of routines common to each one. While you are learning the building blocks of Krav Maga, a specific kind of warm-up is recommended to leave enough lesson time. After all, what is the purpose of stretching your legs if all you will be doing is hand strikes?

I will present you with a warm-up for a comprehensive day of a seminar, and if you are teaching a lesson, you could extract exercises related to the appropriate muscle groups you will be using in your lesson. This is a one of many comprehensive warm-ups I recommend for a class. But if you feel you have other methodical ways to warm up and they work for you, use them.

As an instructor, remember to assess the group's physical ability, and design the lesson and warm-up accordingly. The following warm-up has some very challenging elements. Do not ask your students to do something that they cannot. Remember they are here to learn Krav Maga, and need to stretch to prevent injury during training.

1. Squat to the ground ten times.
2. Keep your knee locked and lean forward while reaching your fingers to the ground, putting all your weight on that leg. Allow your other leg to

either rest on the ground or be lifted up, as long as you do not put any weight on it.

3. Spread your feet apart, keeping your weight at the center between your knees during this stretch. Point one foot upwards, resting on the heel and keeping the leg straight, and bend your opposite knee. Lean your body forward. Switch from side to side. Start slowly and pause, and continue shifting fast. This stretches your thighs and at the same time warms up your ankles. It is important to keep your torso in the middle between both knees to prevent injury.

4. Sitting on the ground, spread your legs forward to the sides as far as you can, slowly trying to touch the ground with your elbow in. Stay in this position and bend your knees. Now shake your shoulders forward from side to side while leaning forward. You are releasing your lower back muscles, making it easier to do the previous stretch.

5. Go back and try the previous stretch again. Now lean forward with your chest getting closer to the ground. If you try to stretch in this position for half an hour you would probably end up reaching the floor with your chest.

6. Grab one ankle with both hands, and extend it forty-five degrees forward and up. Roll on your back and get up to a sitting position a few times to keep stretching your hamstring and calves. Lock the free leg's knee and leave it on the ground, so its weight is used as leverage to pull in the opposite direction of your stretch. Don't forget to switch and stretch the other leg as well.

7. Sitting on the ground and holding your ankles, extend one leg at a time pointing forty-five degrees up to the side. Extend both and try to maintain balance. If you lose your balance, roll back and forth on your back, keeping your legs stretched some more.

8. Standing on your neck and head, hold your waist with straight legs.

9. Continue to stretch your legs gently over your head to the ground.

10. End with pushups (press-ups) while keeping your head alternating to the sides.

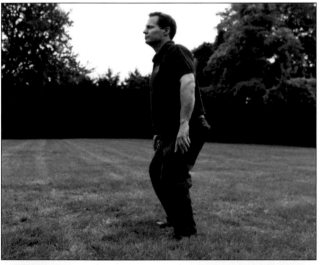

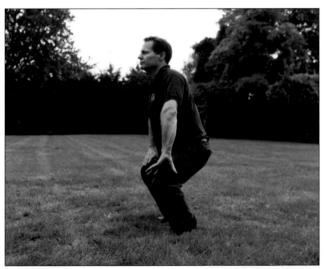

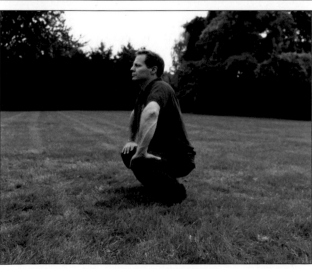

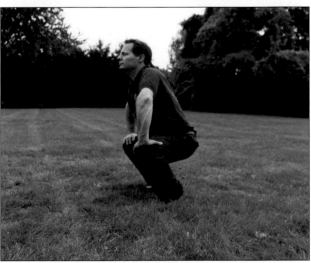

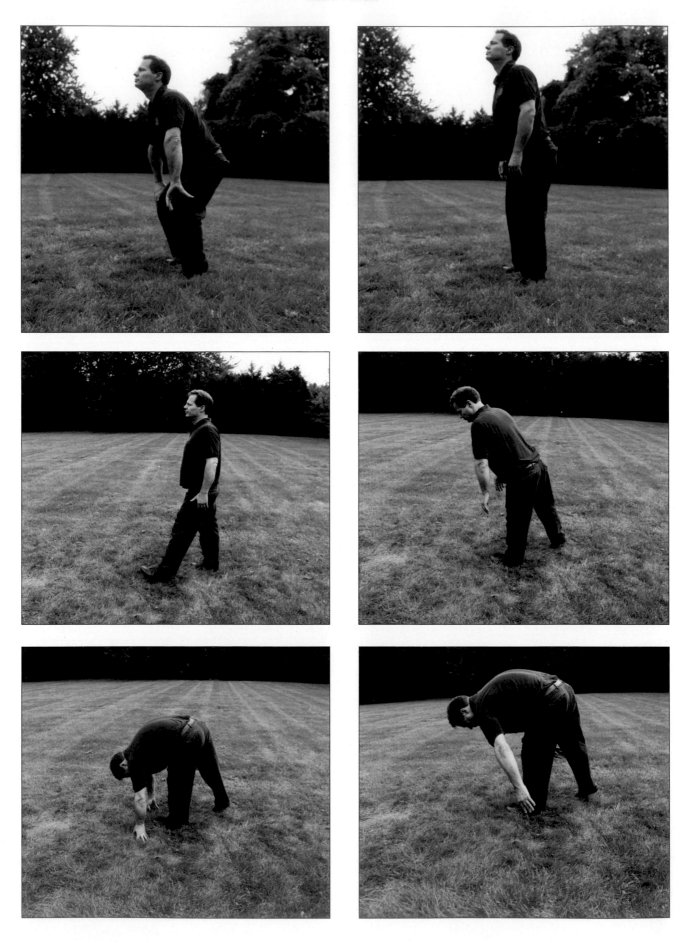

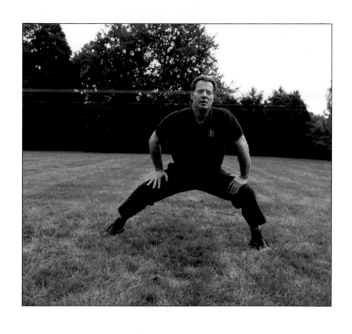
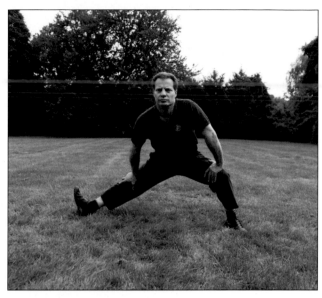

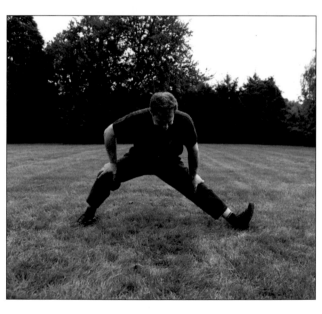
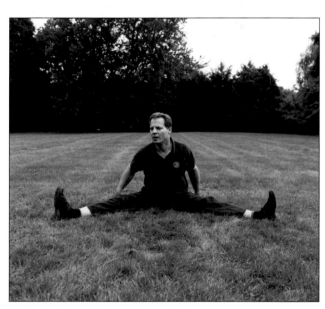

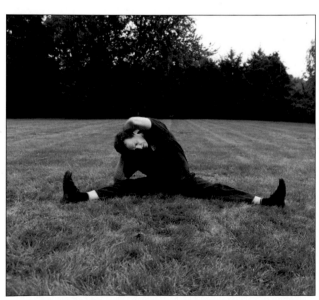
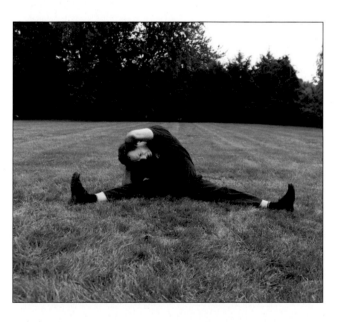

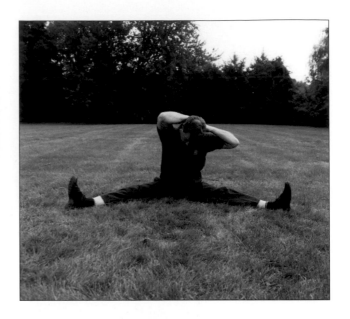

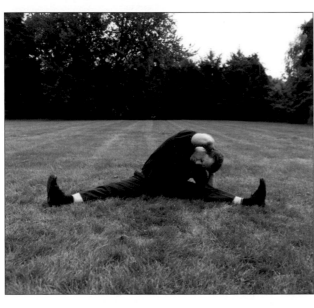

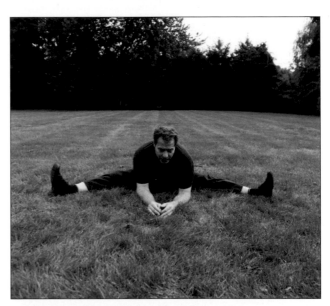

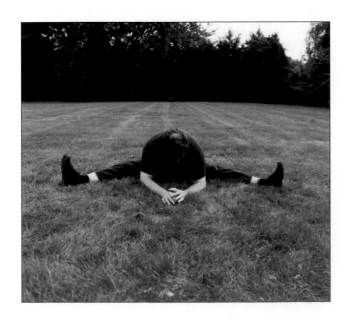

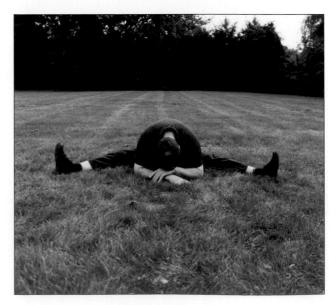

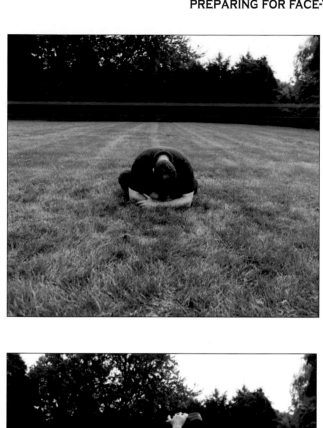

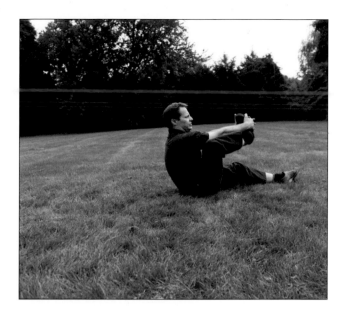

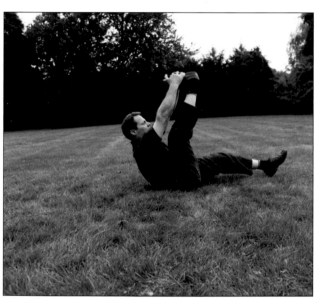

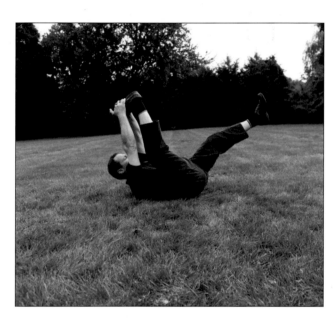

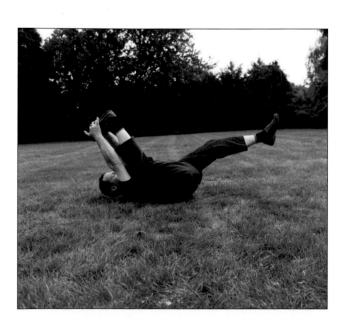

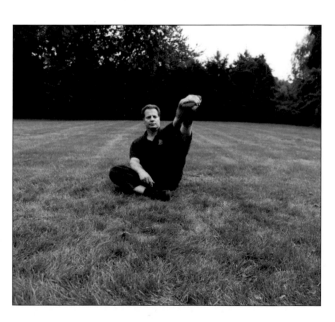

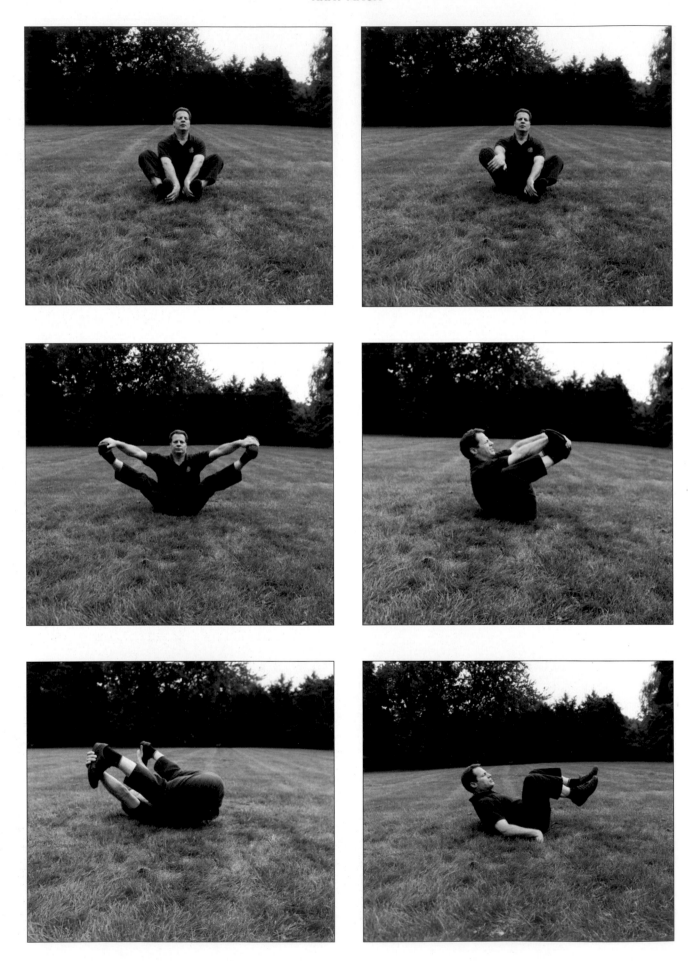

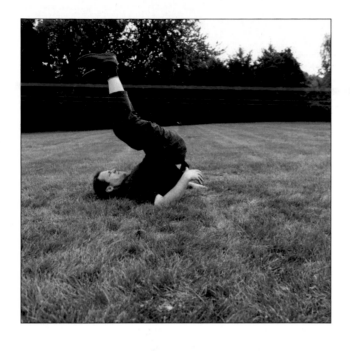

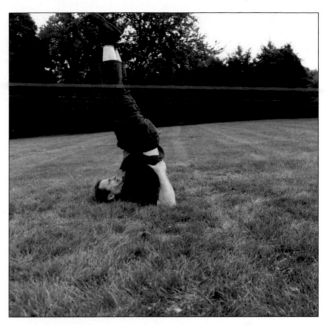

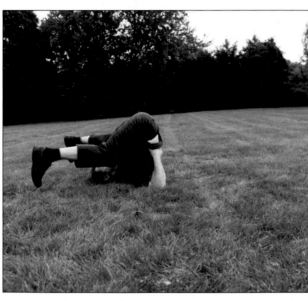

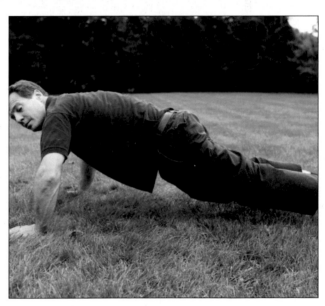

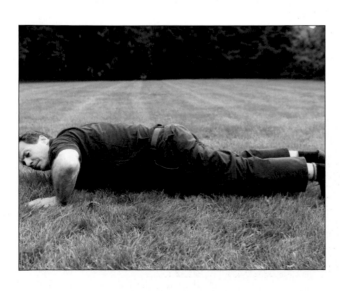

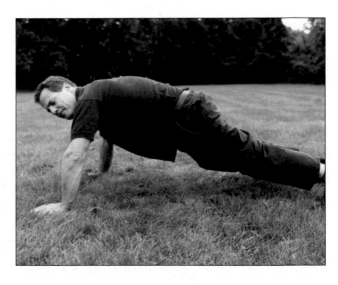

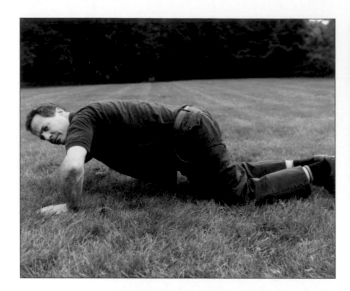
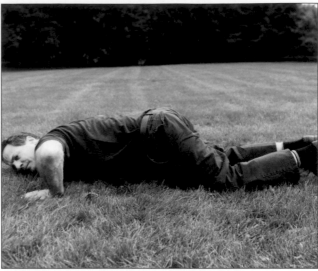
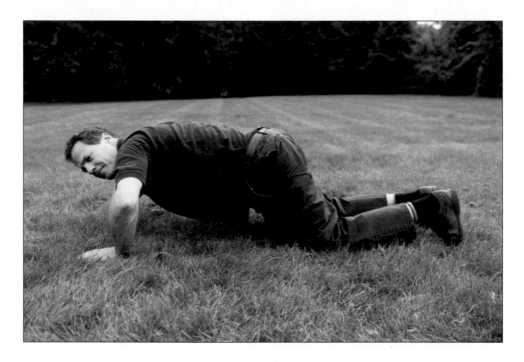

PRIMARY STRIKES AND KICKS

Krav Maga pays attention to the need to close the gap quickly when attacking an opponent. The advance, while kicking or punching, is made with a forward leap. Using gravity to initiate the move, push forward with the toes in an attempt to lodge one of your limbs in the opponent's body as quickly as possible.

Krav Maga training calls for a maximum range of the body's limbs when practicing attacks, and the use of folded limbs to attack in the closer range.

The idea is to gain the maximum acceleration possible with the limb used and to keep the speed at its max when in contact with the opponent's pressure points. Remember that when the motion comes to a complete stop, it must have started to slow down a split second before.

Once a strike is executed we need to maintain full speed if we want to incur maximum damage or if we want to stun him. Therefore we cannot afford to lower the speed of our motion a split second before the strike or a split second after. Aim at the pressure point you want to strike, make sure you use maximum speed, and make sure you do not stop when you reach the range where your target is or will be in the next second.

Take into account that your opponent might start to move forward or backwards, which means he won't stay still exactly where you were aiming for. If your arm or leg comes to a complete stop upon contact with the opponent, it indicates you must have slowed down a second before and the speed was not fast enough to create the desired momentum.

To maintain maximum speed at the contact point with the targeted pressure point, the striking limb should be immediately retracted back. This helps keep up the speed while accelerating. It is faster to retract the hand without the body. We then let the body continue its motion forward while the hand is retracted backward. This sequence ensures that the body weight supports our punch without letting us lose speed.

When executing a front kick, the upper body is used in a seesaw motion to help thrust the foot upwards, against gravity, straight to the target's body. At the same time, a body leaning backwards provides balance to the extended foot.

Kicks are executed in a swing motion where the foot is retracted immediately and at the same speed as the kick. This ensures maximum speed at the contact point, and the continuous balance of the body, which coordinates the upper body and the kicking leg. In Krav Maga, balance is a temporary state during both attack and defense. It does not mean standing in one place, but a rapidly coordinated mobility in a balanced sequence.

To create devastating kicks and hand strikes, Krav Maga attempts to maintain maximum speed at the time of contact with the opponent's body. From a static position, your hand or leg accelerates over maximum distance.

In order to maintain speed that can create the desirable shock to the opponent's head; you cannot stop after you pass the target. The hand or leg is retracted to maintain the speed achieved by the acceleration, rather than arriving at a complete stop once it reaches the target. Reaching a complete stop as we strike indicates an undesired slowdown right before impact.

Training partners execute strikes and kicks in realistic ranges. To control the possible damage to each other, they only extend their limbs to the point where it hits the opponent's body just below the skin. The speed of the attack is what creates enough shock to slow down the opponent's momentum.

If you have ever practiced on a speed bag, remember that it is very different from a full body punch. Since the speed bag always moves faster than your body, you can touch it with your hands or fists, but if you do not use your body fully, the punches are not really effective. While it is a good exercise to practice coordination, it can lead to some lousy punches in real-life situations. However, if the student is aware that all he is doing is practicing his hand-eye coordination, then it is indeed a good training method. Think of it like a trainee trying to catch a fly with a chopstick.

The need to quickly strike from a distance calls for a fast delivered strike. In throwing a punch from a distance, chances are that the opponent will not stand still. This is why a hand strike aimed to the face is preferred.

Great athletes like Muhammad Ali had higher knockout rates than others. Krav Maga would rather teach the mechanics of a knockout punch in the first lesson than leaving it to the student to learn on their own through repeated heavy bag training. A person weighing only 100 pounds could deliver a knockout punch if he learns how to use his or her body effectively. I do not think an attacker can stand still while being hit with a fifty-pound dumbbell in their face. The force generated with a Krav Maga punch is at least one and a half times the person's body weight, with a speed of about 20 miles per hour. While boxers punch with a force of three to four times their body weight, they had the opportunity to take their time for a finishing punch. However without projection one cannot deliver that much force, and the idea in straight punches is to deliver maximum force in minimum time and projection for the most efficient immediate stopping effect.

From the second you decide to move in and strike, all you need is to aim at the face. You then need to accelerate to maximum speed with your arm, and maintain that speed as your fist lodges into your opponent's face. The opponent's skull is sent backward, shaking the brain and nerves to a concussion.

The key to devastating hand strikes is to maintain maximum speed and weight shift at the contact point.

Before we learn defenses, we learn hand strikes since we need to know how to counterattack with our defenses. In addition, we want our training partners to challenge us with the most devastating attacks. At the end of the lesson, a student should be able to execute devastating knockout punches.

Straight Hand Strikes Front (hand closer to the opponent) and Rear

Straight hand strikes can be executed when your body is positioned facing directly at or up to a forty-five degree angle relative to your opponent.

Although the effective range is the distance covered with one leap forward while pivoting your shoulders, you should allow enough room to accelerate your hand and pass the target you are trying to reach.

1. Standing position has your hands down to avoid projecting intentions.
2. Lift your hands up. As your left hand moves forward, your torso is kept at about forty-five degrees toward the opponent. Roll your left knuckles into a tight fist. Keep your thumb bent forty-five degrees over your index finger. Tighten your forearm muscles to support its connection to the fist. Begin and end the punch with the back of the hand pointed to the sides of your body. Upon contact with the target, twist your fist to forty-five degrees where your two big knuckles stab your target. The knuckles should be positioned as a straight extension of your hand. Do not move your wrist once you have it ready for a punch. Keep your elbow pointed to the ground at all times to better deliver your body weight into the punch. The fist is moving toward the opponent's face to hit his chin, and the body follows, pivoting right behind the hand. The key is to lunge forward and only twist your shoulders when your fist is close to the opponent's chin. This will propel the weight shift supporting the punch. If you do it too soon, you will not have your weight supporting the punch!
3. Your left hand is passing the target at maximum speed as your right shoulder aligns your left shoulder.
4. Left hand is retracted to about ninety degrees away from the body. At this point, the punch has ended. Your right shoulder is behind the left. Stay in this position until you notice your opponent's next move.
5. Throw your right hand forward and pivot your body directly behind it in the direction of your opponent's chin. Note that when you execute a

front hand strike your torso leans forward. Now you need to erect your torso, keeping your rear leg extended and your rear shoulder knee locked, pivoting the rear heel and shoulder forward.

6. Your right hand fully extends in a strike with the seam of the pants facing the opponent.

7. Your right hand retracts, while your body is still in a forward motion. At this point, the punch has ended and you should stay in this position until he decides on the next move.

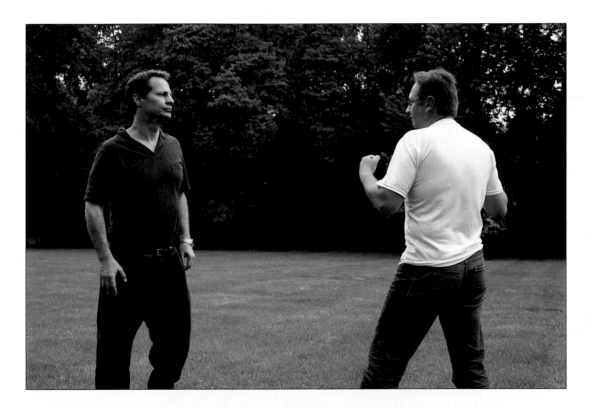

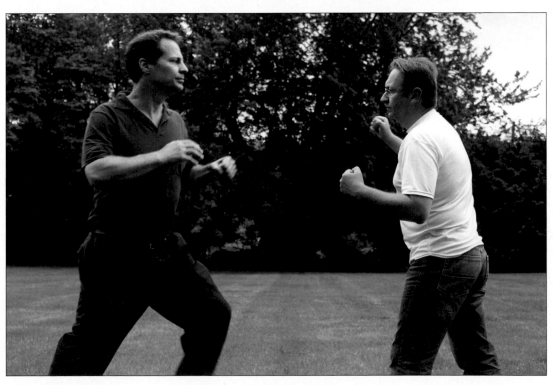

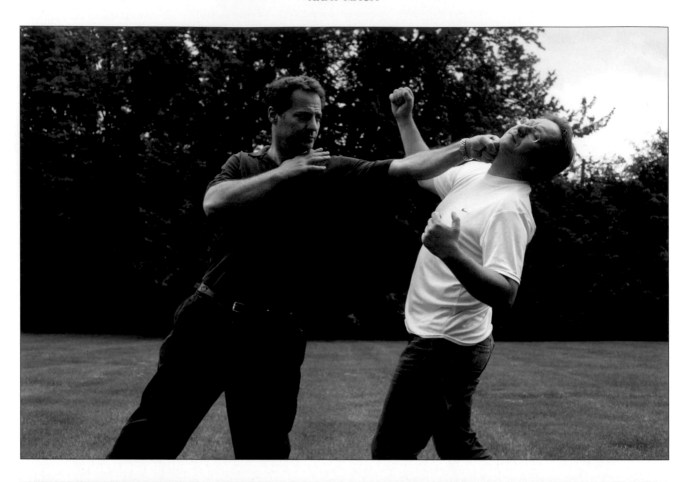

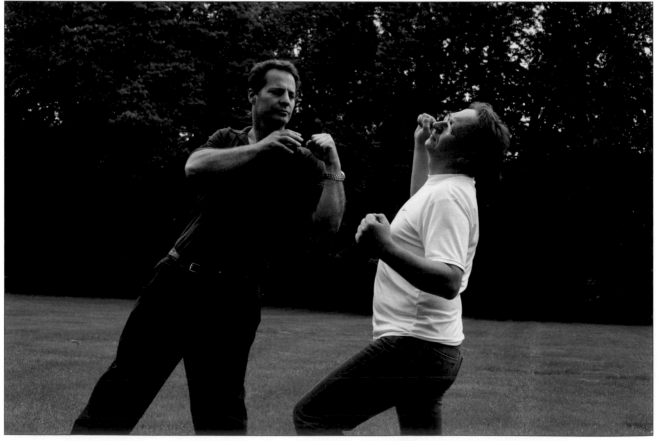

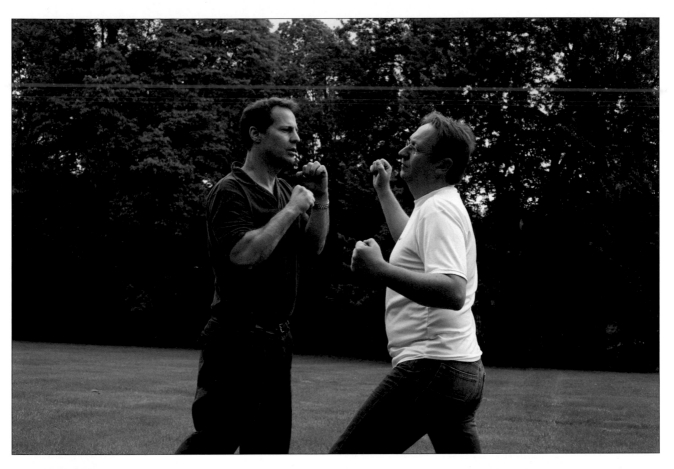

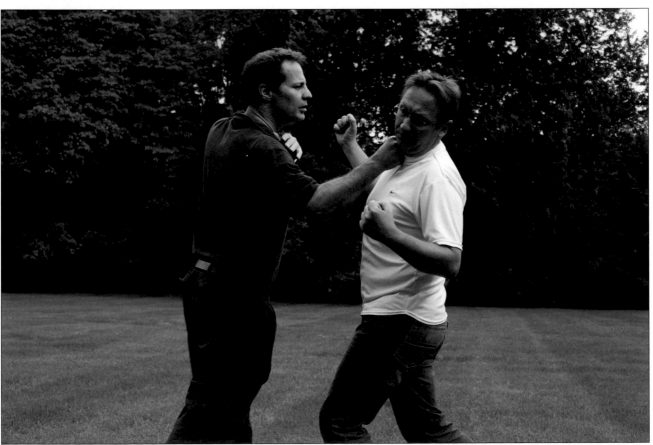

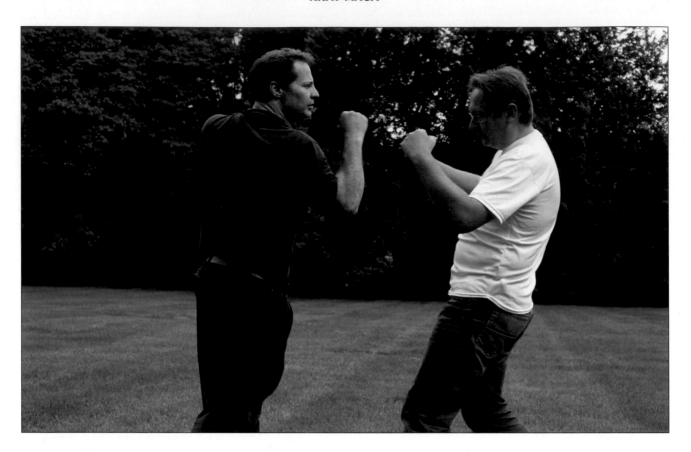

Note that it is preferable to stop the body in a forward position after each strike and wait for the next move, rather than to retract to a neutral position. This helps judge the next move without wasting time. Attempting to start another motion too soon will shift the body weight in the opposite direction, not supporting the previous motion.

The movement is broken into steps to facilitate a correct flow of motion. Each sequence is executed at least ten times until the instructor determines that the student acquired the desired habit. The hand commences the motion in step one, and pulls the body motion on its way to the target in step two, retracting only the hand is step three, and ending retraction of the body is step four. These four steps are gradually combined in an ascending order.

Steps one and two become step one, and step two becomes the retraction of the hand. Step three becomes the retraction of the body. After ten repetitions of each combination, the hand continues in a whip motion when it retracts, as the two steps are combined together, while the body continues forward up to a complete stop. It is essential that the weight shifts into the direction of the strike. If you lunge forward and pivot your shoulders before you contact the target, you cannot shift your weight into him and your punch will not have great force.

To get comfortable with punches, students should stand in a comfortable, balanced position and practice punching with both hands. Let us not forget however, that at the end of each punch the student should come to a complete stop and reevaluate the necessity and direction of the next move. After you practice punching standing up, you need to practice lunging with your front punch and a follow-up punch with the rear hand. A full motion punch would have the body at an angle and the rear leg extended to help keep balance while your weight would be directed behind the striking hand. Generally after you punch you land and retract your hand. Then you retract your rear leg closer, erecting your previously forward-leaning torso. You can then follow with a rear hand strike with the same motion.

Once you have learned these striking techniques, you need to practice them on punching mitts. Following the correct sequential execution will make the mitts fly far backwards. Your training partner should be holding the mitts in front of his face with his elbows locked, using them as shock absorbers. After you practice each hand, execute a combination of three strikes ensuring you finish each one of them. Remember, your first strike ends when your arm has retracted, but your shoulder was kept forward in the direction of the strike.

Practicing Frontal Movement

The following pictures, demonstrate a standing position used for learning principles. In Krav Maga, you learn how to move and execute strikes, kicks, and defenses from various angles. This standing position is basically a stance where one part of your body is closer to your opponent, as you still maintain a frontal position. Remember however, that in reality, you may have to act from an unexpected position.

As you practice the principles of movement, your upper body will aspire to balance itself. With each hand strike, or a kick, your upper body will be tilted forward or backward, supporting your hand strikes and kicks. Here is how to practice your frontal movement.

1. Stand with your feet perpendicular to your shoulders.
2. Pivot your torso forty-five degrees to your opponent. As you pivot, your torso and your front leg toes turn inward and your rear foot is pointed toward your opponent. Your weight is in the center of your body, resting on the balls of your feet. Note that if you are right-handed, you may prefer to keep your right leg in the rear since it is usually stronger and will support your weight better as you land on it while kicking with your front foot. In addition, it will give you greater lunging power.
3. Bring your hands up to where your elbows are in front of your stomach. You do not want your elbows to the sides of your body, since it would take you too long to bring them forward for defensive blocks.
4. Push with your rear foot and lunge forward with your front foot.
5. After you land on your front foot, bring your rear foot forward to the same initial stance. Keep the distance between your knees the same as before.
6. Push with your front foot and lunge backwards with your rear foot.
7. After you land on your rear foot bring your front foot backwards to create the same stance you had before.
8. Move to the left, initiating a movement by pushing with the rear foot to the left.
9. As you land on your right foot, bring it under your right shoulder.
10. Move to the right, initiating movement by pushing with your left foot to the right.

11. Bring your left foot to the right after you have landed on your right foot.

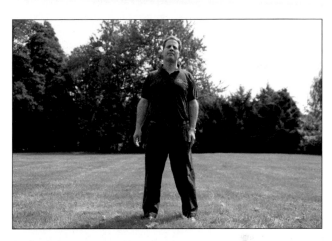

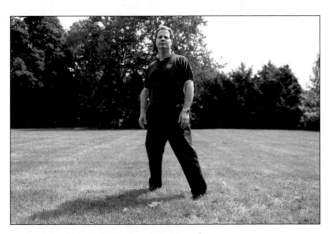

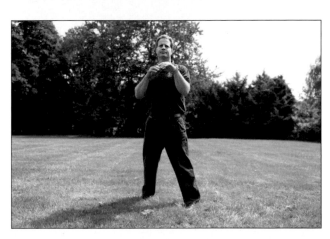

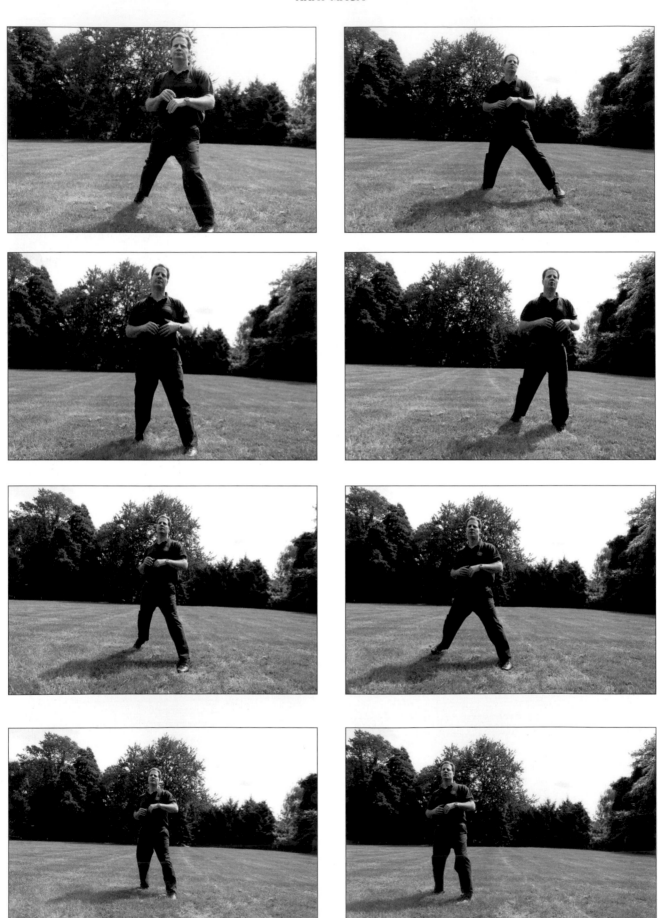

Note: Start slow and control your movement. Once you control your movement, increase your speed and move to all directions faster. You are now getting the footwork of shadowboxing. Add a front hand strike as you move forward. Your punch should be executed before you land, and as you lunge forward, your body will resemble a witch flying a broom.

Refer to the front-hand strike technique demonstrated previously in this chapter. Your front-hand strike should be executed as you lunge before your front leg lands on the ground. Your front hand should be retracted prior to your landing. As you strike with your front hand, your rear leg is extended in the air to balance your upper body that is tilted forward.

After you finish the front-hand strike, retract your hand and calculate your next move. Straighten your upper body, bringing your rear foot closer as you lunge your backhand to a punch. Follow the aforementioned hand strike instructions. Practice combinations of front-rear and front-hand strikes on a punching pad held by your training partner.

Take your time to complete each strike before you move to the next. If you attempt to continue too fast, you waste your initial strikes. Once you cover the gap, keep a distance of a hand and a shoulder as you fist punch your training target to facilitate optimal straight punches. The idea is to make small adjustments to control the range for each technique you practice. In a real-life situation, you may choose to use another technique if the gap has changed. Note that the exact positioning of the feet can be viewed in the Advanced Training Topics chapter.

Low Hand Strikes

Krav Maga low punches are learned for training purposes. Overall, it is faster to strike the face. Although some women have used this technique to punch a man's testicles inflicting great pain, the force of a forward strike instead of kicking upward against the pelvis bone is not sufficient to fold the man in half. Krav Maga uses the most effective low punches to train the student about possible scenarios without putting his face at risk. If you punch the abdomen area, make sure your head is at the same level of your strike. This prevents the opponent from reaching your face before you reach his abdomen. The flow of movement from the hand and body weight is the same as striking the face. Your hand is extended and retracted back while the body weight is being shifted forward.

Front hand low attack punch

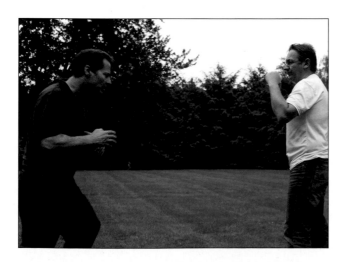 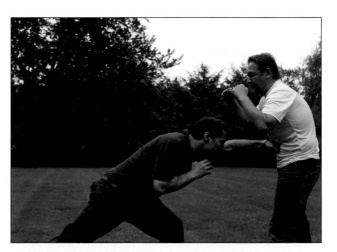

Front hand low defensive punch

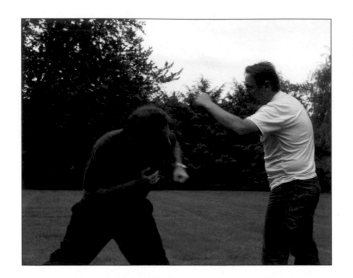 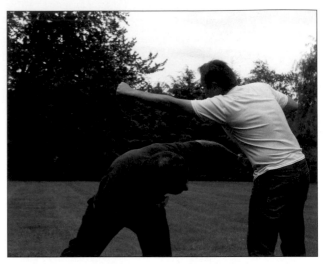

Rear hand low attack punch

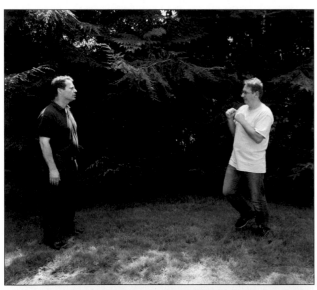 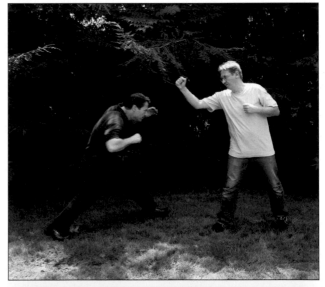

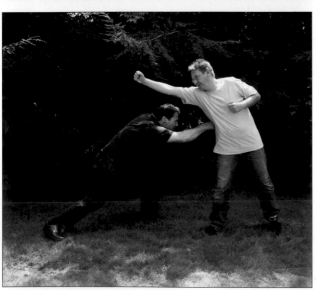 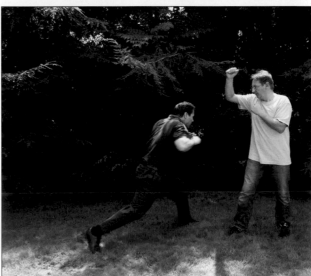

Rear hand low defensive punch

Defensive body movement while executing low punches creates defensive low punches. Using the same principles discussed above, punches are executed and the head now evades a top-down strike. These defensive punches can also be used when ducking down to avoid an opponent's strike. While these might facilitate a variety of opportunities for fighting games at the gym, they are not much needed on the street.

Lower punches help demonstrate the need to use principles of maximum reach with minimum exposure at any angle.

Note: You can continue with a pivot while turning your back to the opponent and executing a back-hand strike to the face.

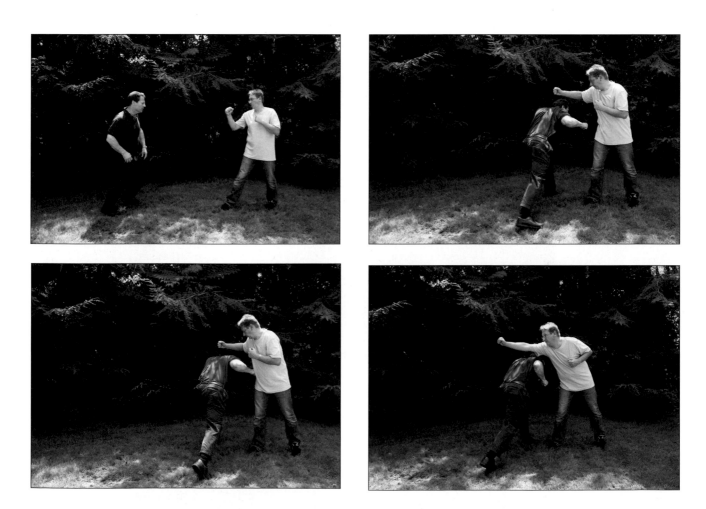

Back-Hand Strike from the Side

When your opponent is to your side within a hand strike range, you can use a back-hand strike to his face effectively. Your fist, with its knuckles inverted, is stabbing the face and your hip is moving forward for weight support. It is like a whip moving forward. Although it may not cause a knockout, it would definitely inflict enough pain to buy you time for your next move.

1. Side-stance with forearm parallel to the ground.
2. Lunge to the side pushing with your rear foot and land with the foot closer to your opponent; you invert your fist, hitting the opponent on his cheekbone or nose.
3. Retract your hand immediately to maintain the speed of the punch as your front hip twists forward to give you maximum balance and your rear leg is locked to balance your extended reach forward.

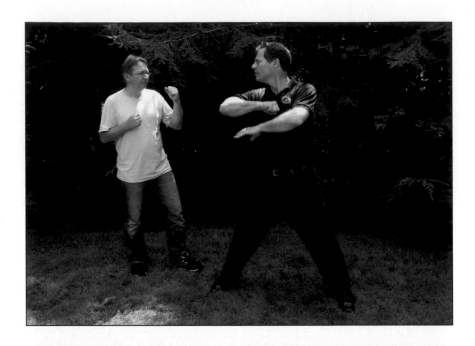

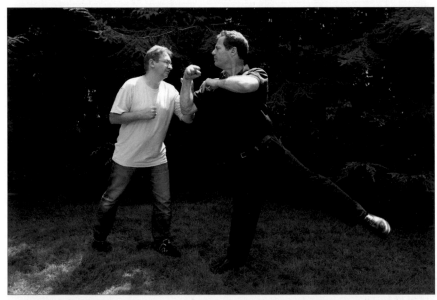

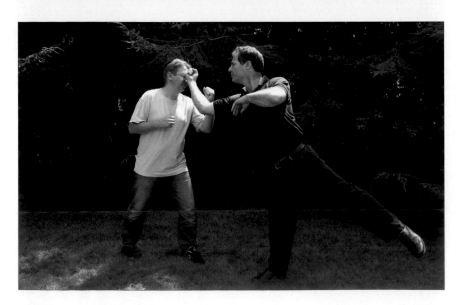

Roundhouse (punch used for training with gloves and learning how to block)

To get a great momentum by having more distance, and to use it as an evasive move, you need to bend your body to the side, then rise and align your fist and forearm to the opponent's jaw. Imagine a train track passing through the opponent's jaw. The blow would be along the track, coming to a stop just past the opponent's far shoulder.

The contact point is the two great knuckles on the fist. If you are using your elbow, the motion is the same, but the contact is the tip of your elbow and forearm. After a complete stop, bring your elbow back to the side of your body and assess your next move as your body stays pivoted.

Fist:

1. Opponent is standing close.
2. Defender bends slightly to achieve a longer distance for acceleration.
3. Defender strikes opponent on the chin or floating ribs.
4. Defender retracts his elbow down to the side of his body without moving backwards.

Note: Front- and rear-hand use is demonstrated in the following pictures:

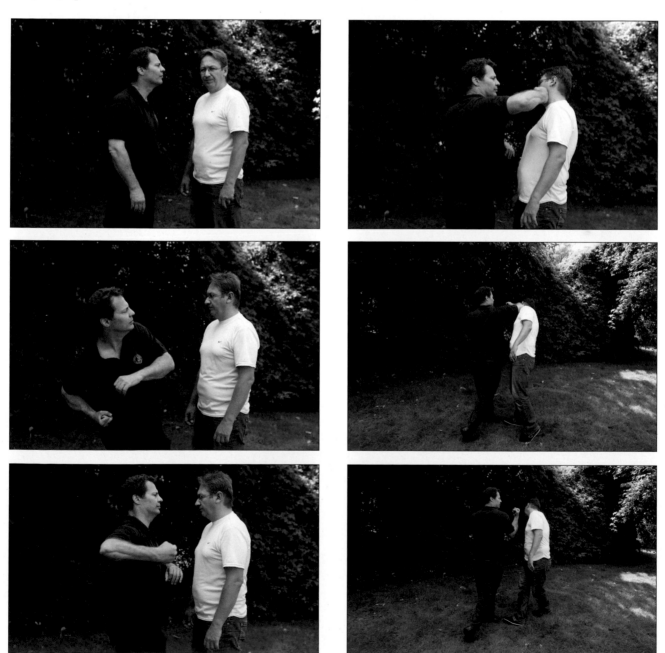

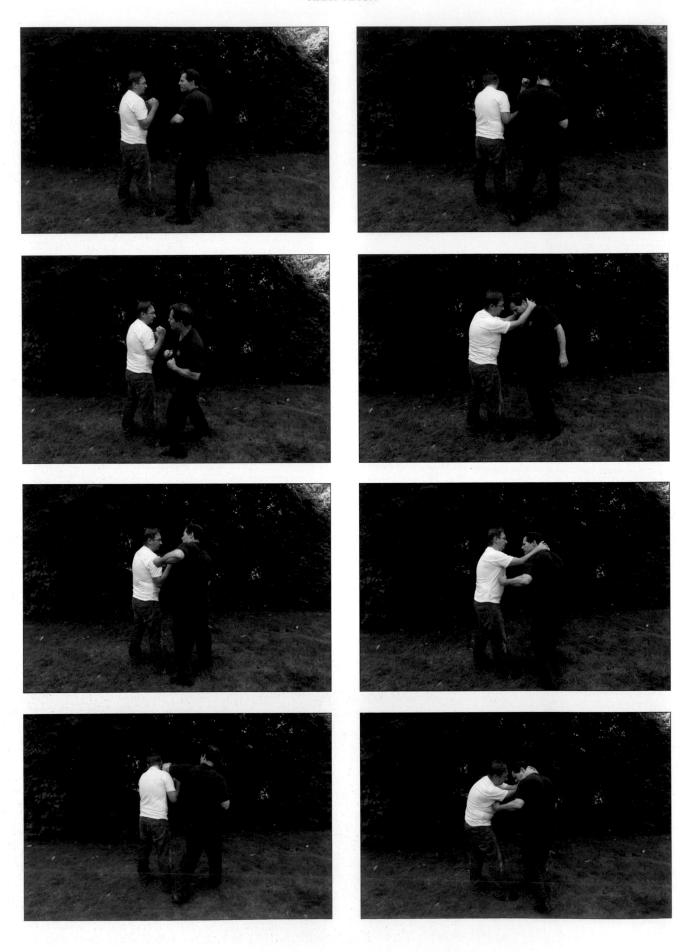

Roundhouse Elbow

1. Opponent is standing close.
2. Defender bends slightly to achieve a longer distance for acceleration.

3. Defender strikes opponent in the chin.
4. Defender retracts the elbow down to the side of his body without moving backwards.

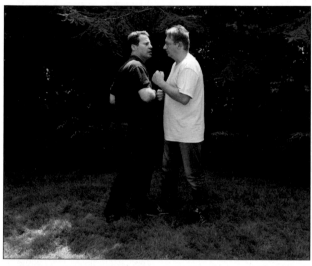

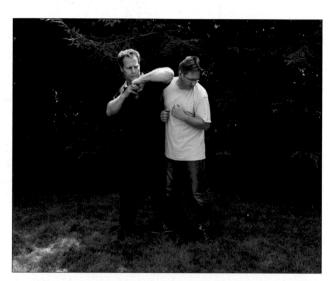

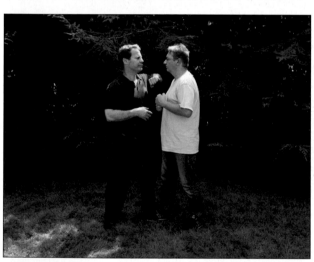

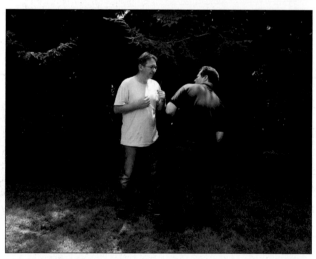

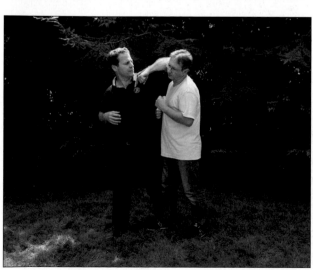

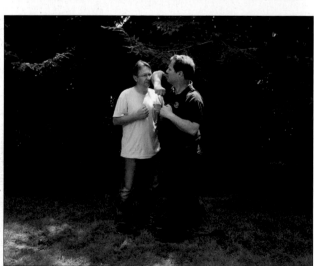

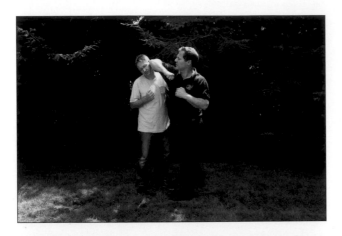

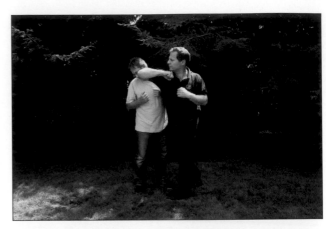

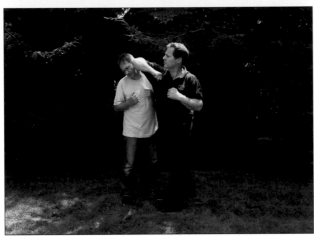

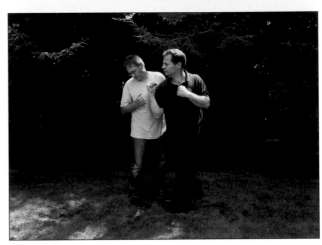

Uppercut: (This punch is used for training with gloves; elbow is demonstrated as a follow-up attack for various techniques in this book).

Lock your elbow at a ninety-degree angle, keeping it pointed backward but slightly in front of your stomach. Duck slightly down, bending your knees to increase the acceleration of the strike. Pivot your body so that your elbow is pointed down in front of the opponent. Strike perpendicularly upward as you rise on your toes. Your two big knuckles impact the opponent's chin as you push your body up in a jump. If you use your elbow, the contact is with the tip of your elbow, and the edge of your forearm hits the bottom of the opponent's chin. For an elbow uppercut, your striking fist is pointing down behind your ear as if you were bringing a telephone to it.

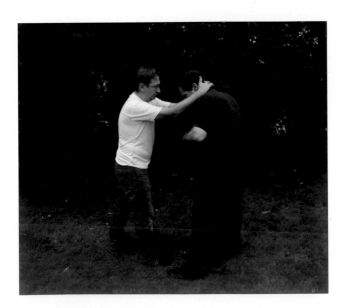

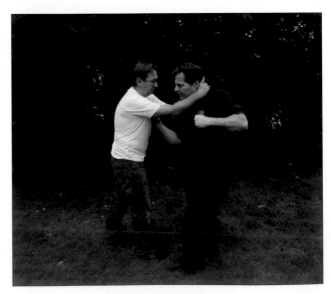

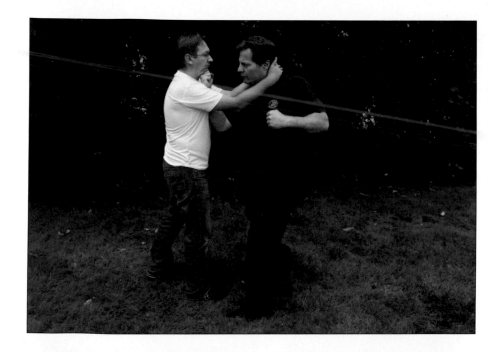

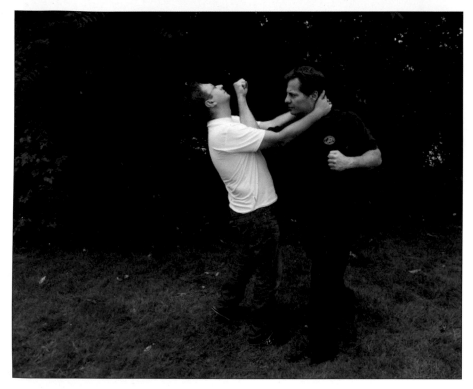

Elbow Strike from the Side

1. As your opponent approaches you from the side, step towards him, bringing your front fist to your opposite shoulder.
2. Shift your weight to your front foot by reaching your shoulder over your knee until you are close enough to pass your target (the opponent's face).
3. Strike with your elbow impacting the opponent's chin, and pass the target.
4. Retract your elbow without retracting your body. (**Note:** Step 3 and 4 should be done fluently in the same speed).

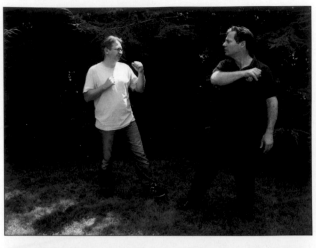 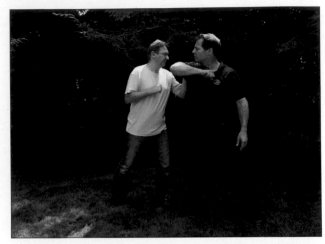

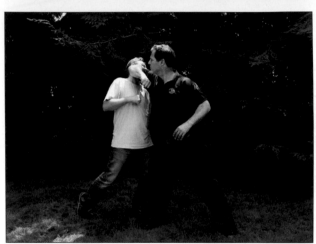 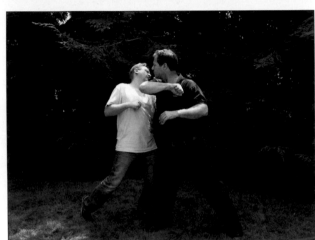

Low-Elbow Strike Backwards

1. You notice an opponent behind you.
2. Step backward and shift your weight to the foot closer to the opponent, as you prepare your elbow for a strike, leaning backwards with your torso. Get into a habit of lifting the opposite foot off the ground. This will ensure your weight is supporting your striking elbow.
3. Strike your opponent with your elbow in the celiac plexus, or the floating rib, shifting your weight backwards as you step.
4. Retract your elbow while your body is still moving toward the opponent.

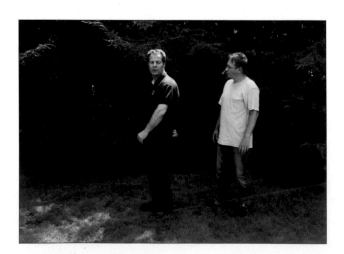 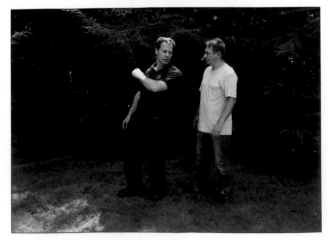

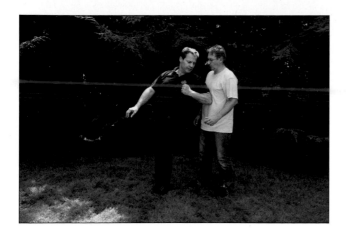
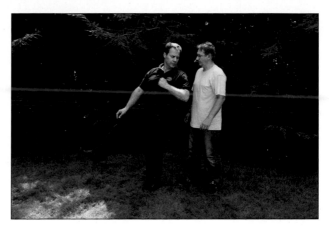

Note: Horizontal backwards elbow strike, backwards elbow uppercut, and elbow-hammer strike are all demonstrated in the close range scenarios chapter.

Knife-Hand Strikes

In using Knife-hand Strikes, one should remember that they require preparation. Your opponent can easily identify your intention since your hand goes slightly back before the attack to gain more force. This motion however could be utilized as a second attack when you think your opponent is preoccupied or disoriented after your initial attack.

Knife-hand Strikes are executed similarly to a slashing motion. The whole hand swings from the shoulder to the opposite waist while simultaneously pointing the knife side of the hand toward the target. This facilitates additional force, and use of the smaller surface with greater force on the opponent's pressure point. The strike point is where the pinky finger is, or the edge of the palm. This motion can be reversed from the opposite hip, ending at shoulder level. Aim toward the carotid artery or the temple. In some scenarios, aim at the opponent's windpipe or kidney.

An outside knife hand can be used to attack an opponent that is approaching you from the side by using the same mechanics of the elbow strike to the side. When you execute knife-hand strikes correctly, you can easily create a whistle of air with a swift slash demonstrating the sufficient force you have achieved.

Rear hand inside knife-hand strike

1. As you move forward with your left leg, raise your right hand.

2. Accelerate your hand in a slapping motion and strike your opponent's temple or carotid artery.

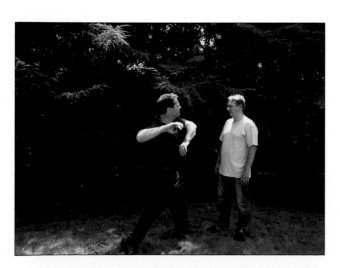
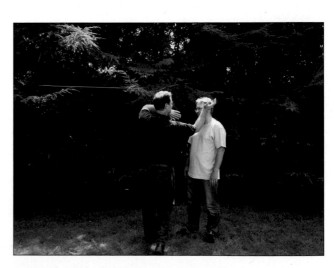

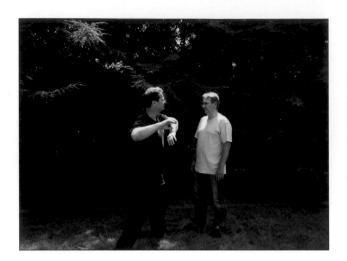 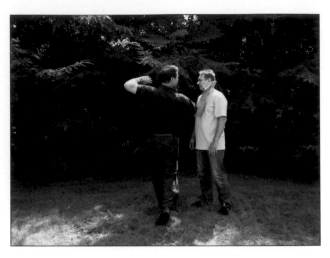

Front hand outside knife-hand strike

1. As your opponent is approaching from your side from behind, step toward him side-wise bringing your hand to your opposite hip for greater momentum.
2. Release your hand and strike him in his throat with your knife-hand. You are shifting your weight to your front leg in the same direction.

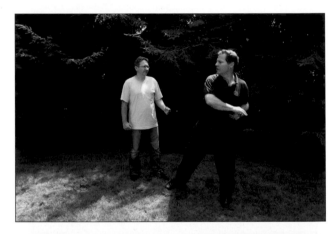

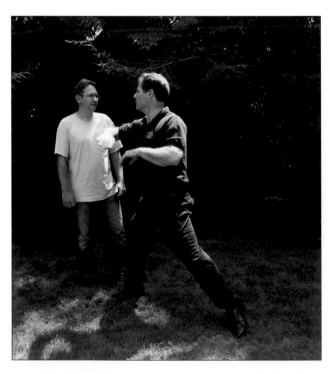 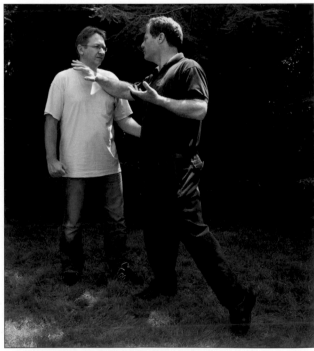

Note: Technically, any part of the arm could be used for striking. Krav Maga training is designed to give the student an idea of the motion of strikes in various angles and their effectiveness.

Front Kick

The purpose of the front kick is to preemptively strike an opponent before he gets closer. When the opponent is at a two-step distance from us, we have enough time to shift our weight to the base leg, and to lift the kicking leg. Depending on the distance, we spring forward and land on the base foot.

We attempt to execute the kick as soon as we close the gap. To cover a greater range, the body should pivot as we move forward, and the base foot should point outward for a greater range for the kicking leg. To initiate the move, we lean forward and push our body forward with our toes.

As we spring forward and pivot our body, pointing our kicking leg in front, we pay attention to keep our leg in front of us at all times. This leg could be used during the movement to stop a counterattack. We close the gap with an erect body and when we reach the target, we land as we kick using the seesaw motion. The base foot will land ball first, followed by the heel, while the other foot will kick the opponent. Attention will be given to positioning the base foot properly to prevent a loss of balance during motion. This will eliminate the possibility of shifting less speed and force into the kick.

Keeping the foot parallel to the ground and the knee at a ninety-degree angle, we drop our head and back backwards, and straighten our leg kicking upward. At this moment the ball of the foot is hitting the opponent's groin. If he turns and we kick his abdomen, the kick will still go diagonally upwards into his body and against his body weight. The retraction will be back to an erect body. The whole kick would be done in a swinging motion. Aligning the foot and the upper body as one unit will keep us in balance during the kick and retraction. More importantly, the upper body will lean backward and downward, helping with extra force for the kicking ball of the foot.

As we kick, we push our hands backwards around our hips, and then throw our hands back to our shoulders in a swinging motion to retract our body.

After retracting, we stay with one knee up ready to kick again, or we block the opponent's leg. This happens if the opponent starts an evasive move backwards and is now returning to kick us back. From this position we assess our next move.

If the opponent is bent from the stunning effect of a kick to the groin, we step closer to him, and strike him on top of his head with a hammer punch. If we kick him in his hip and he is standing erect, we can punch him with our front fist as we land on the kicking foot closing the gap. If the opponent manages to move backwards at a greater distance, we lunge forward and pivot our torso to the opposite direction and land on the kicking leg as its instep is inverted forty-five degrees instep pointing to the opponent, while raising our second leg for an additional kick.

Notes: It is faster to kick with the leg that is closer to the opponent. If we stand straight in front we can choose either leg. Attention: A kicking and retracting motion should be combined into one fast motion.

1. The defender is standing far from the opponent, pushing with his toes and leaning forward.
2. The defender is lunging forward, pivoting his torso and landing on his base foot instep at forty-five degrees to the opponent while bringing his kicking knee up to ninety degrees.
3. The defender kicks the opponent in a seesaw motion.
4. The defender retracts his knee at ninety degrees.
5. Use a hammer strike (rise on your toes and come down using your fist in a hammer motion).
6. Defender retracts his hand only.

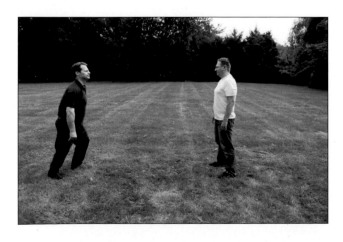
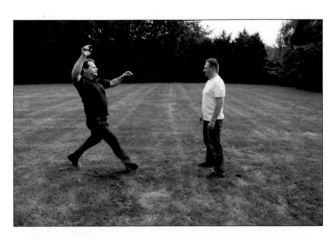

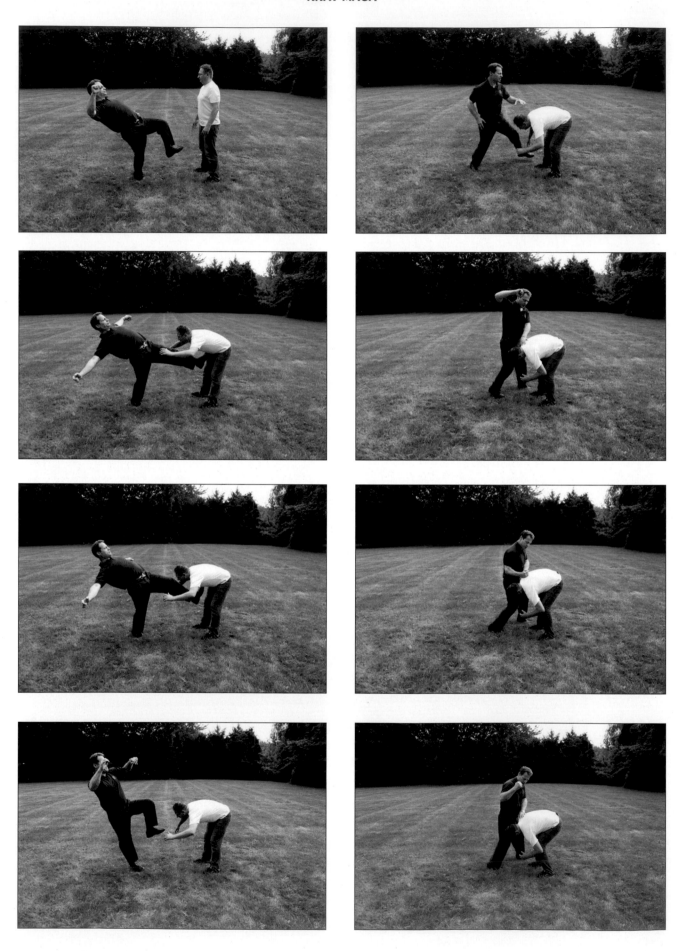

Side Kick

If you notice an opponent approaching from the side and don't have time to face him, use a side attack or stop him. To execute a side kick, we utilize a cork-screw motion where we pivot our whole body into the opponent. The motions of screwing and unscrewing for attacking and retracting help increase the force for the kick.

Turn and look at your opponent as he is on your side. To cover the gap, lean sideways, as you bend your knee. Continue pushing your toes toward the kick and spring to the side to close the gap throwing your rear leg behind your front leg as far as possible. Before you land on the back leg, pull up the kicking knee to ninety degrees.

Our knee and toes are pointed at an angle toward the opponent. The kicking foot is parallel to the ground. We pivot the base foot's toes so that they point backwards to avoid injury to the knee. We point our knee and toe at the ground and lift our heel and point it at the opponent. For correct positioning of your body relative to the target, land your base foot's instep parallel to the direction of your opponent's body.

We pivot our torso and body so that our shoulders are parallel to the ground as we're screwing our foot into the target. Without losing our balance, we swing our leg back and move our shoulders to an erect position. Our kicking leg is back to ninety degrees, ready to go again. We then evaluate how to continue.

Our options include the following; Either the job is done, or we land with a back hand, or we turn our back and kick from the side with our second leg if our opponent has moved backwards with a larger gap.

1. Turn your head to the side and lean.
2. Close the gap and kick.
3. Retract and decide on your next action.
4. Continue with back-hand strike only if the opponent is still standing.
5. Or turn through your back and get ready for another side kick.

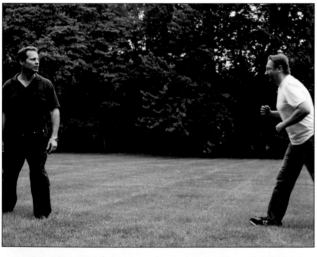
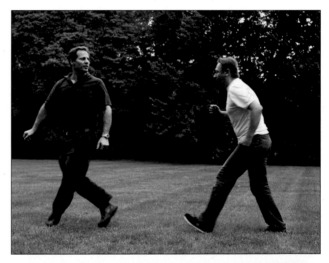
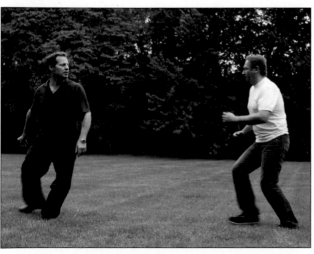
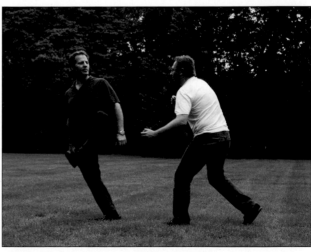

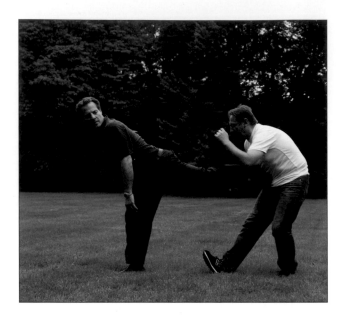
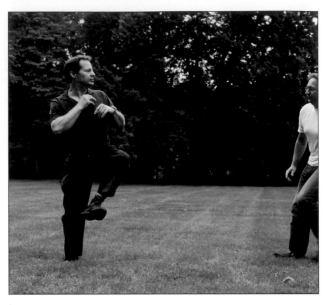

Notes: If the distance is great and you have the time to turn, you should face the opponent and start with a front kick. Or you can run and chase him, and jump on him with a kick.

Once you have learned the basic kicking techniques, you need to practice them on punching mitts. To practice the front kick, your training partner should hold his head perpendicularly above the mitt as he is holding his hands down with elbows almost locked. The mitt is worn on one hand while the other hand is pushed on top of it and is placed in front of the training partner's groin. The placement of the head above the mitt gives the student in the attacker's role the correct measurement of the distance between his eyes and the partner's head, which equals the distance he will need to leap to kick the mitt. When practicing the side kick, your training partner should stand with his side to you and hold the mitt with his back hand in front, holding his front hand above the mitt for the same purpose of giving your eyes the opportunity to measure the realistic distance and successfully hit the mitt. Lunging for a sidekick should be done with the rear foot crossing behind the kicking leg to avoid the crossing foot hitting the kicking foot. It can be done with a short lunge on the spot without even crossing. It can also be done with a forward cross only for a low kick to the knee as your starting stance if facing the opponent with your body.

Other Kicks and Their Usage

Most other kicks are not the best options for self-defense, but since they may be used by other martial artists, you need to learn them to practice defenses and counterattacks against them.

The basic front and side kicks have greater attack range, and therefore are more efficient to use from a distance. Since the hands are faster at a closer distance, you can use them instead of circular kicks.

For fighting sports, when less contact is allowed and no effective defense mechanisms are taught, and when kicking the groin or shin is not allowed, one can attack with a high roundhouse kick without worrying that the opponent will counterattack with a ninety-degree front or side kick to the groin.

There is, however, an advantage to using roundhouse kicks to the groin—they are almost like a front kick, but at a slightly horizontal angle. We use that kick in straight stab knife defense tactics.

Knee Kick

When we grab the opponent we can use knee kicks.

The principles of a knee kick are the same as for the front kick. Remember to lean back with your torso in order to drive the force upward with your upper body weight leaning backwards. As you finish one knee jab, position your foot as you land in a comfortable angle to help your second leg with its knee kick. You can aim toward the groin/ribs, or pull the opponent's head down as you knee his face. The following chapter explains knee kicks.

Headbutts

Headbutts are permissible if you like to use them or have no choice but to use them. Just remember the same principles of passing the target and maintaining speed during contact, and remember to use the middle of your forehead, or the back of your head against the opponent's face, perhaps straight to the nose.

Facing a Karate-Trained Opponent

What if your opponent is trained to stand in a low stance?

While there are still traditional karate schools that try to concentrate all their force on one strike, many that encourage free sparring are a little more evolved. Since you have practiced the maximum range and speed possible for humans, you have the advantage. Get yourself familiar with some of the basic karate strikes. Traditional karate moves with a low stance, requiring the use of the back hand for attacks.

Traditional karate is not geared toward simultaneous defense and counterattack. Its kicks, executed from a low stance, would come from the back leg. More evolved schools might have better motions, but you can still see remnants of years of unresolved errors in traditional training. A trained karate attacker can knock the wind out of your lungs if he hits you, but you should know enough by now not to let that happen.

Facing a Boxing-Trained Opponent

Krav Maga hand strikes are modified boxing-style punches. They are modified to get maximum reach while entering the hot zone. Krav Maga students learn to shift their weight with each punch, including the jab. Boxers, however, learn to quickly jab for distraction and gain an extra split second for the knockout punch. The Krav Maga philosophy is that you have no time to spar with a threat and need to resolve it immediately. The combination of strikes, defenses, and kicks facilitates a totally different strategy than boxing does. This is why Krav Maga hand strikes are modified. Assuming your opponent is accustomed to taking gloved strikes to his face and deflecting them with evasive body motions, you need to give it your best shot. If in kicking distance, use kicks and then throw a front hand punch followed with a forward elbow. This will catch an evasive opponent.

Krav Maga students do not tuck their chin since they need to learn to maintain good peripheral vision expecting possible kicks and other opponents. Finally, while boxing tactics include combat motion to evade your strikes and surprise you from all directions, they do not take into account how you can strike to the sides, using kicks and elbows. Remember, your hand is always faster than the motion of the whole body.

Defenses vs. Strikes and Kicks

Attack as defense is not possible when an object is moving at a threatening speed toward your body by surprise. Your instinct is to deflect the object or move your body away from its direction. Krav Maga defenses utilize various moves and principles that are based on minimum motion and maximum reach according to the positioning of your body relative to your opponent.

In Krav Maga, the student learns to improve his instinctive defenses. These defenses later become automatic moves during a hand-to-hand combat scenario. As a Krav Maga attacker throws a knockout punch with one hand, he keeps his second ready to deflect a strike.

As the range between attacker and defender decreases, the reaction time equals the time it takes for the attacker to complete his strike. That does not leave time for the defense move.

To execute a defense, one needs sufficient distance from his attacker. The distance is a barrier that the attacker has to cross to reach the defender. With the defender standing at a sufficient distance from the attacker, he can take advantage of the time the attacker spends on covering the gap.

The defender could see the attack and immediately execute a short defense simultaneously with a counterattack. During this time, it takes the attacker longer to complete his motion than it does for the defender to defend himself, leaving enough time to recognize the attack and to send a defense command to his limbs.

Since counterattacks in Krav Maga are usually done during the window of opportunity where the aggressor is attacking instead of defending, the attacker is not able to block precisely timed defense and counterattack.

The execution has to be quick to minimize the chance that the target will move to a different position. During this process, the attacker does not have enough time to stop and defend himself. As the attacker gets closer to the defender, he takes the risk of failing his attack, and the defender can block and counterattack him simultaneously.

The attacker becomes too close to have sufficient time to see the counterattack, send a command to his body, and have the body execute the command. He is simply out of time. This risk cannot be avoided; if the attacker hesitates in his attack, he loses the window of opportunity needed to produce a devastating attack. In addition, if the attacker delays it, he is risking the opponent counterattacking him. In closing the range with no attack, or a hesitated attack, the attacker is serving himself on a silver platter.

Once these possibilities are explained, there should be an understanding of the entire detailed process between the training partners, that they are training each other and not taking advantage of the attacker role. Since it is impossible for the attacker to block a correctly executed counterattack, both training partners should know that their roles will switch during the class.

Consider the following scenario: Let's say an attacker closes the range and advances toward us with no intention of immediately attacking, but instead forces us to subconsciously attack. His intention is to wait and block our counterattack. If, however, we time our preemptive attack or preemptive defense according to when he closes the gap, he will lose his opportunity to prevail. As the attacker closes the gap without immediately attacking, he has one chance to execute either an impact or a distraction. Once he is close he would lose his reaction time. If we time our counterattack to the moment he enters our territory, we would leave him defenseless.

As the attacker attempts to set up a trap by closing the gap in anticipation of a counterattack, an experienced defender can initiate a defense and counterattack based on the attacker's initial standing position. The defense involves deflecting the attacker's hand, leg, or weapon nearest to the defender, combined with a counter-strike.

The mere deflection of the attacker's hand or leg breaks the attacker's train of thought. It is a nice try, finding a way to handle opponents that have the same skills, but if both have learned the same method to perfection, the loser would be the first to make a mistake. What then happens, hypothetically, if both of them have exactly the same skills is that the person who attacks loses.

For an attack among people who have the exact same skill level, try to gain an advantage from a longer distance. If the attacker throws an object or spits on the defender while initiating kicks and hand strikes at the same time, the defender could be confused for a few seconds.

However, the defender could escape the object, or try to deflect it by changing his body position. I would compare my opponent in this scenario to a person that has to fight two opponents at the same second. It would not be very easy for him.

Krav Maga scholars have made an attempt to have the upper hand while utilizing the concept of a continuous attack. However, I must stress that while this concept works during a defensive move when combined with a counterattack, it is dangerous to use it to initiate an attack unless you are stopping after each move and reassessing your next move.

This, of course, would not utilize a planned series of attacks, but instead the awareness of a need to continue, and choosing the logical way to continue each time.

I believe that while a defensive use of this method is acceptable, and lets the defender buy time, it is not acceptable as an attack method. Rather, it is a successful manipulation and buys time only if the defender is not equally skilled.

If you attempt to continuously attack using kicks and punches with both legs and hands, a skilled opponent would be able to block your first kick or strike, and counterattack it. Training in continuous attack is only good for practicing how to continue from a new position you are in, after your last move failed to achieve or complete your goals. The nature of being at the correct distance from the opponent and of understanding the principle of reaction time does not give the attacker the luxury of completing more than one strike before being counterattacked by a skilled defender. Once you have created the distraction with your first strike, you need to continue and attack appropriately. Therefore, when you train, students need to gain a complete understanding of what they are drilling and the training drill should be designed accordingly. Be aware that the human mind is constantly trying to create imaginary connections between motion possibilities without always seeing the whole picture.

Shortening the range from a kick to a hand strike cuts down on time between the first and subsequent attacks. Such an attempt does not recognize that a good defense against a kick eliminates the option for a continuous hand attack since that was already taken into account.

Executing multiple attacks on the defense however would break the opponent's train of thought and give the initiator another second to hit again. If you have reached the target through the first strike, with no obstacles, you are buying time for a more devastating attack. You must recognize that with less devastating strikes, you buy less time, and in a real fight it is measured in splits of a second. It should only take a few seconds to finish the opponent.

Krav Maga principles dictate a perfect relationship in which a counterattack requires the same speed as the block, but sometimes the distance can be too close to accelerate the hand to a maximum speed—and then you are just buying another second and must follow up with a more devastating attack.

If you deliver attacks of medium strength, your opponent might get the message and stop attacking you. However, while it is a good practice to change an attacker's mind and habits, you may not want to risk your own life protecting your attacker from extensive harm.

Finally, when executing a counterattack, please be as precise as possible, so you do not need to rework. I personally would not spend more than two seconds on one opponent, since it would occupy and distract me from other dangerous changes that might occur in the environment. If you break glass in a store, you would want to get out of there as quickly as possible instead of waiting around in the same spot.

I'd like to remind the reader that the above paragraphs elaborate the dangers and safety in both training and in reality. By understanding safe training, you need to understand the dangers of reality. To master the process, you need to train in simulated scenarios that are as close as possible to a realistic fight for survival.

Keep in mind that when you identify a threat, you should set your boundaries, and decide that if the opponent gets too close to you, you should attack him by kicking or punching according to the distance between you two. If however the attacker attacks you by surprise, not giving you enough time to think, your body instinctively defends itself. This means that if you are at the point where you notice an attack coming at you, your primary instinct is to defend as opposed to attack.

In summary, two well-trained Krav Maga experts do not leave the outcome of a possible fight in the hands of fate. The one that makes the first mistake would be at a disadvantage.

Defense vs. Hand Strikes

Efficient motion is very important for defense. You cannot waste time deciding whether or not you want to block your opponent using your inner forearm and palm or the outer forearm above your waistline. You use the area that is closer to the opponent.

Furthermore you cannot afford to waste your time reacting to your opponent's front-hand strike or rear-hand strike. You need to block his front-hand and counterattack even as he is thinking about using his rear hand. Training methods that attempt to improve your reaction time never consider the limitations that the range brings in. Therefore, the attempt to improve your reaction time is insignificant and will never succeed. The training emphasis should be on blocking the front hand only, when it is within reach.

In the process of blocking, you start from a neutral position where both the opponent's hands are the same distance from you. This gives you the opportunity to practice blocking with both hands, and the concept of proper distance to help reaction is initially ignored. The student should understand that this scenario is only a step in the training purpose.

The instructor should note that a block should have been initiated before the attacker completely closes the gap for a hand strike. In a scenario where an attacker stands in front of you and you have no clue what direction he will go in, you should realize he is far enough away from you that you can kick him first. At the same time, you can also move toward one of his hands, block it preemptively and counterattack.

If your hands are to the sides of your body and an opponent has tried to punch your face, you should reach for his wrist with your palm and slap it so that it slightly passes your sternum. That will deflect his motion away from your shoulder while not blocking your other hand's counterattack. If he tries to slap you from the same position, stop his attack away to the side of your body using your outer forearms.

If your hands are folded on your chest, all your defenses would be in an outer direction. When you do not have enough distance to stop the strike, you should thrust your forearm diagonally while pivoting your hand simultaneously. This would deflect the attack, like a rock hitting the water at an angle.

As you use your palms to deflect a punch, you do not want to move his hand too much away from your body as it may block your attacking hand.

Elbows can be used to block as well. A back-hand strike can follow a horizontal elbow block.

Outside Defenses

The human body has an innate instinct to sacrifice an outer limb for a more vital organ, should such a situation arise. That can be noticed when a child or an adult's hand jumps to protect their head. In Krav Maga, we take the body's instinctive motions and train the student to improve his posture and angles to create more effective responses.

In executing outside defenses, it is important to keep the elbow at an angle slightly greater than ninety degrees. This maintains a sufficient stopping force. Remember, you do not have to fully extend your arm, since your opponent can easily slide his attack to other parts of your body.

The 360 degrees outside defense drill

The purpose of this drill is to learn to utilize the most efficient and effective block and execute it in the correct angle. Memorizing numbers is not essential but instead the drill is designed to teach principles. For ease of learning, defense is practiced separately from the intended attack. For the purpose of demonstrations, the final stage is shown in pictures.

In this drill, students pair up and get the feel for shifting force to forty-five degree angles to block round circular attacks. While the training method is designed to teach the student to trust his arms to stop an attack, it also gives the student a handle on reaction time.

The attacks should be directed to the body and not to the arms. Otherwise it would defeat the purpose of learning how to counter realistic attacks. Remember to use the middle of the forearm on the opponent's wrist to the side of your body where your arm has a slightly greater angle than forty-five degrees at the elbow for greater force. When using this defense against a round-house kick however, you must rotate your forearm so that the back of your hand will be perpendicular to the attacker's shin. This will create more support needed to counter the greater force of the attacker's shin.

After the student has sensed the strength of his forearm, the technique should be practiced from a distance creating a need to close the gap in each attack and defense. This part of the drill incorporates the aspect of the reaction time.

1. Outside No.1: Forearm above the head with the thumb pointing down:

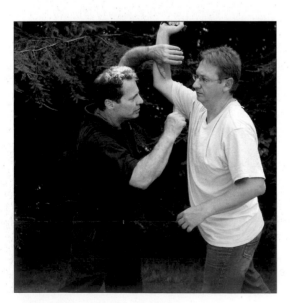

2. Outside No.2: Forearm forty-five degrees across the clavicle:

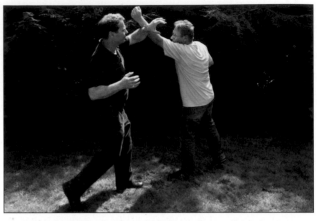

3. Outside No 3: Forearm forty-five degrees to the side of the head:

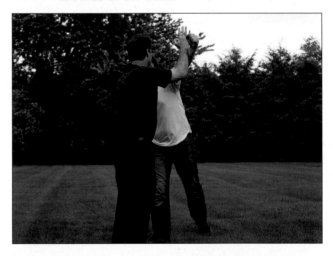

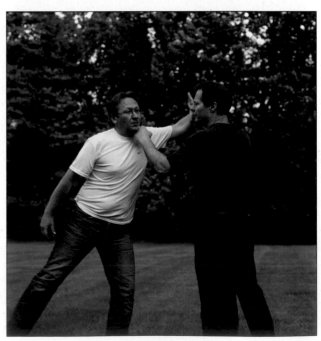

4. Outside No. 4: Elbow leaning on the rib and forearm pointed forty-five degrees forward: This block protects the rib area.

5. Outside No. 5: The elbow of the arm raised up to the side of the body:

The forearm is parallel to the side of the body. This defense is demonstrated in the defense vs. kicks chapter in the toreador outside defense technique.

Defense no. 5 and no. 4 protect the same area. Choosing which one to use depends on where your hand is prior to the defense. If it was hanging down to the side of your body, you would use number 5 since it calls for a shorter execution. However, if you are defending your ribcage and your arm was initially across your chest or raised above the shoulders area, it is quicker to use defense no. 4.

6. Outside No. 6: Defense no. 6 differs from no.5 with regards to body position. If attacked by a knife, one must block the wrist holding it, while also moving your body away from the blade. See the chapter on knife techniques and defense.

7. Outside No. 7: This is used for instinctive defense against a bottom-up knife hold.

As you bend your torso away from the blade, slide your feet slightly backward.

Notes: These defenses, when used against round-house strikes, should use the inner or outer forearm contacting the two bones with the blocked kick instead of one bone. You will see these defenses in the close fighting sections and defenses vs. kicks sections.

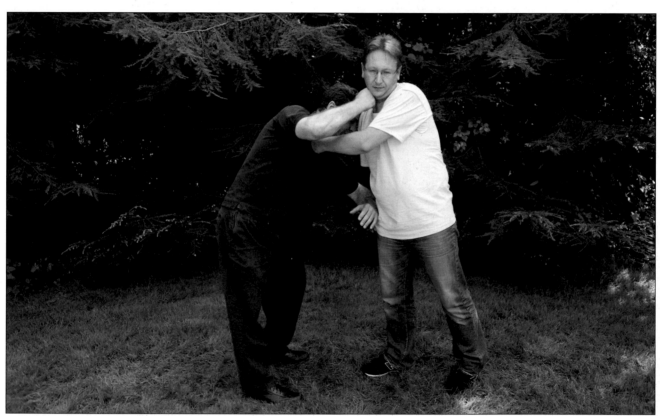

Fighting game drill

After the students have practiced the angles of outside defenses, they should practice with training partners at a gradually increasing speed to improve their reaction. The attacks should start by announcing where the partner is going to strike and what hand he is going to use. Further training attacks should be random, forcing students to react to the attack naturally and instinctively.

The counterattack should then be combined, and for training purposes should be limited to an open hand tap on the opponent's nearest shoulder. The instructor should stress that in real life, or when sparring with gloves, the counterattack is actually aimed at the opponent's face. Continue to the next step and add a combination of four palm taps to the training partner's shoulder using maximum body motion with minimum penetration. This will discourage your training partner from executing a follow-up attack or completing his planned combination.

Outside defense vs. straight hand strike

Earlier in this chapter, we discussed outside defenses vs. roundhouse strikes.

In this scenario an outside defense is used against an opponent's direct straight hand strike:

4. The attacker is attempting to strike defender with a straight punch. The defender's initial position is with his hands crossed in front of his sternum.

5. The defender blocks the attack by engaging his forearm with the attacker's wrist and pivoting the thumb down to grab it. At the same time the defender steps forward and pulls the opponent's arm down and counterattacks with a Knife-Hand Strike. The strike could be directed toward the back of the attacker's head or to his kidney.

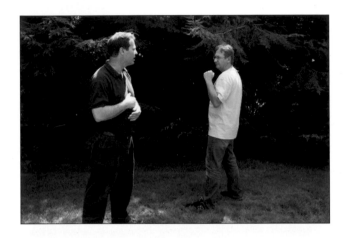 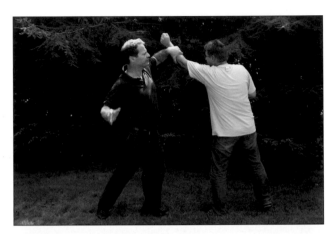

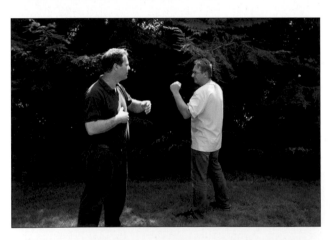 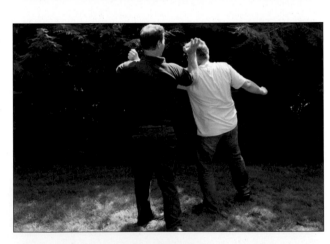

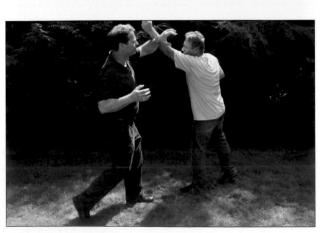 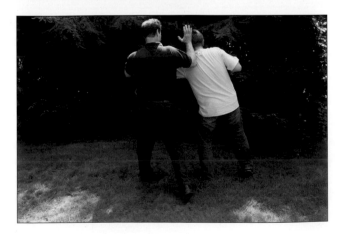

Outside defense vs. low punch

Outside defense can be used against a low punch when your hands are crossed over your chest or perpendicular to your shoulders. You simply stab your hand, sliding your forearm down the opponent's forearm, and follow with a counterattack by striking the top of the attacker's head.

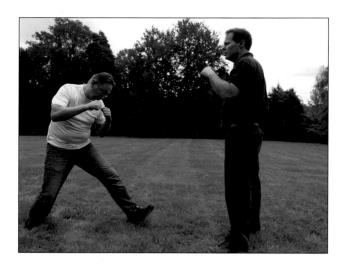 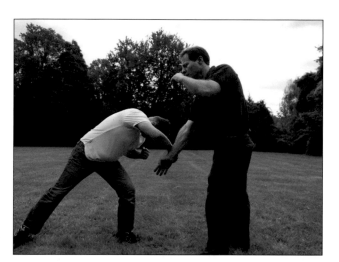

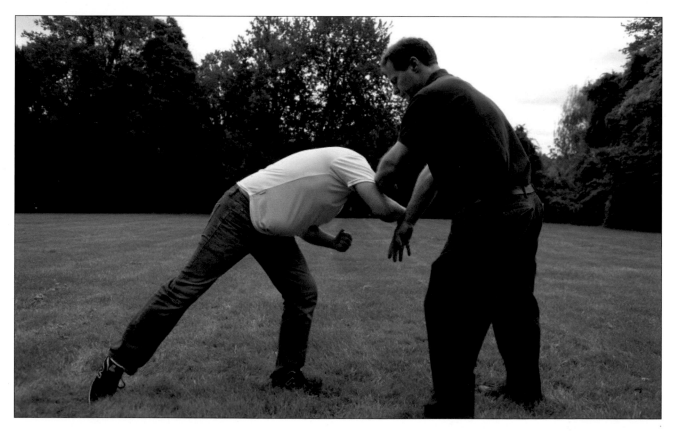

Inside Defenses

The category of inside refers to deflecting or sliding in an inward direction. In the starting position, the defender's hands are either hanging to the sides of his body or are raised up in front of his shoulders. The defenses would be executed by a horizontal motion toward the opposite side of the defender's body.

Fighting game drill (inside defenses)

1. Training partners stand in front of each other and the attacker attempts to touch the defender on the forehead.
2. The defender blocks the attack with the opposite hand.

Notes: When the attacker is facing you with the center of his body, you can use either hand for defense. Use whatever hand you want, since you may not have enough time to identify which hand the opponent is attacking you with.

When practicing, both partners need to test to see that their striking distance is realistic. In other words, if no defense is employed, the target will be hit.

Note: When you see the opponent's body approaching you, note which side of his body is closer. If he is a step away, all he needs to do is take one step and lunge forward with a hand strike. You need only to consider which shoulder of his is closer to you. He will not be able to use his other hand before he completely closes the gap. Since you are not waiting for him to complete any of his attacks, you attempt to block the fastest and nearest threat only. If he had his back hand on his

mind, his attack would come after you are done with your defense and counterattack.

Never wait to figure out which hand he is going to use. Deflect the hand that is the easiest for him to use in the fastest manner to reach you. You should execute your defense on his front hand and simultaneously execute a counterattack.

To make your life easier, consider the following scenarios and their solutions:

Consider you are standing where your left leg and left shoulder are closer to the opponent, and your opponent is standing with his left leg and left shoulder forward. You should always block or deflect his front hand, which is his left hand in this scenario, and simultaneously counterattack with your free hand. To block his hand, use your right hand, your back hand, to block while you counter strike with your front hand.

1. The attacker and defender are standing in front of each other with the left sides of the body in front.
2. As the attacker lunges with a left punch, defender deflects it with his right palm and counterattacks with a left punch.

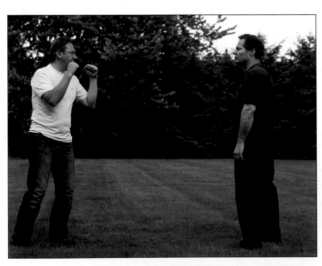

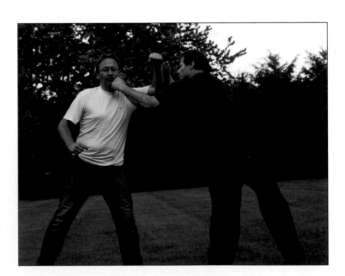

If, however, he is standing with his right leg and shoulder in front while you stand with your left leg and shoulder in front, you should block his right hand with your front hand (left hand), and counterattack with your back hand (right hand). In this scenario, you would need to cover the additional gap as you are using your rear hand to attack. From that distance, it would be more comfortable to attack the opponent's rib area first. A second attack might be needed to finish the defense.

Common sense should tell you to follow reversed instructions for reversed scenarios.

1. The attacker is standing with his right side in front, while the defender remains in his previous position with left leg in front.
2. The attacker throws a right hand punch with his front hand.
3. The defender blocks with his left hand and delivers a right punch to the opponent's floating ribs.

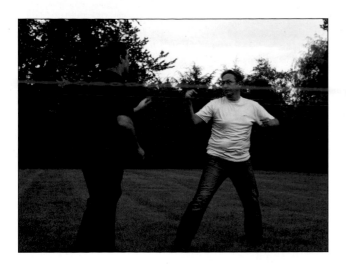 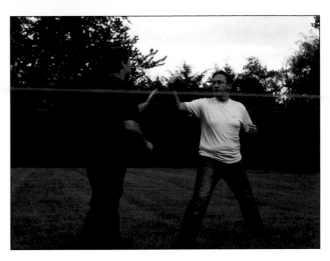

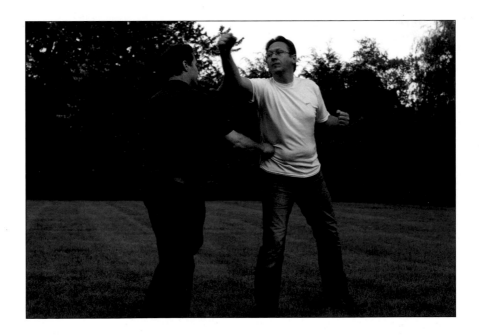

Inside defenses vs. lower punches

If the attacker is docking a lower punch to the ribs or celiac plexus, you can block it with the inner side of your forearm and then continue with the back hand to counterattack. Rotating your thumb forward bringing your palm facing yourself, you move your forearm to deflect the strike from you.

1. The attacker strikes with a lower punch and the defender blocks it with his front forearm.
2. Counterattack with a back hand.

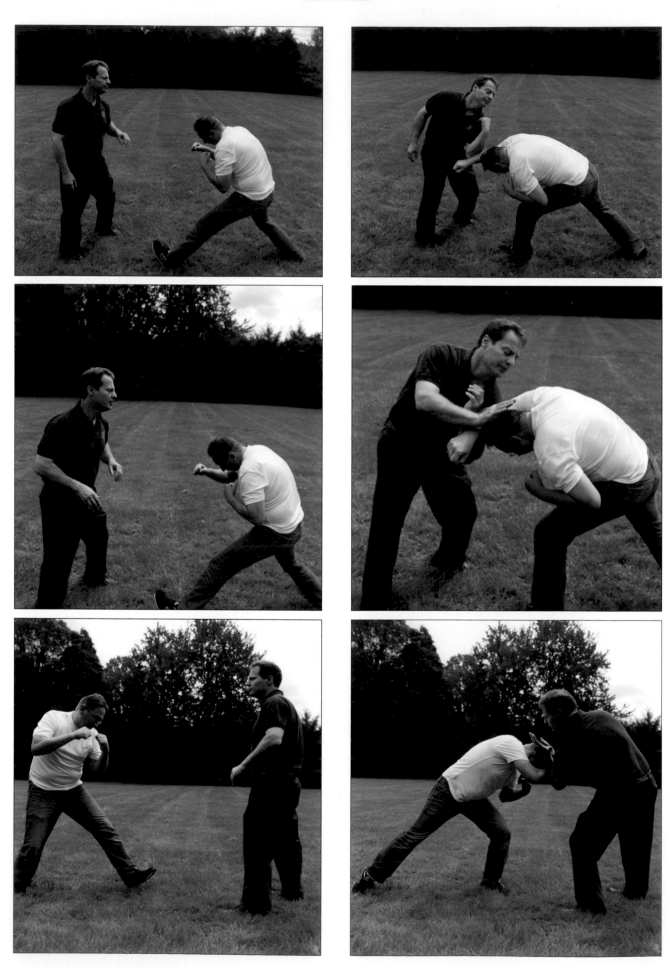

Inside defense with the elbow and back hand counterattack

The attacker throws a straight punch and the defender blocks it, executing a roundhouse elbow strike followed by a back-hand counterattack with the same hand. This technique could be very useful if you are carrying an expensive bottle of wine in your left hand and do not want to waste it.

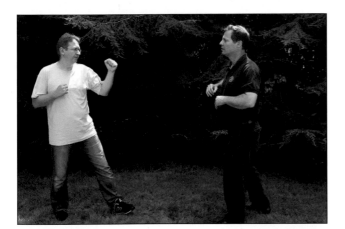 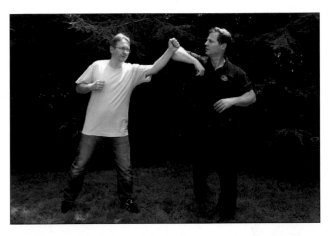

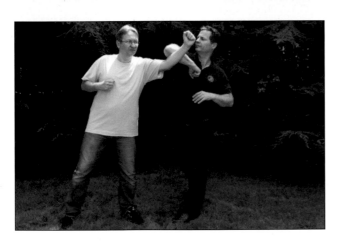 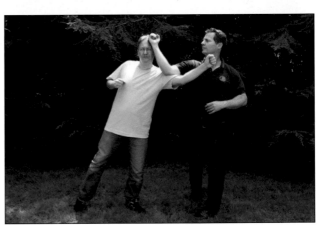

Defense with body lean backwards vs. consecutive hand strikes and return with hook defense down

The following option, although risky, can be attempted when the attacker moves into your territory and tries to punch you. If you hesitate and do not move forward, but lean backward instead, you should wait for him to finish his second-hand strike and come back forward by hooking his fist down and counter-striking.

Defensive Kicks vs. Kicks

Remember that a kick is expected when you identify an opponent at a two-step distance from you. Your opponent can then close the gap with one kick. Choose the leg that is closer to the opponent to block the kick with.

In defensive kicks, you should remember to have your foot on top of the opponent's shin or knee. You need to start the block kick on time to let you lock your knee before contact so it would take the impact without throwing you off balance.

Defense vs. front kick:

1. The attacker lunges to kick and the defender blocks it with the inner side of his foot pivoted forty-five degrees outward. This helps catch the opponent's shin or ankle better.

2. The defender executes a counterstrike, delivering a front punch followed by a rear hand punch finishing the combination with a front punch.

Defense vs. front kick

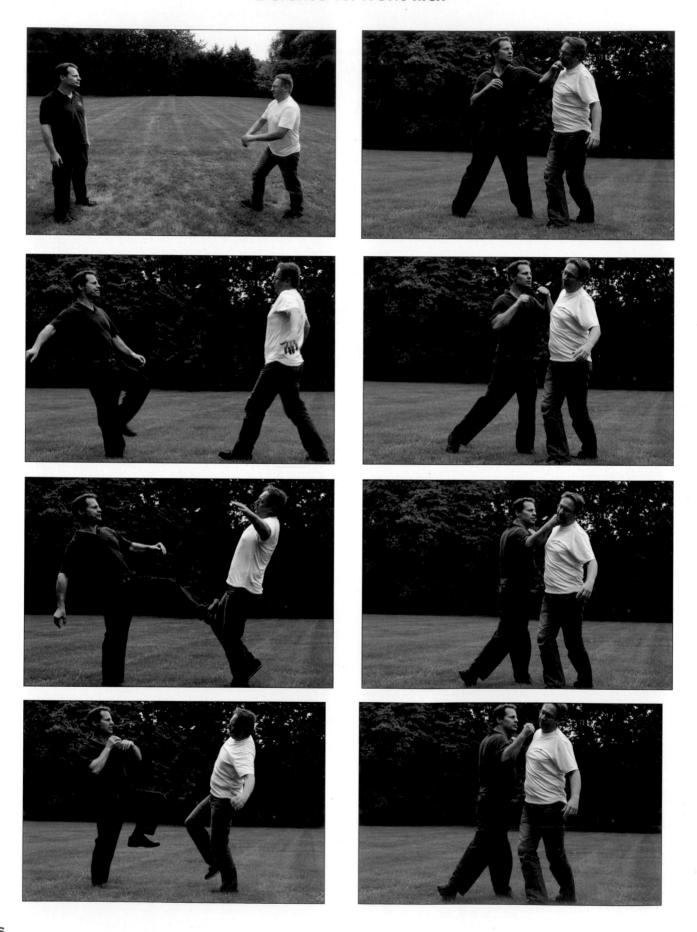

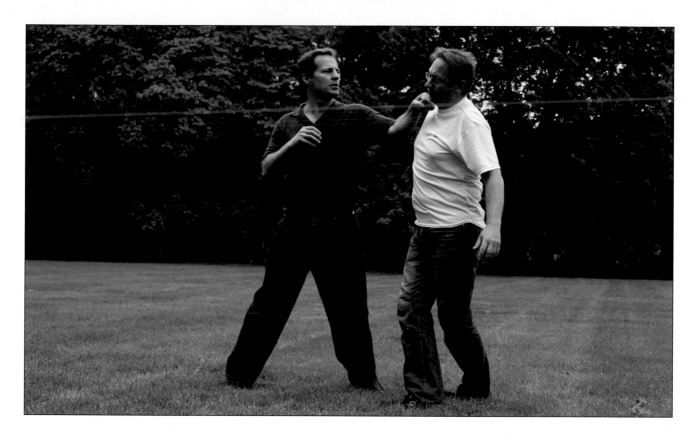

Defense vs. side kick:

1. The attacker approaches the defender from the side.
2. The defender advances toward his opponent if there is time left.
3. The defender intercepts the attacker's kick with a side kick, keeping his foot on top of the opponent's knee.
4. The defender executes a counterattack with a back-hand strike.

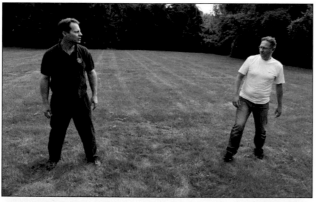

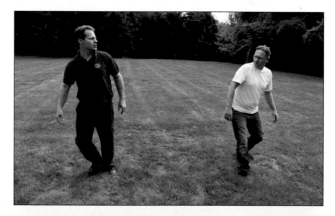

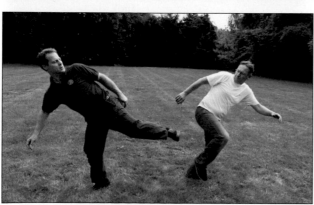

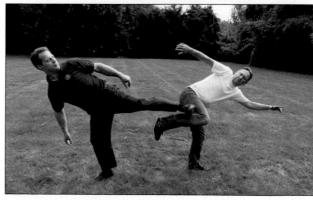

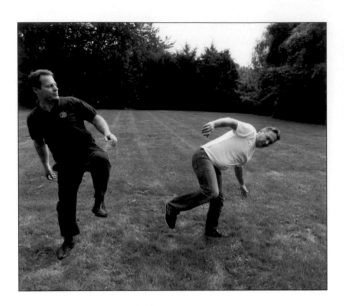
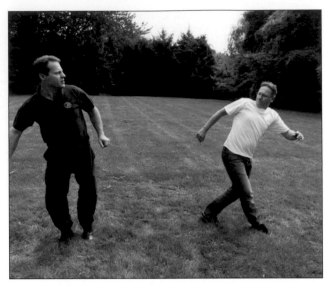

Note: Stopping a full turn roundhouse kick is done with a kick to the rear end (coccyx), followed by a hand strike to the back of the opponent's head.

Inside Defense vs. Kicks

If using your hands for an inside defense, remember to have the middle of your forearm or palm on the opponent's side of the lower leg, ankle, or shin.

If you are executing an inside defense, you should use your front hand for defense and back hand for counterattack. However, there is a chance that your opponent is planning to continue with a hand strike, or fake a kick to distract you while closing the gap and then deliver a hand strike. This is the reason you should cross your back hand to your front shoulder as you block with your front hand. It lets you deflect any additional attacks as you and your opponent close the gap.

Your front hand, after blocking the kick, is lifted to prevent a roundhouse hand strike from your opponent.

1. The defender is lowering his left shoulder to calibrate his hand and forearm to meet the attacker's kick. The defender positions his right hand on his front shoulder, preparing to block a possible hand strike. The defender's body pivots clockwise to evade the kick.
2. The defender leaps forward, closing the gap.
3. The defender pivots his body counterclockwise with a counterattack.

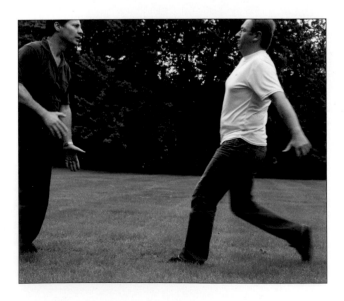
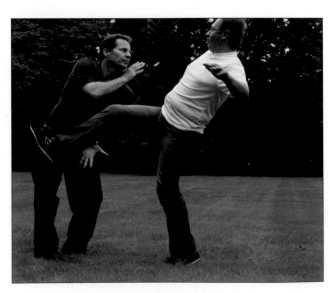

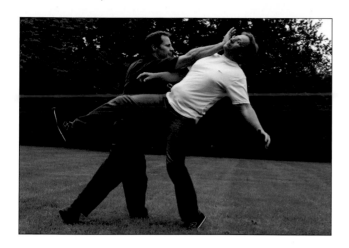

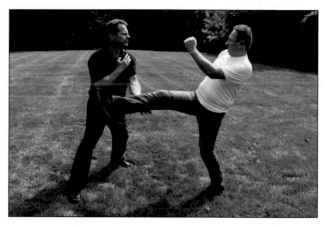

4. The attacker kicks and continues with a front-hand strike, as the defender continues to slide his counterattack punch, deflecting his opponent's strike and continuing with a back-hand strike.

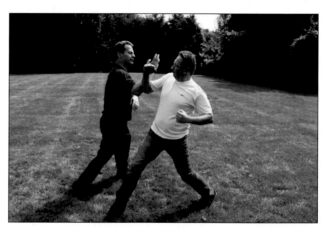

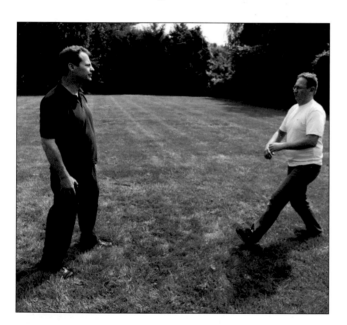

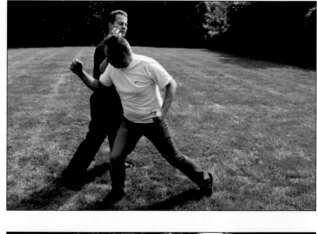

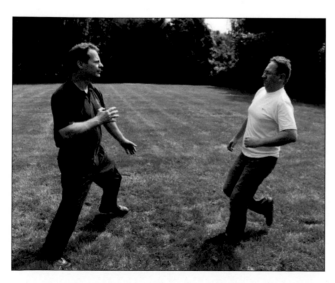

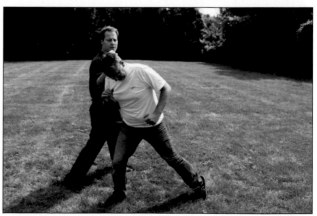

5. The attacker kicks and continues with a round-house. The defender's left hand immediately comes up after the initial block, ready for this possible scenario. The defender strikes the attacker at the back of attacker's neck.

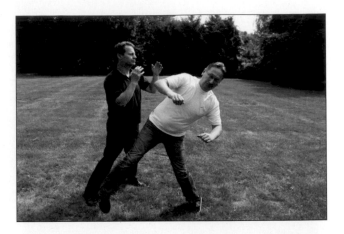

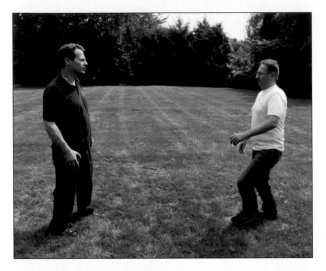

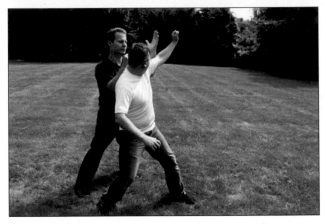

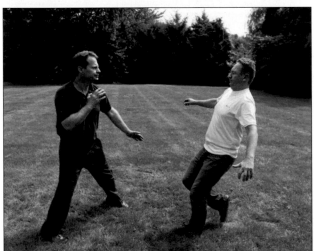

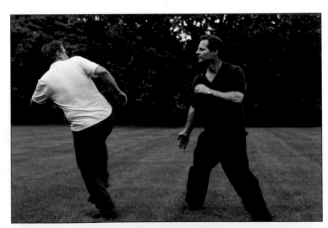

6. Variations of inside defense vs. side kicks where you face the front of the attacker's body while defending.

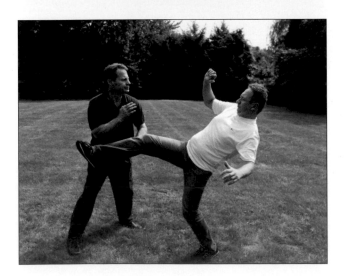

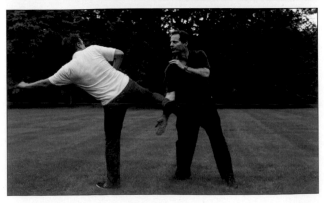

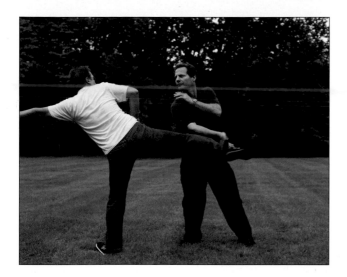 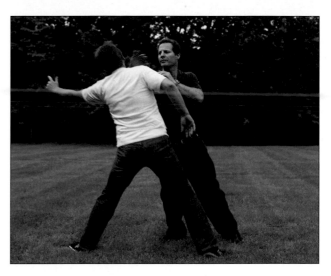

Outside Hand Defense vs. Kicks

At times you have the choice of getting ready for an approaching opponent with a stance that helps outside defenses. It could also be that you happened to be standing with your hands crossed over your chest before you noticed the opponent kicking.

1. The defender is standing with hands crossed over chest as the attacker lunges with a kick.
2. The defender smacks his hand down, pivoting his body clockwise. The defender's forearm slides on to the attacker's side of the leg, deflecting it. The defender simultaneously strikes with left punch.

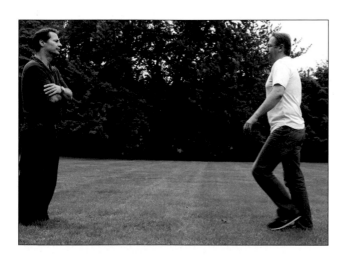 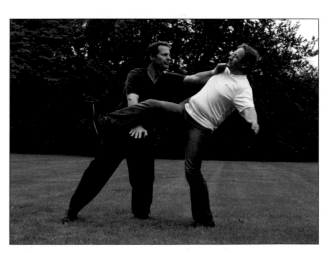

Note: If the opponent uses a hand strike, the defender blocks the hand strike with his front hand and counterattacks with the same fist hitting the opponent's face.

Outside hand defense vs. side kick

1. The attacker is approaching from sideways.
2. The attacker is executing a side kick and the defender slams his back hand down behind the attacker's knee, leaning his torso down to meet the attacker's knee before the kick is done. The defender attempts to strike the attacker in the face or to grab his groin and throw him to the ground.

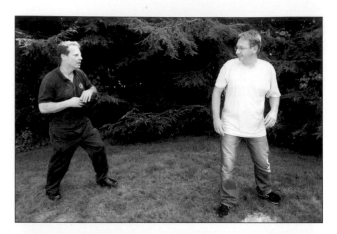

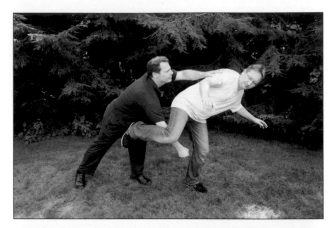

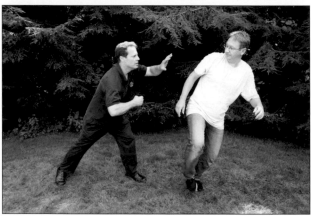

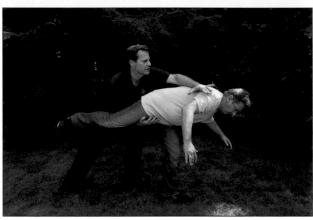

Notes: Outside defense for a side kick is executed by stabbing your fist into the loop created by the opponent's leg as it is lifts from the ground for a kick. The attacker is forced to extend his kick outside the direction of the defender's body.

If the attacker executes a full spinning roundhouse kick, the defender can move to block with his hands and counterattack to the back of the attacker's neck.

Outside defense vs. roundhouse kick

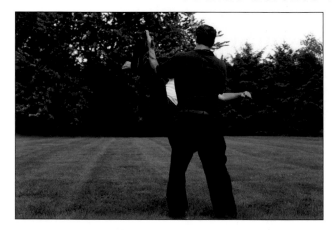

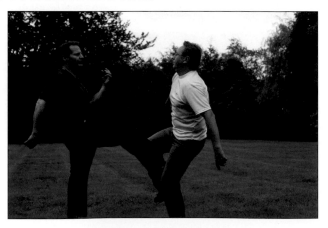

1. Attacker executes a roundhouse kick and defender blocks it with the outside of his forearm. Note that the back of the hand is facing the kick to distribute the impact on both bones in the forearm.
2. The defender counterattacks with a front kick to attacker's groin.

Notes: Stopping a roundhouse kick with inner forearms and counterattacking with a back-hand strike is optional. Attempting to throw the opponent is not ideal since you lose the opportunity for a simultaneous counterattack, and if the opponent retracts his kick, you lose the opportunity to throw him as well.

Toreador Pass Behind the Back

The last motion for defense vs. kicks to be learned can be seen in bullfights. We call it the toreador pass behind the back:

1. The defender stands with hands crossed in front of his sternum or even to the sides of his body with his body positioned forty-five degrees toward the attacker.
2. The attacker executes a front kick and the defender protrudes his stomach forward curling his back away from the kick. This propels a forward fall and the defender lands on his rear leg, lifting his front leg to ninety degrees to avoid exposing it to the attacker's possible low kicks. The defender blocks the kick with his front forearm inverted where the soft part is the contact point.
3. The defender attempts to pull on the opponent's leg backwards to make him lose his balance and land on his front foot, which will become a target for a follow-up kick.
4. The defender kicks the attacker's leg from the side.
5. The defender follows with a back-hand strike.

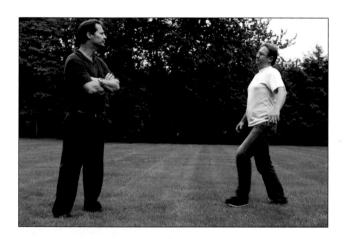
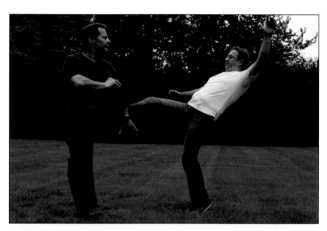
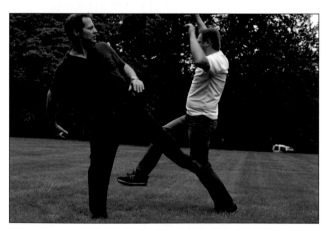
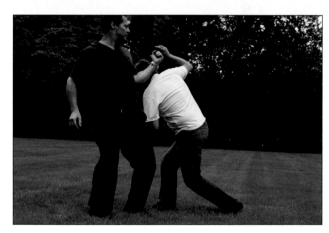

Notes: The same defense can work when the attacker executes a side kick. Your body is moving sidewise to avoid getting a low or a high kick.

Your front hand is aligned to the opponent's kicking leg, and is pushing your body sidewise. You give a little tug to the attacker's leg behind your back to make him lose his balance. He is now susceptible to getting hit with your side kick.

Never attempt to grab the opponent's leg as if he retracts it will pull you down backwards and you will expose your face to his continuing strike.

Tactical Consideration in Strikes and Kicks Used in Attack and Defense

When you have enough time to identify a dangerous scenario before it starts, the primary attacks are kicks and secondary attacks are punches. In the short range it is faster to reach with a punch than to shift the body's weight up for a kick. In the long range it is faster to leap one step and lift the leg for a kick instead of leaping two steps. Therefore in the long range, kicks are considered to be primary attacks.

If you block a fake kick, attack at the same time. If your opponent tries to punch you, he would not succeed since he would have closed a two-step gap before reaching you while you were moving to block his kick as he started to move. Since he initially planned to lunge two steps forward to close the gap, he would not expect you to meet him halfway and it would break his train of thought.

Another tactical move would be to move forward and close the gap without immediately attacking, and waiting for the opponent to attack first so that you could follow with a block and counterattack. However, your opponent could preemptively kick as you try to move in.

Krav Maga defense techniques are designed to automatically counter a kick with a follow-up hand strike. First, the right hand goes to the left shoulder before it strikes, therefore catching the outside of the forearm in any such possible attack. During training and practice of that particular defense, the student should practice the defense with all the possible follow-up scenarios as well.

Reaction Time Consideration

Remember that you are a human being and your skeleton is designed for use in a unique way. If you try to crawl like a snake, or walk like a monkey, you will never reach the speed and balance of your natural movement. Therefore as a Krav Maga fighter you have the upper hand. If a martial artist attempts to get into a particular stance, or makes an opening statement with a few threatening moves and screams, or tries to fake an attack, you should know by now that he is wasting his energy and attacks and you should really react to his initial standing position when he is about to close the range, or preemptively attack if you think he is serious about hurting you. At times ignoring a person at the right time but yet being ready to counter him with the right timing will discourage a bully through the messages your body and actions deliver.

From a distance, you can see that his closest limb, according to the striking distance, is what you should be concerned about. Follow your training and counterattack by blocking only the closest limb. If he fakes his first move, it should not be a great concern. While he is doing this, you should block the fake attack and counterattack him at the same time. He should never be able to get to his second planned attack.

How to Practice Defense and Counterattacks Realistically

I've noticed that during the first few years of training, Win Tsun (an offshoot of Chinese boxing) practitioners dedicate their training drills to punching and blocking at close range their training partners. They start their sparring from an arm wrestling position. This method may be suitable for two opponents in complete darkness relying only on their sense of touch.

If in the bright daylight, an opponent striking from a further distance would have an advantage over someone trained only to fight at a close distance. In that close of a distance, knowing the Krav Maga principle of reaction time, there is no point in reinforcing close scenario defense and attack.

In reality, from that close of a distance, there would not be enough time to see a swift attack and block it. A defender in this scenario would always be one step behind. That type of training, while promoting a slower speed, would never work at maximum speed. Moreover, students are getting false perceptions of reality, and are training the wrong reflexes for an extended period of time before they have enough subconscious experience to realize what works and what does not.

I've encountered some martial artists who waste their time attempting to get into an animal position and imitate the animal's sound. The whole motion is a waste of time; the time spent on getting into the position is time that could be used to attack the opponent. A stance that attempts to mimic a natural stance of another animal would definitely not contribute to a fast mobility with a human spine. Making a monkey face is fine, but dropping to a monkey stance and expecting to move forward as fast as the monkey is ridiculous. As a matter of fact, any wasteful movement could prove fatal since if you flail your arms to block, your brain needs to have the time to send them a signal to move and this takes up time, since first your brain needs to find their current location and direction of motion before it can redirect them to execute a block.

CLOSE RANGE SCENARIOS 5

Let us think about how we got into this situation first, and see if we could've avoided it. We must have been caught off guard, allowing someone to get that close, or we must have been sharing a small space with other people. Before we start, let's think about our options. If we got punched first, we may have a slight concussion, and the opponent might take advantage of it by swiftly trying to break our neck. We would have very little chance to execute any reaction. We need to keep perfecting our previously learned material to avoid these scenarios.

However, if an opponent attempts to grip our bodies to execute his favorite wrestling technique, or attempts a type of sexual or kidnapping assault, then we have some sort of an advantage. Since the opponent tries to throw us off balance, get a hold of our bodies, or inflict pain with his grip, our instincts are fully functional. In addition, we have the advantage of having our "prey" right at our disposal, occupied with trying to grip our bodies. We usually get a better sense of justification when we use all our resources to get rid of the attacker as well.

While wrestlers and jujitsu-trained fighters perfect their ground fighting techniques through years of training, Krav Maga allots only a few hours for close range scenarios. Sports martial arts base their training on their rules. Krav Maga, however, prioritizes training time based on levels of vulnerability.

While sports martial arts train to inflict pain or discomfort leading to controlling the opponent, Krav Maga cannot afford to give too much attention to one opponent where there is a great chance he is part of a group of attackers. Therefore, attackers should be neutralized in a matter of seconds. A quick strike to a pressure point, or a quick leverage on the neck, finger jab to a nerve, or quick squeeze to the testicles would end a fight much faster.

Finally, if your opponent grabs your body, he probably feels confident in his strength and fighting skills. You really do not have the luxury of slowly testing his skill to compare it to yours. Instead, you need to take advantage of the scenario and end it in a way that there is no more danger of strikes, chokes, leverages or anything that puts your body at risk.

You need to get him under control in a swift second. You definitely do not want to give him a chance to attack you again. To emphasize this point, I would like to present what could happen if you did not react with the maximum amount of force. If you did not take the opportunity, your attacker could hit you and have you unconscious, and in the next scenario you would find yourself being kicked, punched, kneed, or choked, leading you to a quick or slow death. Anything can happen quickly when you are not in control. You need to regain your mobility immediately.

It is easier to strike the weakest accessible pressure point that leads to the most damaging results in the swiftest option possible in each scenario.

Keep in mind that in close scenarios you do not want your opponent to run away and attack you again.

So do not push him too far and lose your window of opportunity to strike him. Always maintain a grip on his body or arm as you strike him.

Generally, with a wrestling or jujitsu technique, keep in mind that if you let someone tie you with a rope, you will be helpless at the end. Never allow yourself to get into this situation. Understand that while sports martial artists are trained not to go for the immediate and most devastating blow, they expose themselves in their attack. You should be able to use the principles you will learn in this chapter to foil these attacks.

In Krav Maga, the techniques chosen give students principles of approach with consideration to prioritizing all involved. In the real world, every situation is different. Therefore, if you understand the principles, you can adapt them to the situation.

An overview of body holds from different directions teaches the students to identify how to overcome opponents by understanding risks and pressure points.

Defense from Body and Arms Hold from the Rear

1. The attacker grabs the defender's arms and body from behind and lifts him up.
2. The defender spirals his leg around the attacker's leg, stopping any possible sway attempts. Note the knee is locked.
3. The defender is using his free leg to kick the opponent's groin and to land on the ground immediately after.
4. If the attacker doesn't lift, the defender tilts his hips to the side and executes an open hand slap to the groin.

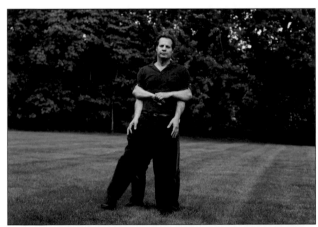
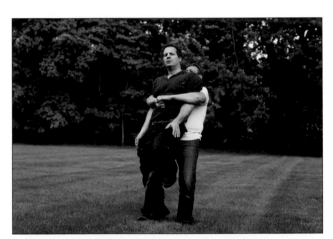
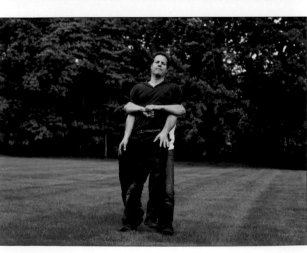
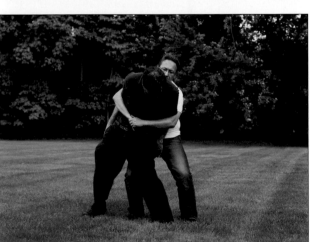

Note: The defender continues to use the space between his body and the attacker's body to execute a kick to the attacker's groin. Kicking the shin is optional as well and elbowing the opponent's center of the body is also an option.

Defense from Body Hold from the Rear

1. The defender elbows backward to the attacker's head, and elbows the other direction to surprise the attacker's possible attempt to escape. Remember, if the opponent is trying to take you off balance, you may have a short window of opportunity. Note that in a static hold, where the opponent has gripped you or is standing next to you from behind, you can utilize a backward headbutt to stun him and hence buy yourself time.

2. The defender grips the attacker's arms with his forearms, sensing where his hands are and paying attention to which hand is above the other.

3. The defender slides his hands forward on to the attacker's forearms gripping the upper forearm and sliding his fingers to extract one of the attacker's fingers with his free hand. creating a leverage on the finger.

4. The defender pushes both hands toward each other, keeping them under his center of gravity, around the belt with all his weight. The defender breaks the attacker's finger.

5. The defender pivots to face the opponent (note that the pivot should be a jump where the defender adjusts his distance to be comfortable enough to execute a kick).

6. Defender kicks the attacker's groin from the front.

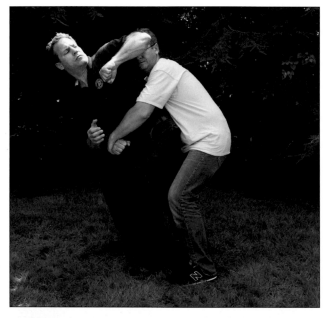

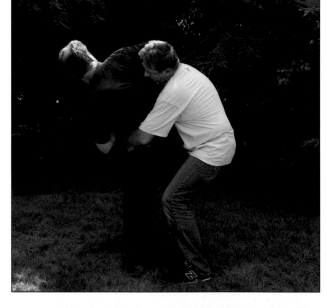

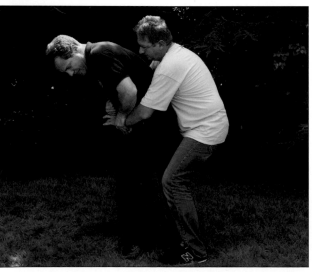

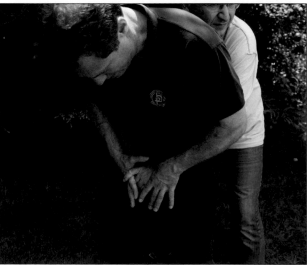

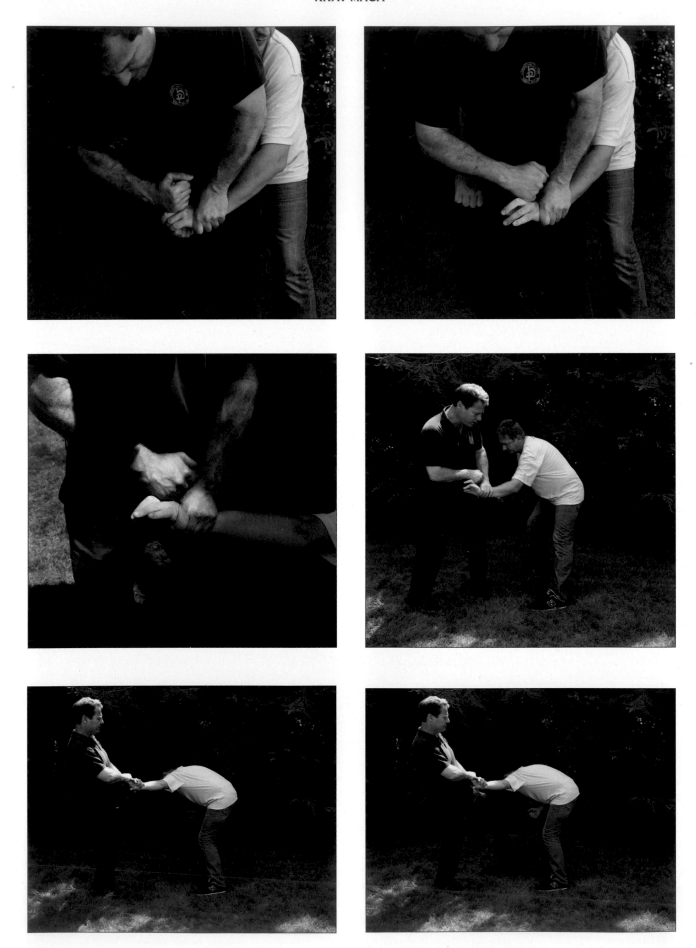

Release from a Front Body and Arms Hold

1. The attacker captures the defender's body and arms from the front. The defender cannot use his knee since the attacker is too close.
2. The defender jabs the attacker's groin using the back of his fingers, giving him an instinctive evasion move.
3. The defender grabs the attacker's shoulder blades as he knees him in the groin. The defender leans his torso slightly backward, using his hands to pull the attacker's shoulder blades down to support the knee kick.
4. The defender stomps the top of attacker's foot.

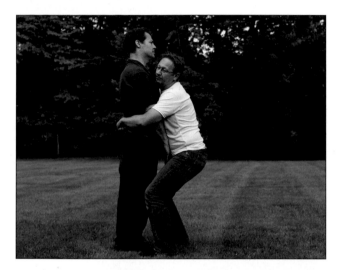
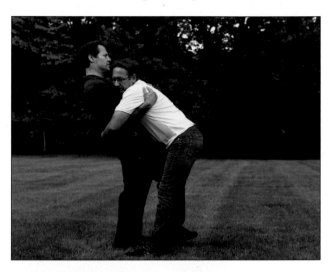

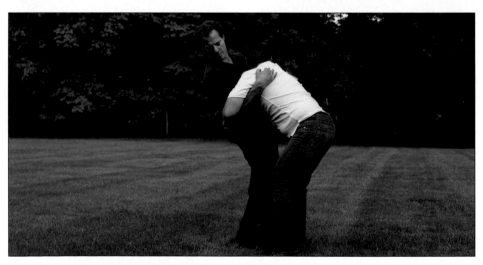

Note: Screaming into the opponent's ear would hurt his eardrum and set you free. You could bite a nerve in his neck or his tongue, but you might not want the exchange of fluids so it should be used as a last resort.

Release from a Front Body Hold

The defender pivots the attacker's head in a clockwise direction and down toward the ground, creating pressure on the neck while keeping his hands close to his body so the body can assist in the force. A swift execution will cause the attacker to fall to the ground. The result could be a stiff or broken neck. To get comfortable with the correct angle of the motion during practice, you need to slowly control your training partner as you bring him to the ground and ensure he is not able to escape throughout the motion. In real life, remember to give his head a spin like a globe, and watch his world turn upside down.

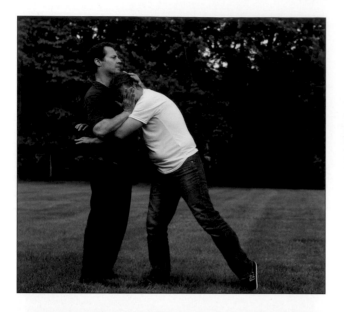
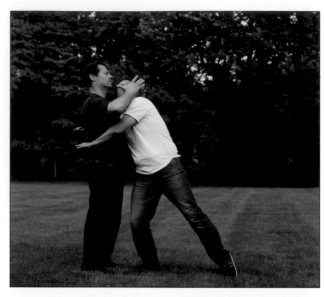
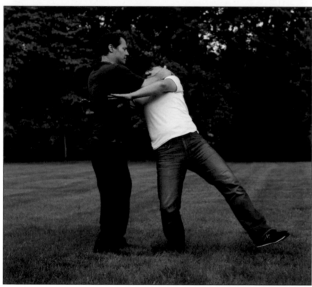
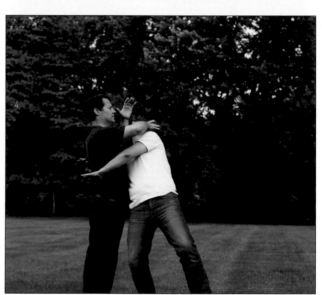

Note: Other optional methods not shown above:

With the side of your thumb, find attacker's nose without even trying to look and push underneath his nose forty-five degrees upward to move him away from your body. Follow with your free palm and hit your opponent.

Or, you could also shove a thumb to his eye where both your hands are wrapped around his cheeks to make sure he doesn't escape. You can control this motion slowly in training, but in a real situation, the faster you do it, the more immediately you get your result.

Release from Low Front Body Hold

1. The attacker grabs the defender's body in a low body hold from the front.
2. The defender sends a roundhouse punch pointing his middle finger to the attacker's temple.
3. The defender pivots his body, executing an elbow blow to the top of the attacker's head.

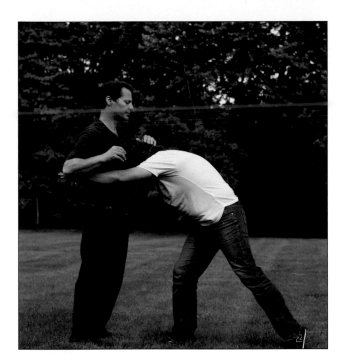 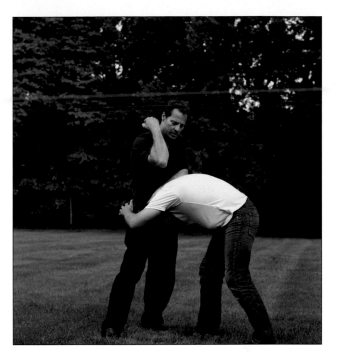

Note: The above practice should give the student a direction in scenarios where punches and kicks end in some sort of a grab scenario. For example, if you kick and the opponent grabs your leg with two hands, you can retract your body forward by folding your leg back to ninety degrees and bringing your upper body close to your opponent. You then punch him in the face, or grab his head as an anchor to your stability. You can twist his head, leveraging on his neck.

Release from Neck Chokes

Choking is an attempt to push your windpipe in and limit or stop your air intake by breaking it. Some chokes are designed to tear your windpipe down with a singlehanded grip. The result could be loss of consciousness and possibly death if it goes on more than fifteen minutes.

The windpipe can be broken with a punch or a knife-hand strike as well. In a chokehold, your opponent needs to get a hold of you first to choke you.

That takes at least two seconds, not giving you a lot of time for action, but enough to execute the correct technique.

While you can kick or punch your opponent as he puts pressure on your windpipe, your immediate reaction would be to release his grip before you think to strike. Remember: all you need is to move your opponent's thumbs or fingers away from your windpipe.

Release from a front choke

1. The attacker, using four fingers in each hand to leverage the back of the neck, pushes his thumbs into the defender's windpipe.
2. The defender uses all five fingers to pluck the attacker's wrists. Never insert your fingers between your throat and the opponent's hands, since you would have no room to react to the pressure.

3. The defender executes a knee kick to the attacker's groin.
4. The defender elbows the attacker's chin quickly after letting go of one hand. Remember to keep both your legs on the ground before executing the elbow blow. Attempting to knee kick and elbow at the same time detracts from the effect of each separate counterattack.

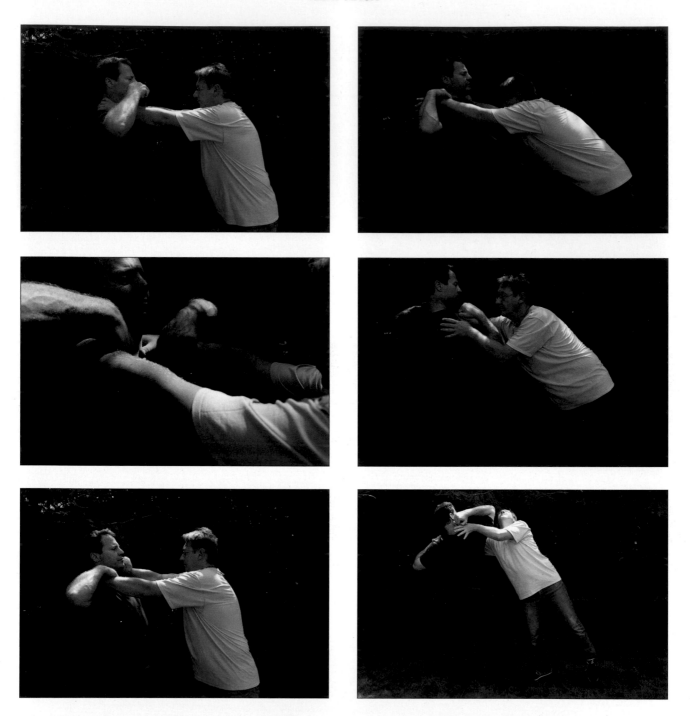

Note: If the opponent chokes you from the side, you can release his choke taking down the hand in front and ignoring the hand on the back of the neck since it is not choking. You then execute a counterattack with a slap to the opponent's groin followed with an elbow strike to his face.

Preemptive defense

When you see an attacker reaching with both hands reaching to grab or choke you, you can extend your hand as far as you can reach and strike his chest with your palm, pushing your fingers into his throat. A kick is not considered in this scenario, since an opponent usually will raise his hands for a throat grab as he is get-

ting near you, not before. If, however, you have enough time to realize your opponent is attacking you when he is two steps away, you should immediately kick him.

1.   The attacker is reaching his hands to grab the defender's throat.

2. The defender throws his palm toward the opponent's sternum, pivoting his body directly behind his arm. The defender lifts his rear leg for balance. The key in this technique is to lock your elbow before impacting the target.

3. As the defender thrusts his palm on to the attacker's chest, the defender's fingers continue to push into the attacker's throat. The body and shoulder pivot with one hand, which helps create a longer reach than the attacker's two-hand reach.

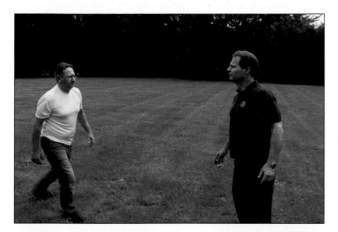 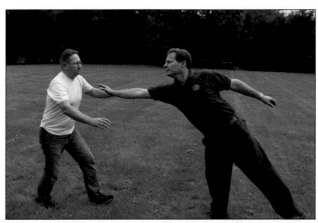

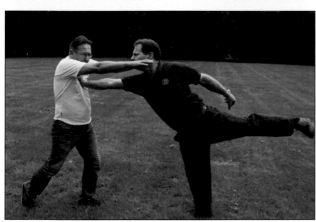 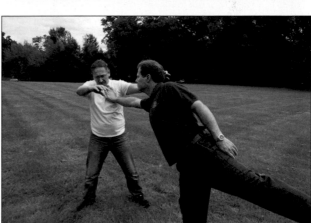

Front choke (attacker is pushing)

1. The attacker is choking and pushing the defender.
2. The defender lifts his arm to the side of his ear and pivots his opposite shoulder back and down towards the ground. This creates pressure on the opponent's wrist.

3. The defender pivots backwards, landing on his rear foot as the opponent's torso is tilted forwards.
4. The defender returns with an elbow to the attacker's face or with a knife-hand striking at the attacker's throat.

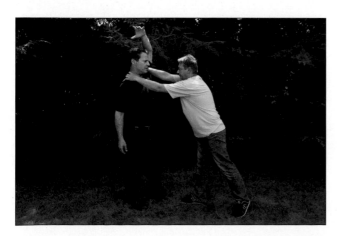 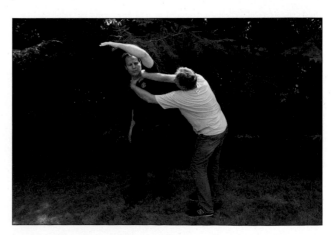

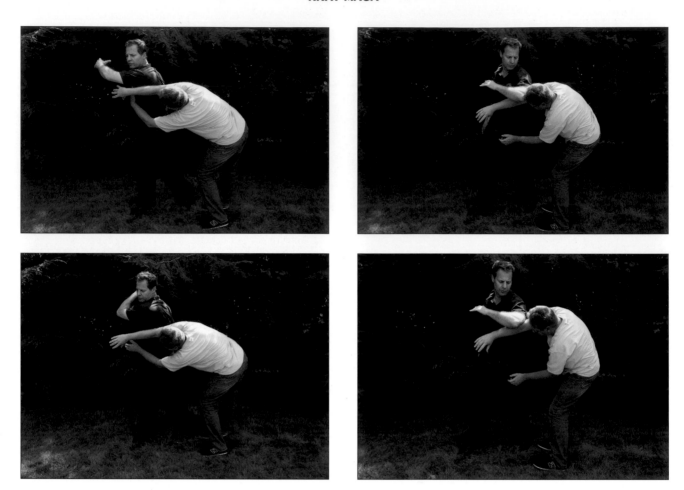

One-handed choke with attempt to pluck the windpipe

1. The attacker grabs defender's windpipe.
2. The defender immediately immobilizes the attacker's hand by hitting the back of it and attaching it to his chest with one or both of the defender's hands.

3. The defender executes a counterattack with a knee or a foot kick.

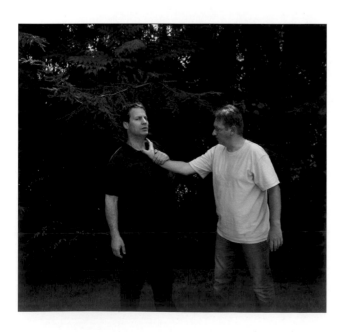

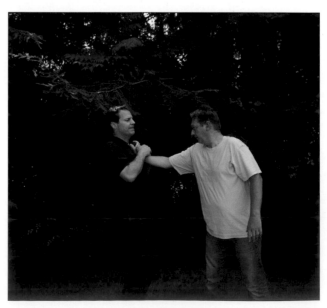

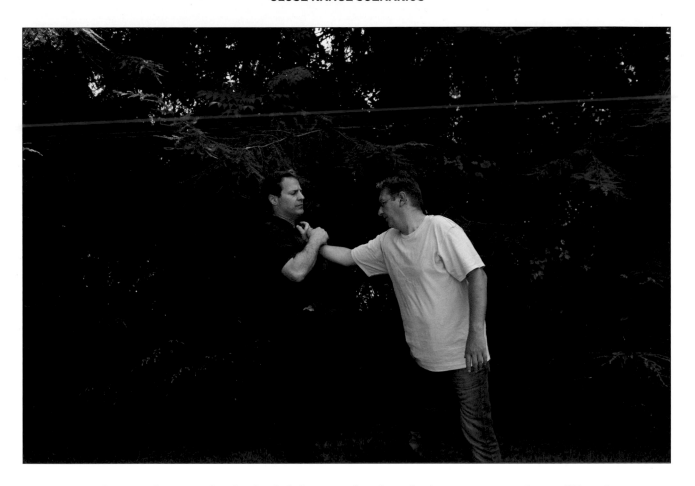

Release from chokehold from the back (opponent is pulling)

1. The attacker is choking the defender from behind.
2. The defender reaches behind his neck, cupping his hands and plucking the attacker's wrists.
3. The defender steps backward diagonally away to break the pull.
4. The defender releases one of the opponent's hands and swiftly hits attacker's groin. The defender continues to hold the attacker's second hand to prevent the attacker from escaping the counterattack.
5. The defender follows with an elbow strike to the attacker's chin as the attacker bends over in pain.

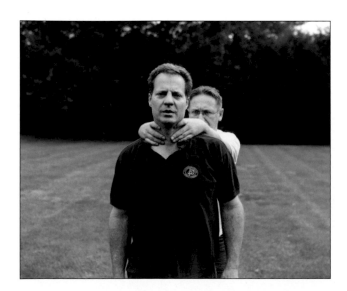

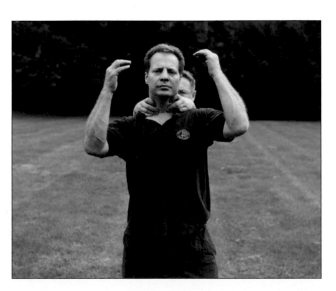

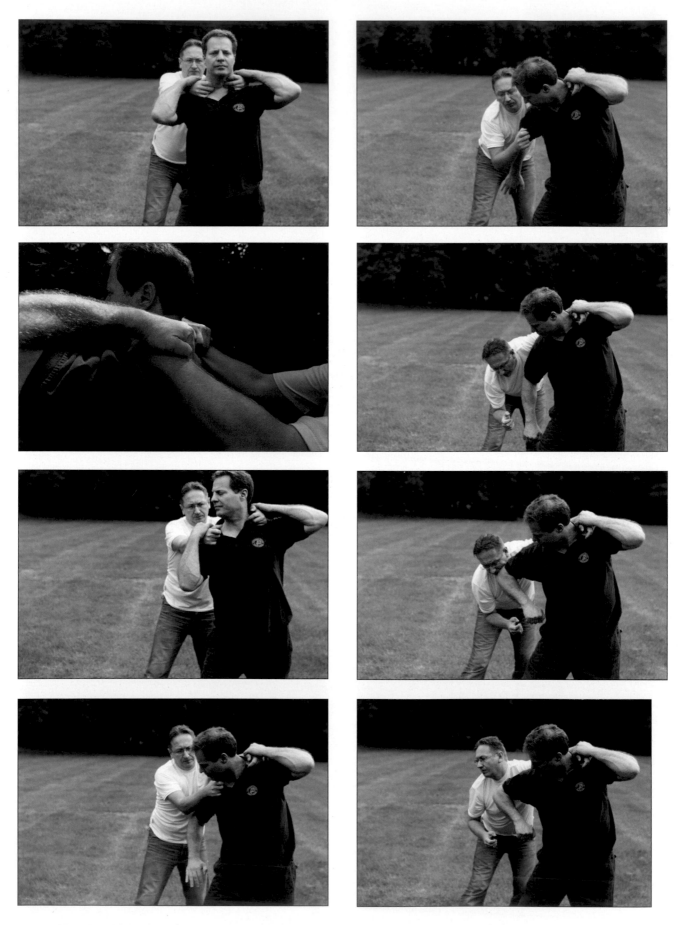

Note: This should be practiced in steps to achieve a chain reaction.

Release from a chokehold from the rear (attacker is pushing)

1. The attacker is choking the defender from the rear and pushing him with the same motion.
2. The defender puts pressure on the attacker's wrist using his biceps.
3. The defender drops his opposite shoulder down to the center of his body using gravity and a shoulder throw.

4. The defender uses his shoulder throw to escape the grip, landing sideways to the attacker.
5. The defender shifts his weight back as he strikes the attacker in his kidney with a knife-hand strike, or an elbow blow to his face if attacker is too close.

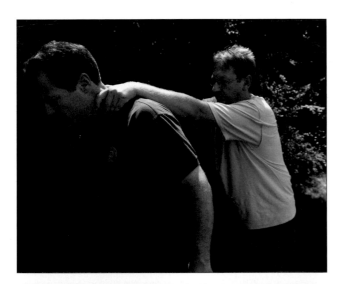
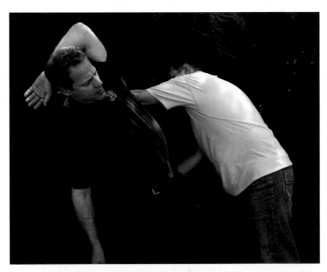
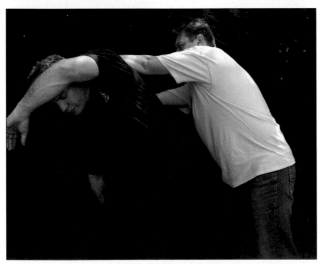
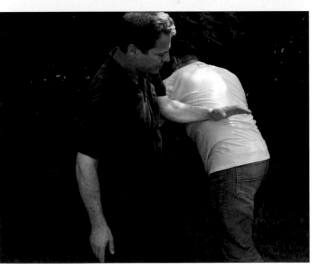

Countering Front-Knife Threat to the Neck

1. The attacker puts a knife to defender's throat.
2. The defender spoons his opponent's wrist and attaches it to his chest.

3. The defender joins his free hand to his opponent's wrist that's holding the knife, and uses his whole body to move the attacker's hand.
4. The defender throws the attacker off balance, kicking his groin or face.

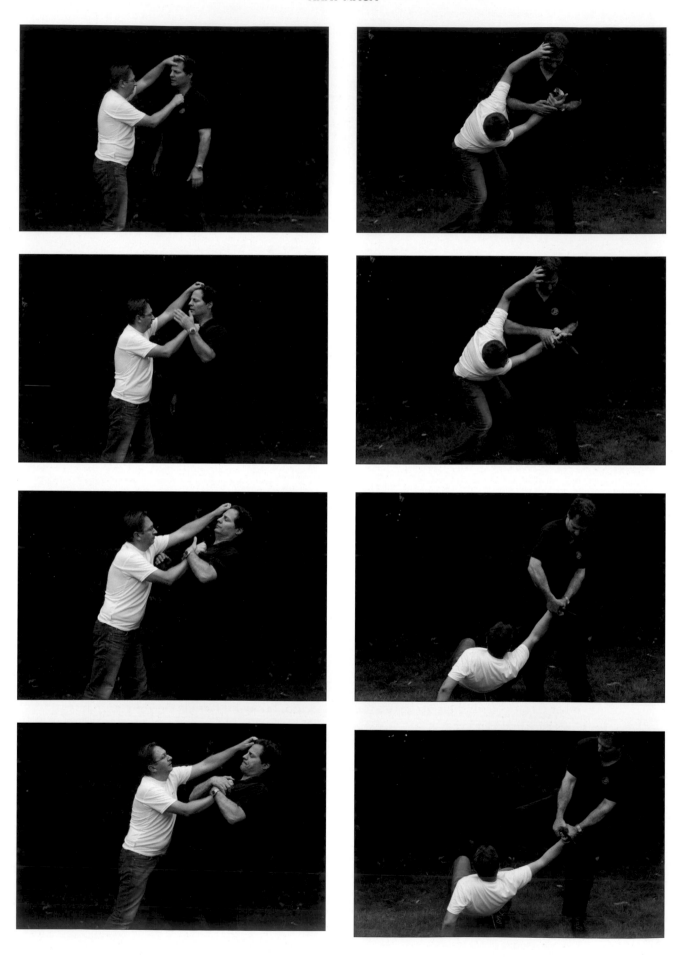

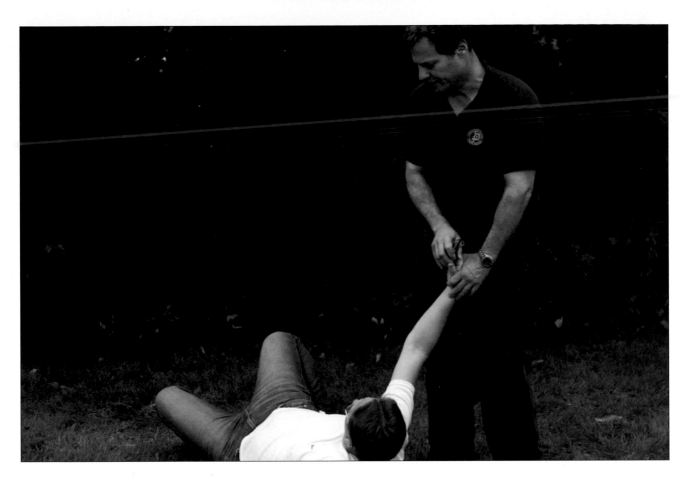

Release from Head Locks

Head locks can be used to control your body or to strangle you at the same time.

Strangling can limit the blood flow of the arteries in the neck that provide oxygen to the brain. If this occurs, you can still breathe, but there is no oxygen supply to the brain, and if you do not react you will faint within a few seconds.

The hanging technique

1. Approach and strike to the opponent's kidney and wrap your other forearm around his neck.
2. Pivot your hips back and bend your knees, joining your hands and locking them together.
3. Roll your opponent on to his back, to the opposite hip, lifting his feet off the ground. In this position it is very hard for your opponent to escape.
4. Look at his heels and wait for them to drop. When they drop, he has probably fainted.

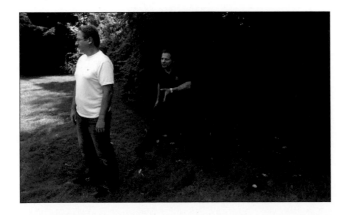

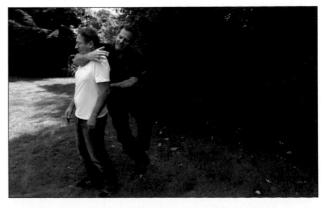

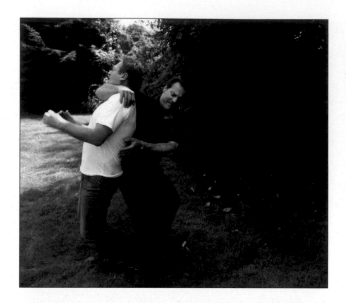 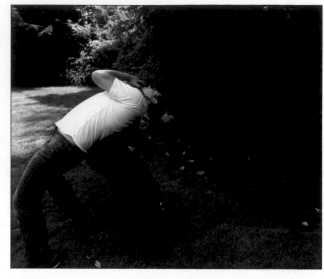

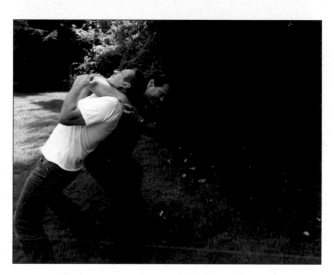 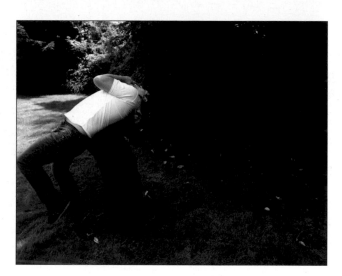

Note: This is a favorite skilled technique. While there are easier, more effective, and less risky techniques, I wanted to use this technique to stress the importance of a quick reaction. Many times, this hold can end on the ground, or be accompanied by a knife threat. However, anything less conclusive would make it easier to escape. Keep in mind that if your opponent is grabbing you with one hand while holding a weapon with the other, he cannot strangle you, and you should concentrate your efforts on preventing injury before thinking of escaping the hold.

Release from neck hold from the rear

1. First move both hands towards the opponent's eyes in an attempt to poke them.
2. Land your hands on the opponent's wrists, pulling them down as you gain your breath. If the grip is too forceful to pull down, use your hands to attach the attacker's hands to your chest and lean your head backward to release the pressure on your neck.
3. Pivot your body and your chin to the direction of the opponent's hands, easing your head out.
4. Push with both shoulders, making room for your head to exit.
5. Let go of your right hand and use it to grab the attacker's elbow before standing up. That would surely keep him down. Hold the opponent at the wrist and elbow and kick to his face.
6. You can kick his coccyx bone or the groin according to his position.

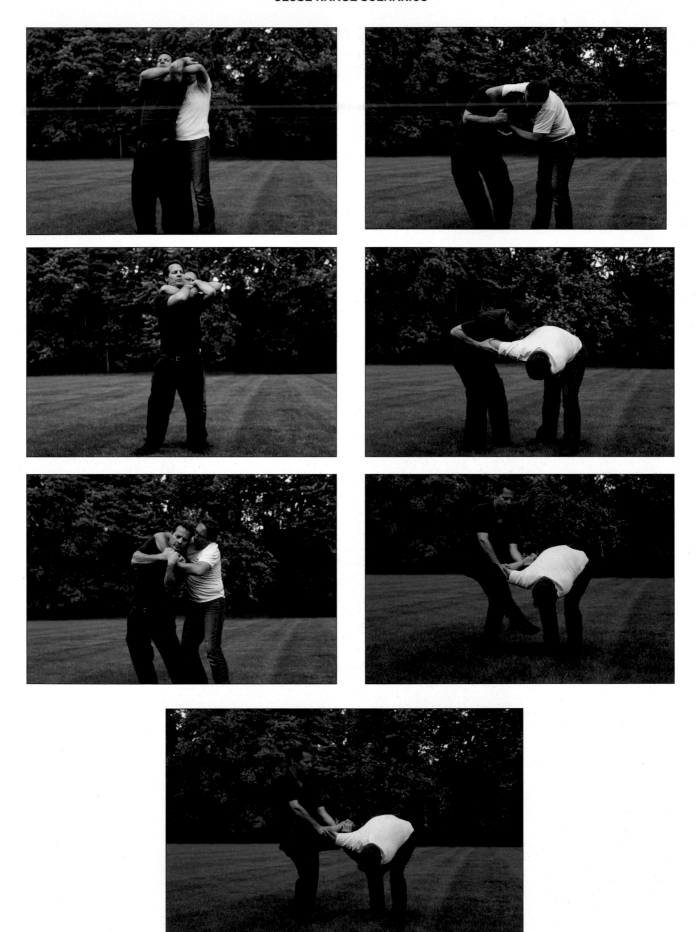

Escape from head lock with a knife to the throat

1. The attacker grabs the defender with a one-handed head lock and a puts a knife onto the defender's throat.
2. The defender hooks both his hands on top of the attacker's knife-holding hand's wrist. The defender continues using his hands to hook the attacker's wrists and pulling them down as he leans backwards to breathe.
3. The defender steps diagonally backward toward the attacker's pull. The defender can stomp on the attacker's foot to weaken him before proceeding to the next step. The defender releases one hand to grab the opponent's shoulder. This limits the attacker's knife-holding hand.
4. The defender twists his body and gets out of the hold safely.
5. The defender finishes with the counterattack; same as in the prior scenario.

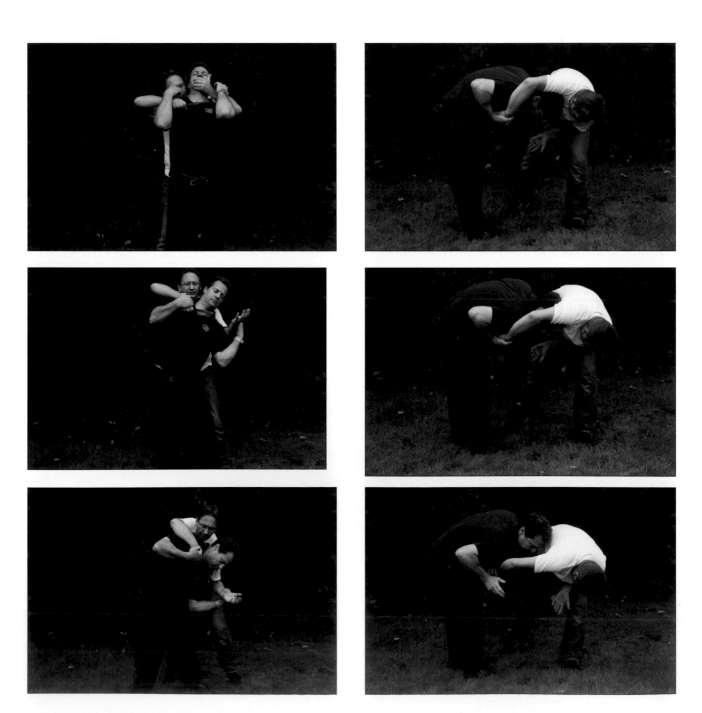

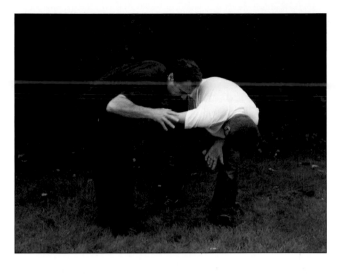 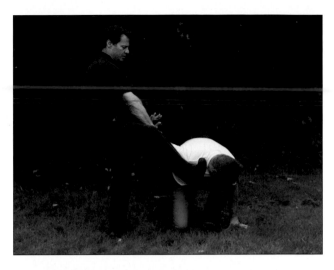

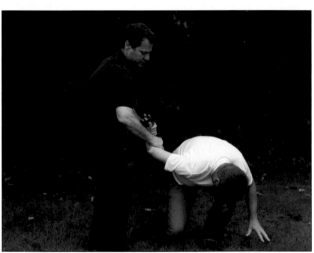 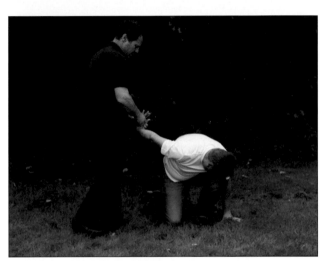

Release from head lock from the side

1. The defender punches or grabs the attacker's groin.
2. The defender pushes down on the bridge of the attacker's nose or his vagus if he can't reach the attacker's nose.

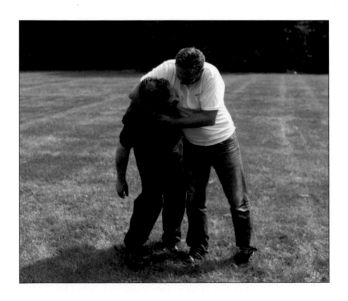 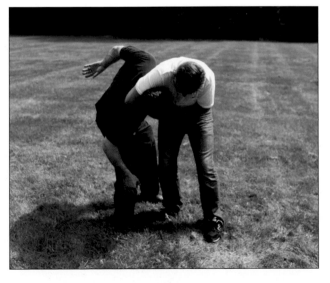

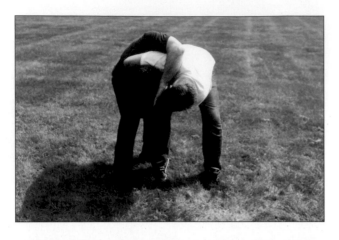

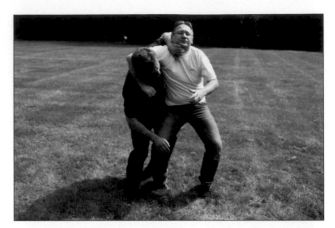

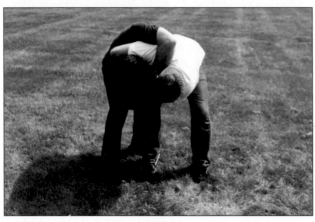

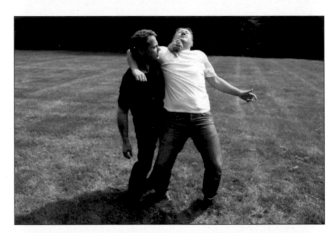

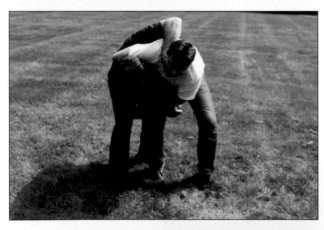

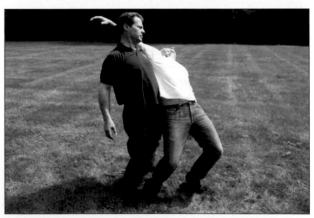

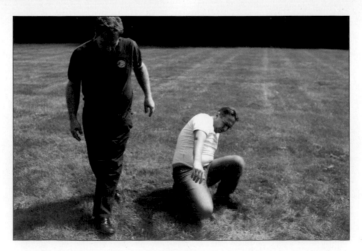

Release from head hold from the side while rolling to the ground

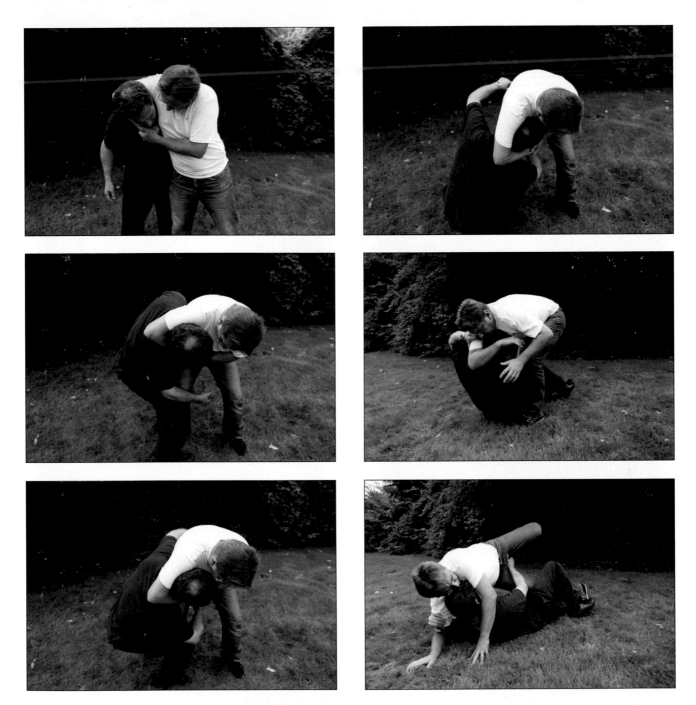

Release from neck hold from the front

I would like you to stop for a moment and think about how you got to this position, and how you could have prevented this. You probably tried to pull back from another position and run away without counterattacking. But since you are there, I will show you the way out.

1. The attacker locks his arms around the defender's neck, and defender prepares to block a possible attacker's knee kick.

2. The defender grips the attacker's wrists and punches his groin.
3. The defender pivots his head to the direction of attacker but without letting go of the grip.
4. The defender twists the attacker's arm behind his back and kicks the attacker's groin, face, or coccyx bone.

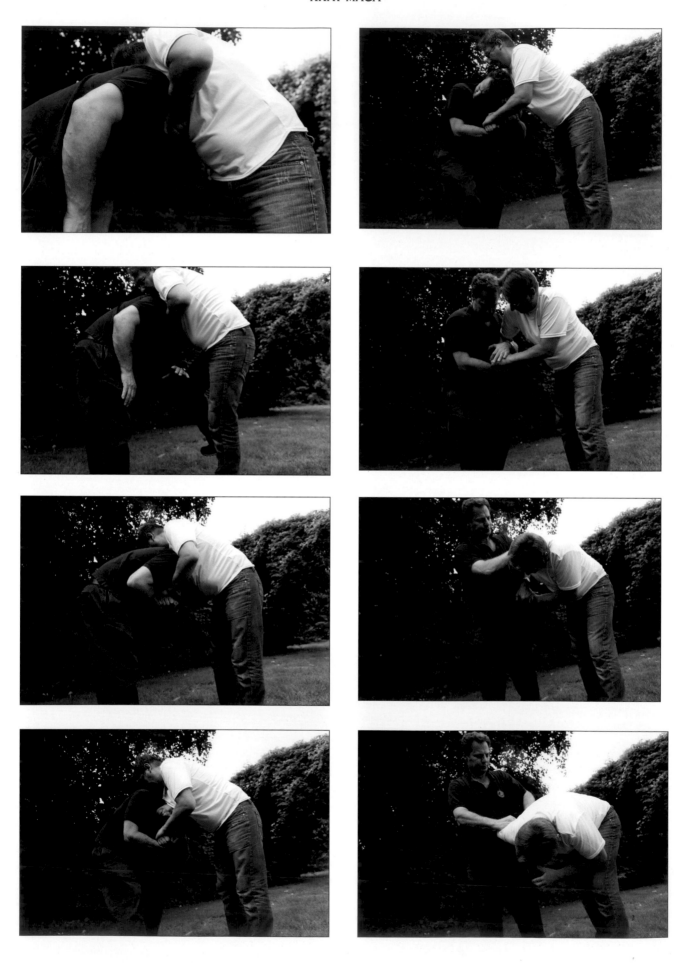

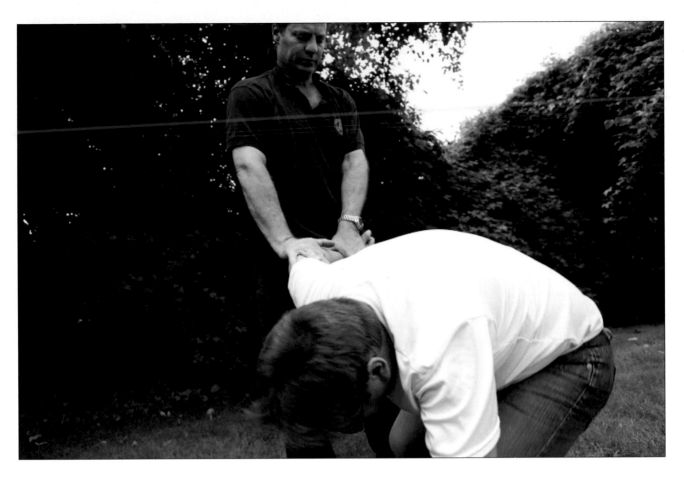

Release from a Front Hair Pull

Hair grabbing is often used to pull someone's head for a knee kick or to get someone close for a sexual assault. If you move toward the direction you're being pulled, prepare to block a knee kick with one hand as you attack the opponent's groin or face with the other.

1. The attacker grabs the defender's hair and pulls it down, attempting to knee him.
2. The defender blocks the attacker's hand and executes a counterattack.

Hair Pulling from the Side (when the attacker hesitates)

1. The attacker grabs the defender's hair from the side.
2. The defender hits the attacker's wrist. This would relax his grip.

3. The defender counter-strikes with a punch.

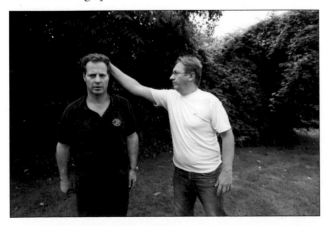

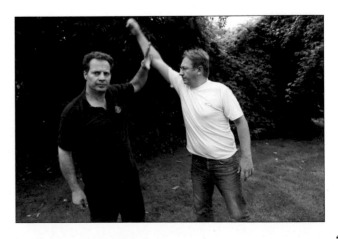

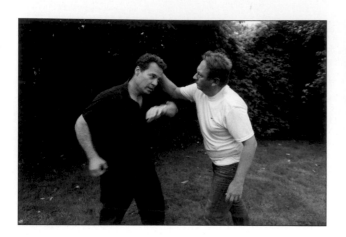 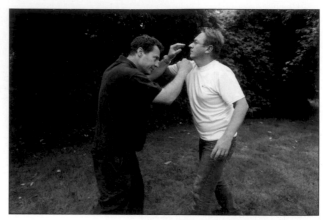

Release from the hair pull

1. The attacker is grabbing the defender's hair.
2. The defender closes the gap by turning towards the attacker's pull.

3. The defender attacks by smacking the groin (if the attacker is wearing jeans, use your fist instead of an open hand; it hurts more).

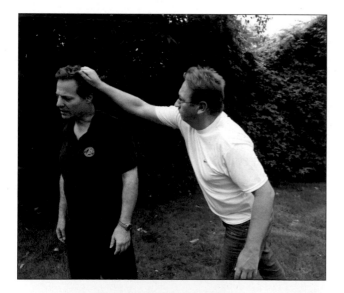 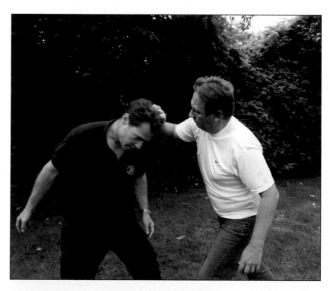

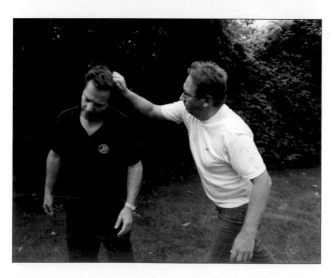 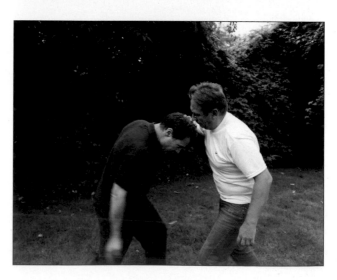

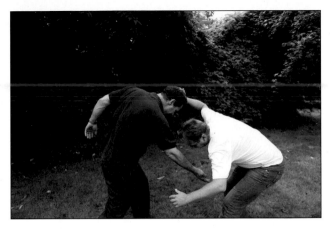
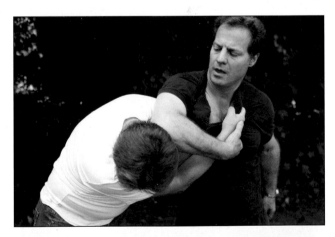

Release from Shirt Hold Counterattack with Pressure on the Elbow

If someone grabs your shirt, be aware that they may try to headbutt you. To prevent this, throw your elbow between you and your opponent as you turn sidewise. Then grip his wrist and pivot backward. Counterattack according to your judgment. This technique would stop your attacker from taking you off-balance for a throw or a leg sweep as well.

1. The attacker grabs the defender's shirt.

2. The defender pivots backward striking with his elbow forward to block a possible headbutt. Defender grabs attacker's wrist.
3. The defender returns to the other direction.
4. The defender applies pressure to the attacker's elbow to take him down, or continues taking him down in the opposite direction.
5. The attacker can kick the opponent in the face or chest.

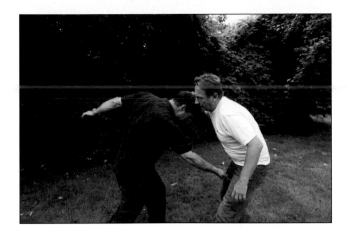
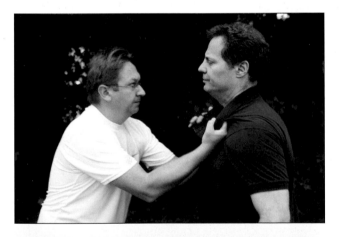

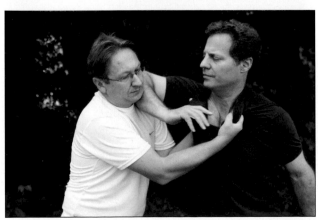
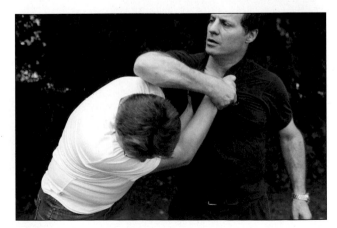

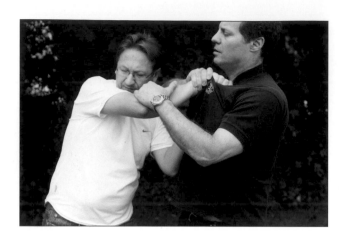 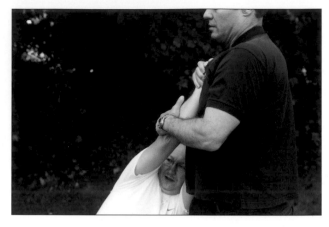

Release from Shirt Hold Counterattack with Pressure on the Shoulder

1. The attacker grabs the defender's shirt.
2. The defender throws an elbow strike to foil a possible headbutt as he pivots backwards.
3. Defender grabs the attacker's wrist and pivots back to the opposite direction.

4. Defender slides his hand on the attacker's elbow reaching to his shoulder and taking him down. Then he twists his wrist.

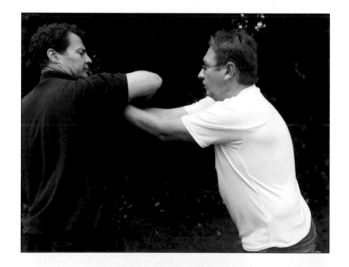 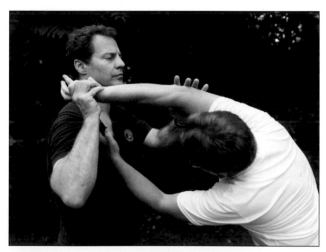

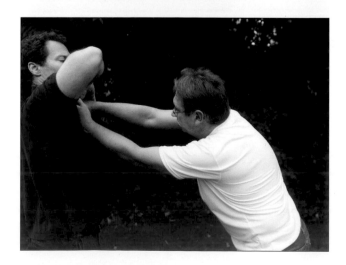 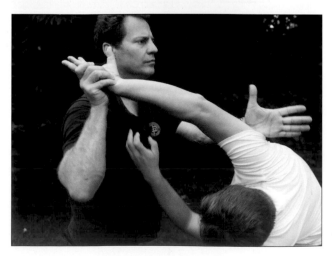

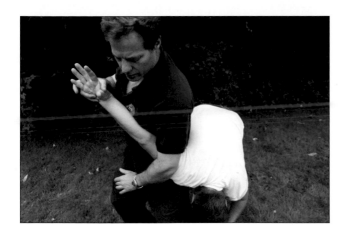 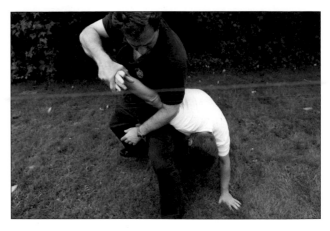

Taking an Opponent Out of Balance for Leg Trips and Hip Throws

The purpose of these techniques is to build confidence in the principles of grappling and to let training partners practice defenses against realistic attacks. In addition, students need to learn how to break their falls in worst-case scenarios and how to continue fighting from the ground if they have to. Note that an attacker using any of these techniques should be countered by releasing from a shirt grab technique. See Chapter 13 for further analysis.

Leg trips

1. As you grab your opponent's clothes, wrists, or waist, shift his weight on one foot by twisting his torso.

2. Follow by sweeping the leg he is standing on.

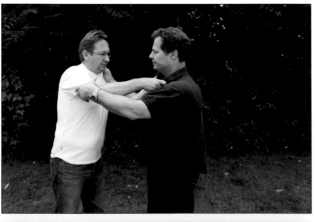 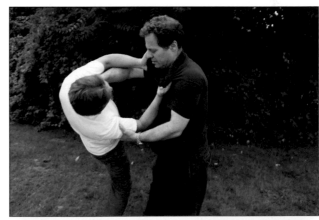

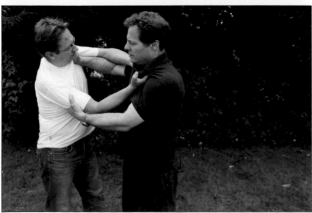 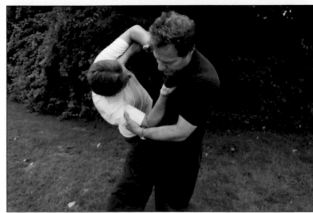

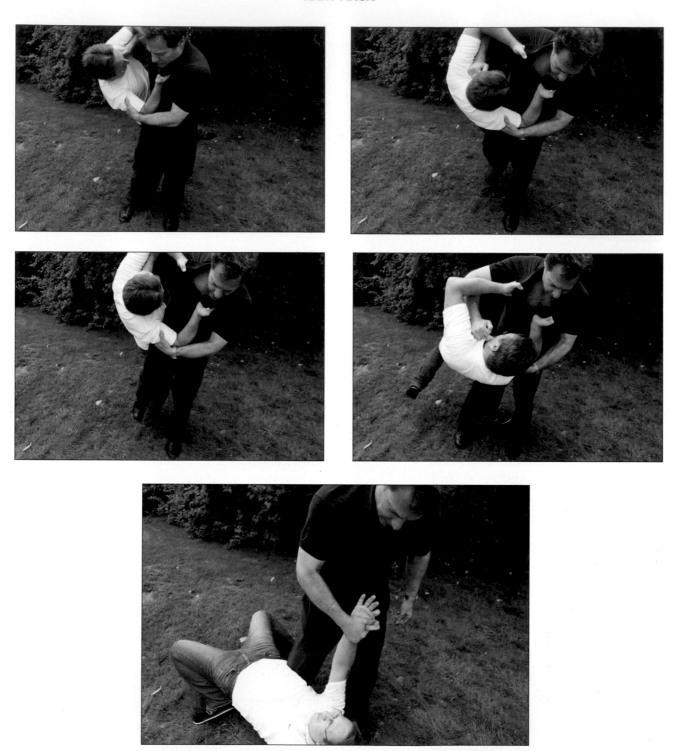

Note: You could strike someone in the face with an open palm and sweep his legs at the same time. A strike is a quicker method to throw someone off balance, but the foot sweep could be helpful in throwing him down on his head. In my opinion, it is too risky since you can't predict your opponent's skills.

Hip throws

1. As you grab your opponent's clothes, head, wrists, or waist, shift his weight on one of his feet by twisting his body. You can also bend your knees as you hold him tight and lift him off the ground for a hip throw.

2. Follow by pulling his shoulders toward you as you turn your back to him and let your waist collide against his hips while keeping your knees bent.

3. Straighten your knees and roll him over your waist and onto the floor.

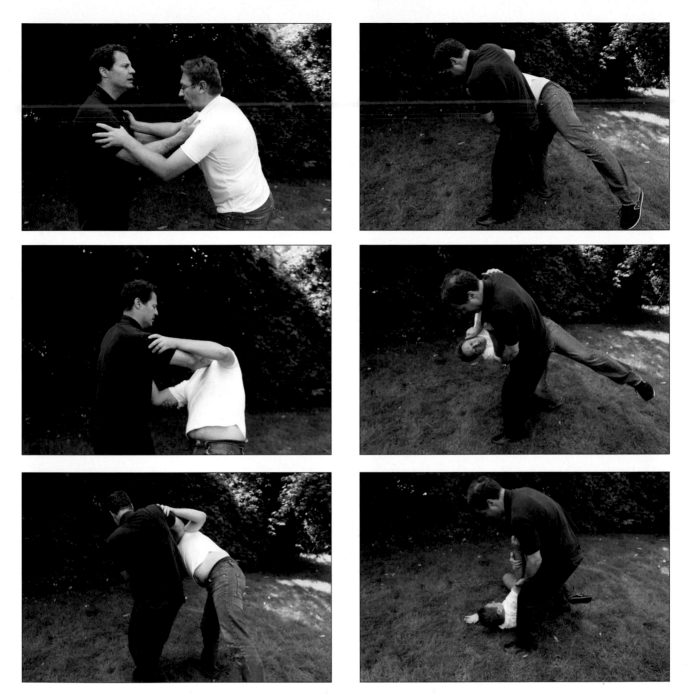

Note: You can use this hip throw against an opponent trying to wrestle you by turning around as soon as he is approaching.

If Your Opponent Tries to Grapple

Consider kicks and punches to the head or groin according to the distance. Consider a release from a shirt grab as demonstrated earlier.

Your opponent may move back on your first kick and try to grab your lower body. Your Krav Maga kicks should not allow for that even if you missed the kick. Retract your limbs quickly to maintain maximum speed during contact with your target. This also gives your attacker fewer chances to grab you. Kicking with the same leg another time would catch a returning

attacker. Switching to another kick with the other leg will chase an attacker that is moving back.

If, however, your attacker does grab your leg, you can in turn grab ahold of his head and take it down with your fall. Retraction of a kick aimed to the center body will bend down and off balance an opponent that tries to grab the leg. The Krav Maga close scenarios approach and techniques should have provided you enough training to prevail in any of these scenarios.

Release from a Nelson Hold

1. I am not sure if the nelson hold was created by Hollywood for the movie *Tarzan* or if it was actually in use by some form of wrestling sport. However, if your opponent attempts to use this hold on you, relax your arms down, and there is no way he will be successful in clamping his hands down on your neck. You can also use the surprise element: keep your arms down, spiral your body, and fall forward with your back on top of your opponent as he hits the ground.

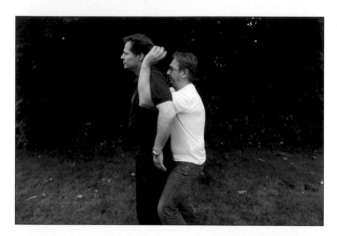 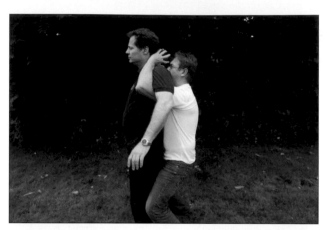

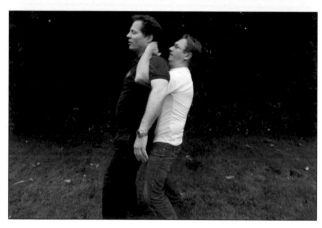 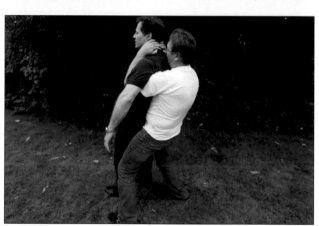

Release from Hand Grabs

Generally if someone grabs your hand, it is easy to use that to your advantage and fall toward and attack him with your free hand. Hand grabs generally do not put you in an immediate reaction, although they should.

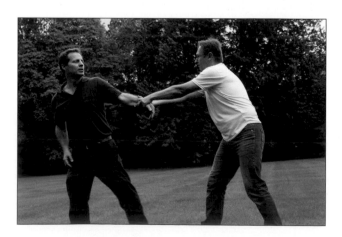 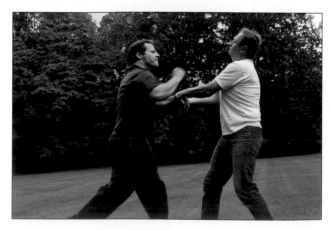

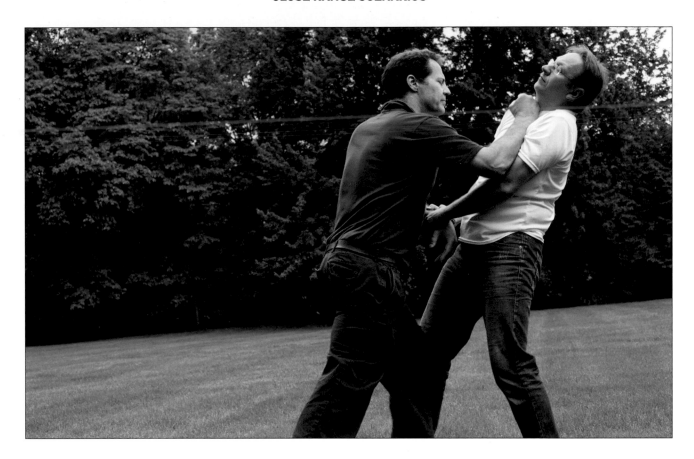

Release from a Mouth Cover and a Wrist Grab

Hand grabs can be used with a mouth grab to keep a person quiet. This could be done with chloroform as well. You may need to hold your breath while getting out of this hold quickly. Note that in this scenario, the attacker's wrist grab is ignored as we do not want to waste time wrestling out of it.

1. The attacker grabs the defender's hand and mouth, pulling him backwards.

2. The defender scoops the attacker's wrist, pulling it down while the defender twists his chin away from the attacker's palm.
3. The defender steps away from the direction of the pull to avoid ending up on the ground.
4. The defender stomps on top of the attacker's foot.
5. The defender releases the attacker's wrist and quickly punches him in the groin.
6. As the attacker bends, the defender hits him with a hammer punch or elbow on his head.

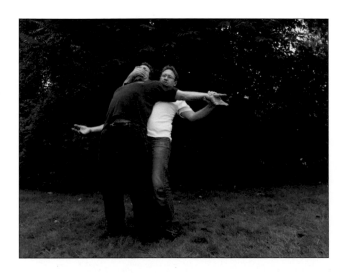

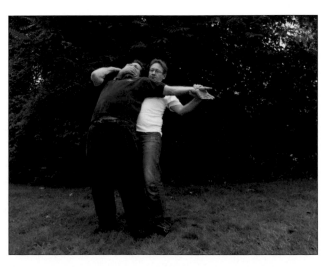

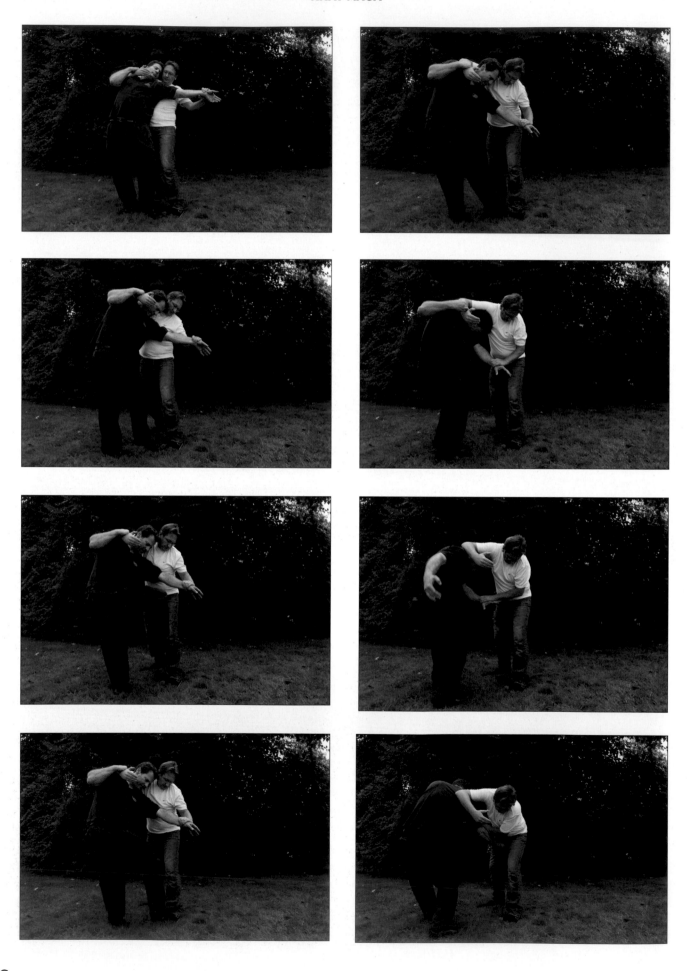

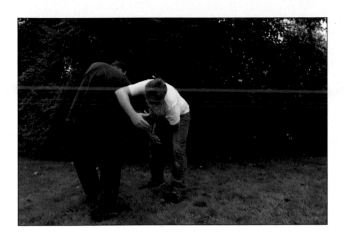
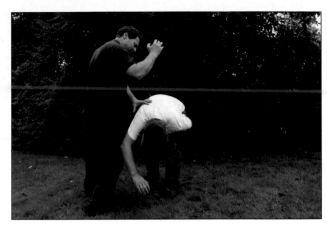

Release from Wrists Pinning Behind the Back with a Forward Lean

1. The attacker grabs both the defender's hands behind his back.

2. The defender pivots both hands forward and kicks the back.

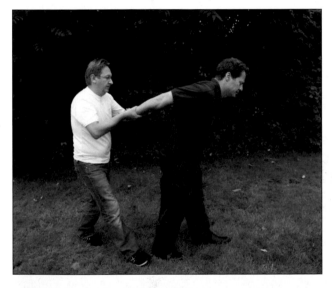
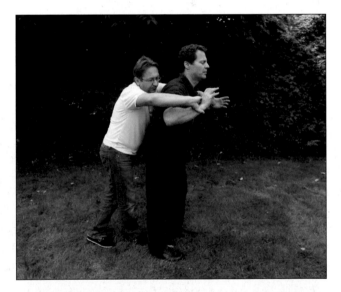

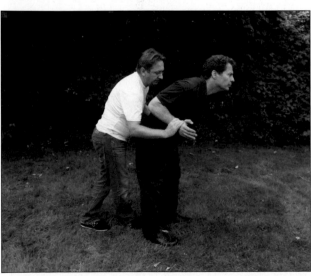
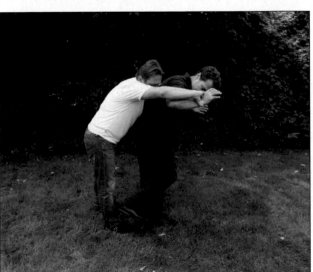

Release from Wrists Pinned Behind the Back with Side Pivot

1. The attacker grabs both the defender's hands behind his back (demonstrated in the previous technique).
2. The defender turns his right palm to face the side of his body as he pivots his left hand while simultaneously attaching its forearm to his back, aligning it to his belt. The defender pivots his body to the right. This can be done with a small jump turn to the side.

3. The defender brings his right elbow over his head as he turns his torso to the left, letting his left wrist get out of the grip.
4. The defender grabs the attacker's wrist with his left hand, sliding his right hand to pressure the attacker's elbow or shoulder, bringing him down to the ground in the style of a carousel.

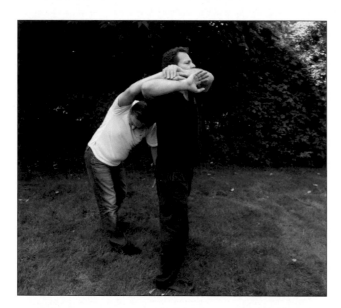

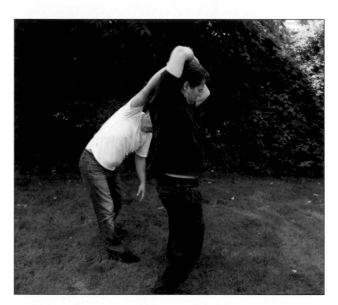

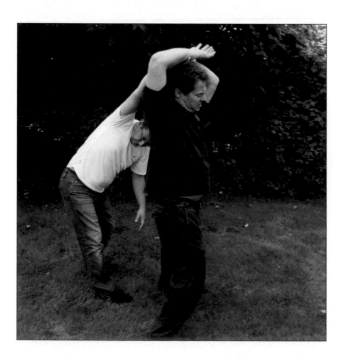

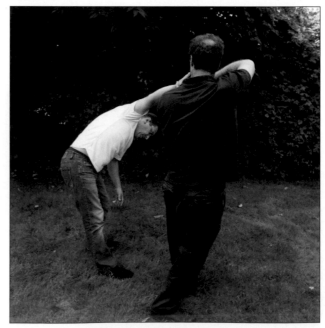

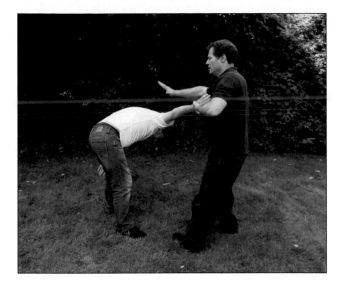 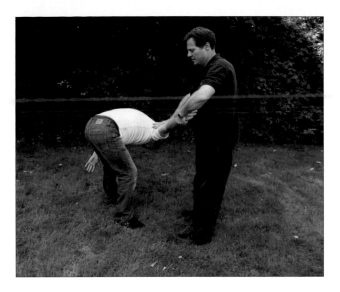

Note: Aikido practitioners build their training by gripping at their opponent's wrists. Trained in wrist manipulation, they can quickly shift the direction of the force by turning your wrist in various directions. This can stun you so you cannot even try to punch back.

The key is to pull your arm quickly before the grip takes hold, punching your opponent quickly as he attempts to grip you. At times going with the force of pull can help too as you can try to find a window of opportunity to escape, which buys you time so you can strike him.

Cavalier

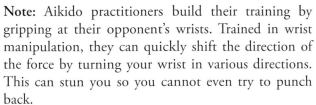

The word cavalier comes from the French word for gentleman. This move comes from the manner of a gentleman who escorts a woman by giving her his arm to lean on. You grab the opponent in the same hold, and then manipulate his wrist to control his body. Your control comes from you throwing him to the ground, or by inflicting him with enough pain to restrict his movement.

1. The defender grabs attacker's arm in a cavalier.
2. The defender rolls his wrist and bends the attacker's arm like a motorcycle throttle.
3. The defender uses his right hand to twist attacker's fist to the left.
4. The defender throws the attacker on the ground.

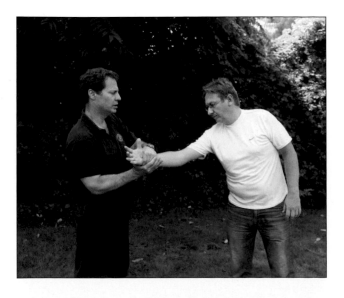 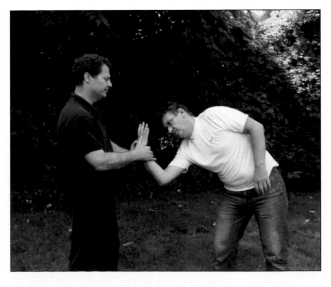

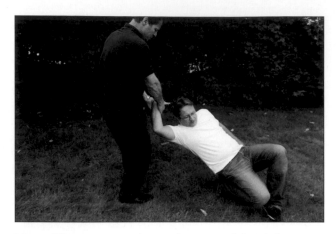
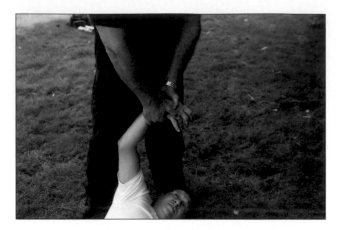

Note: This move can be used in any of the defense moves if we want to throw the attacker to the ground. But as a Krav Maga trainee, why would you want to waste time? The best method to execute a cavalier move from a tactical point of view is to keep your elbows locked, switch your stance by bringing your forward leg back, and pull the opponent, while holding his fist at your belt level. This will put his balance on one leg and force him to a twist, where he will not be able to reach your pressure point with his free hand or leg. In addition, you will use your whole body weight to counter any resistance attempt.

Arm-Wrestling Tricks

Changing directions of resistance to the weakest point:

1. Your training partner assumes an arm-wrestling position.
2. The defender twists his wrist to apply force at a new angle to obtain an advantage. The defender should continue to initiate change, causing the attacker to follow behind until the defender wins. Otherwise, the defender ends up teaching the attacker how to win. Note that you can also loosen your resistance up. After he almost brings you down, you can put your resistance back on when he expects it the least. You will be surprised to see his arm coming down to your direction.

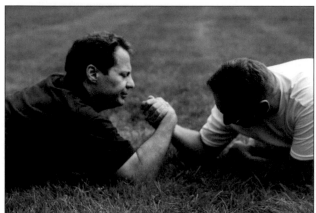
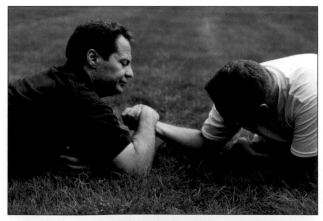
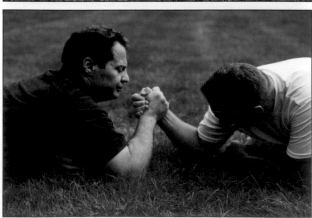
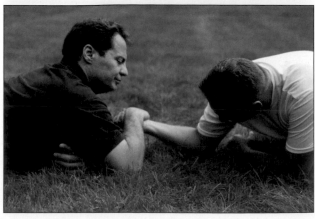

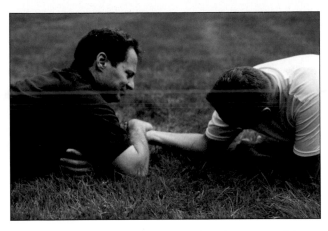 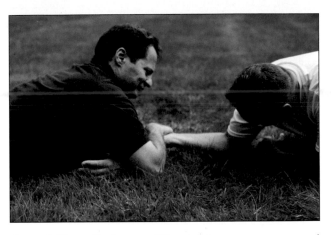

Note: Remember that you can take advantage of this principle, and if you find yourself in motion, you can control your opponent's body for a few seconds. However, you should try not to rely on it since it is not an efficient approach and not the most efficient technique.

Redirecting the Attacker's Force

1. The attacker is pushing the defender forward.
2. The defender applies just enough pressure under the attacker's elbows, not letting him realize what the defender is doing.
3. When another attacker assists, he ends up being lifted in the air. This trick was used over the years by many martial arts schools, claiming supernatural levels of energy. While scientists study the various forces of energy, a simple leverage trick should not be presented as supernatural energy.

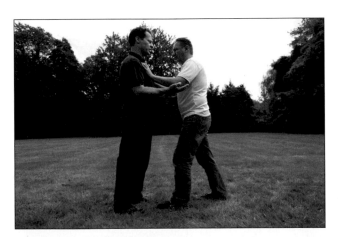 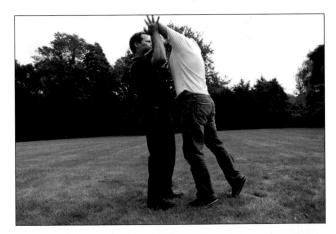

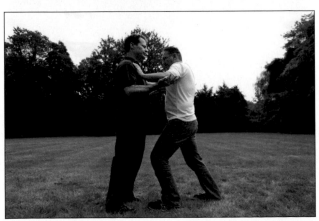 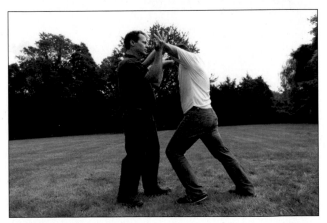

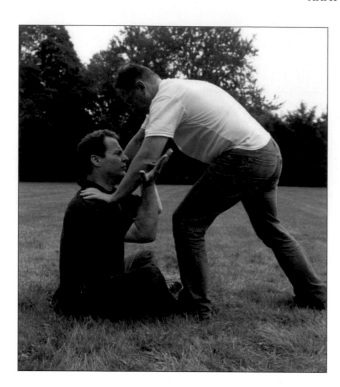
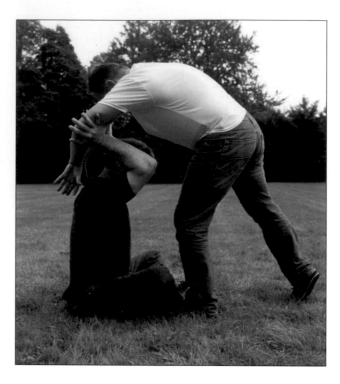

Taking an Opponent Out of Balance to Stop Knee Kicks

In grappling scenarios, if your opponent attempts to knee you, pull up his body to force his knee down.

1. The training partners hold each other's necks.
2. The attacker is trying to knee kick the defender with his left knee.

3. The defender is pulling the attacker's shoulder to his left.
4. Repeat attempts and foil attempts. Switch roles and use this as a fighting game.

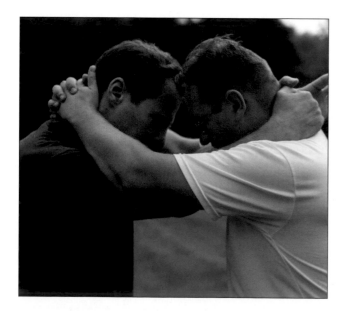
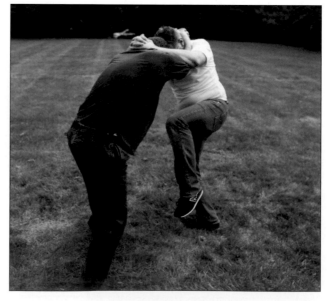

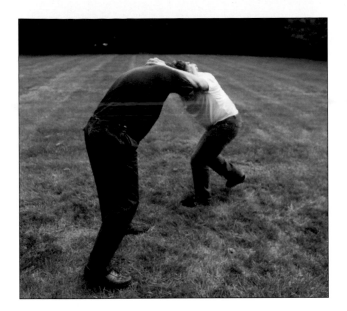 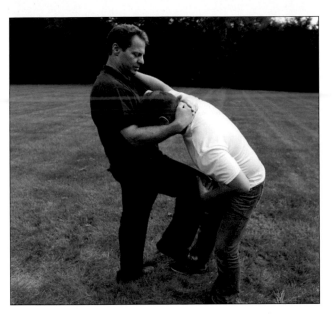

Note: When in a grappling scenario, you could find yourself off-balance in trying to push and pull. Instead, you could immediately reach for a pressure point in a continuous move, or try to divert this direction and stay balanced on your feet and then reach for a pressure point. You definitely cannot afford to hesitate and end up with your arm or leg twisted behind your back. It could be too late then. Obviously, in Krav Maga there is no point learning techniques on how to turn an opponent around to face you. You would rather hit him on the back of his head.

GROUND FIGHTING

In the previous chapter, we learned how to prevent ground fighting. However, we may find ourselves inadvertently on the ground, so we better learn to overcome any obstacle and get up as soon as possible. We really cannot afford to take the risk of being on the ground and more vulnerable to other hostile opponents.

In ground fighting, Krav Maga prescribes not more than six techniques. These are used to teach principles of action according to the opponents' position and center of gravity. In fighting sports, for example, striking the testicles, neck, or head is off limits, and fighters must keep repositioning their weight to have a hold on their opponent. While this principle is not neglected in Krav Maga, it is not often used. Instead, students learn to throw a quick punch to the testicles, or to shove a finger into a nerve in the neck, in the eye, or on the bridge of the nose.

Breaking falls means getting to the ground softly.

Break Fall on Your Back

You are falling on your back from, let's say, the first flight of a building. In the first scenario, you probably use your hands to tap the floor; in the second, you do not really need to. You are pushed into falling backwards. You need to keep important information on your mind. First, you want to avoid sending your hand backward, since you can easily dislocate your shoulders doing this. Second, you do not want your head to hit the ground as it may cause a concussion or smash your skull. Third, you do not want to fall on your ass, breaking your coccyx bone. In Krav Maga, students learn to fall on concrete floors while avoiding damage to their bodies.

1. Lying on the ground, keep your hands at thirty degrees to the sides of the body. Lift your head and look at your belt. Apply pressure to the ground with your palms, leaving elbows locked and lifted off. Lift one leg off the ground, bringing your knee to your chest. In this position, your head and shoulders are not touching the ground. In addition, your coccyx bone is not touching the ground. The only contact you have with the ground at this point is the large muscles in your lower back. This is the position you will end up in when you finish softening your fall. Relax and put your head, shoulders and leg back on to the ground. Repeat this step about ten times. You are getting accustomed to instantly reaching the desired position. Keep one heel on the ground to prevent anyone from kicking your groin.

2. From a squatting position, cross your hands over your knees. Sit backwards, close to your heels, and lift one leg. Continue to the position described in step one. As you sit and roll your body backwards, keep your torso leaning forward. Release your hands only after completing the fall. Repeat this step about ten times.

3. From a standing position, step backwards on one foot, and squat on it close to the heel. Keep your hands crossed over your chest, lifting one leg as you come down. Continue to get through all prior steps until you come to a complete stop on the ground. All through your fall, you need to shift your weight forward as you roll your torso forward to soften your fall. Avoid reaching your hands backwards since you could dislocate your shoulders this way.

4. Your training partner is pushing you and making you lose your balance.

5. Step backwards, as you lower your center of gravity forward while falling.

6. Land close to your heel, keeping one knee up to avoid the coccyx contacting the ground.

7. Keep your head forward by looking at your belt.

8. Your elbows should be locked if your hands are touching the ground, and your shoulders lifted up.

9. Kick up from the floor.

Keep in mind that the only contact with the ground should be your heel, and your wide lower back without the coccyx bone. You are now in a perfect position to kick your opponent upwards, if needed.

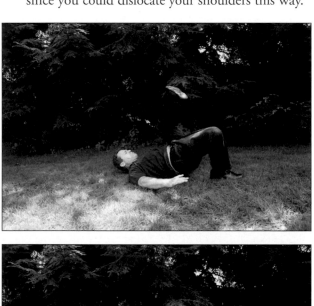

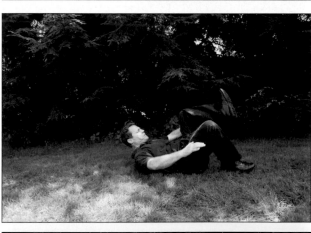

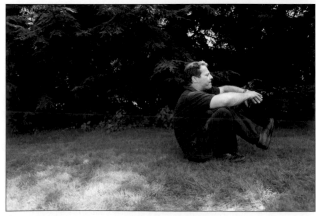

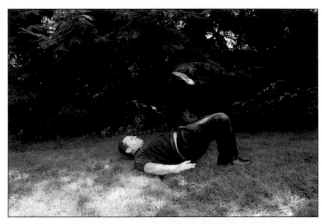

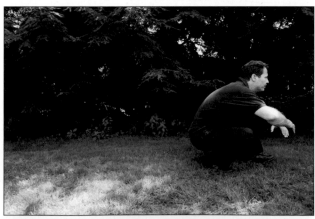

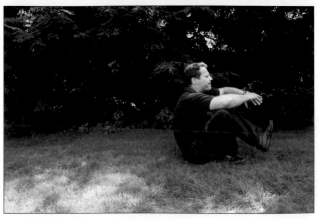

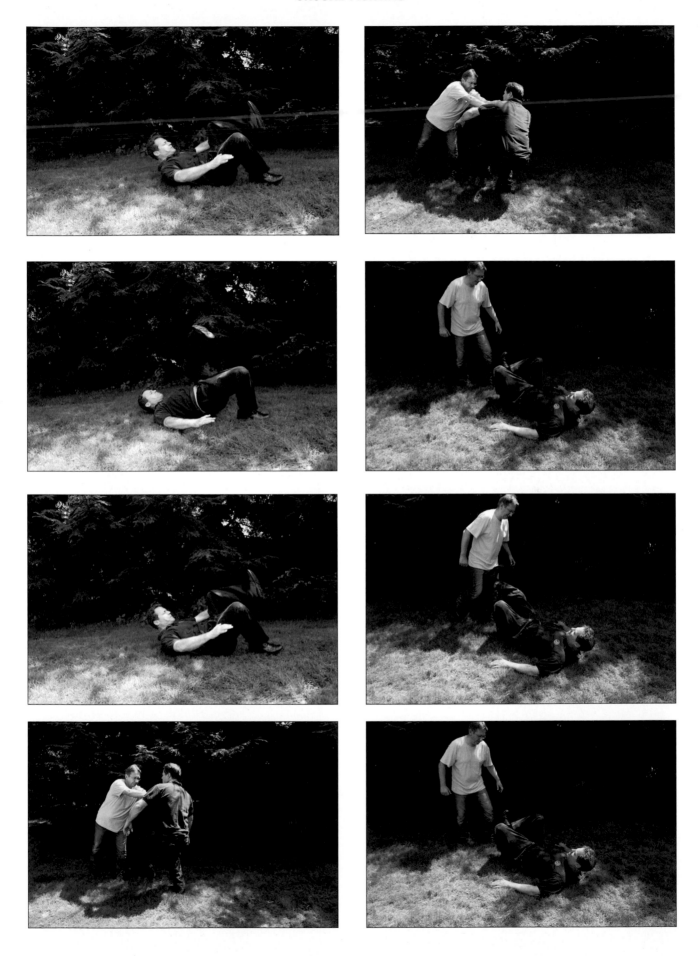

Training notes: First, start by lying on the ground and lifting your head and knee while applying pressure with your palms, elbows locked. Second, fall back from the sitting position, getting down to the final position. Third, squat and fall backwards from this position. Fourth, stand up straight, step back, sit on your heel as you are squatting, lift one knee up and fall back to the ending position. Finally, ask a training partner to push you so you can do this instinctively. Rehearse every step a few times until you feel comfortable moving to the next step. Have your training partner move forward above you in an attempt to kick your groin. You should have one leg on the ground and in front of your groin. As he moves toward you, kick him with your free leg. He should have a punching mitt in his hand for practice. You can also do this on a concrete floor.

Side Scissor Kick While Lying on the Side

If your opponent is approaching you from the side, your best possible move would be the scissors kick:

1. The opponent approaches from the side as you are on the ground.

2. Turn on your side and wait until he is close enough, and kick with your top foot while the bottom foot pulls his leg in the opposite direction.

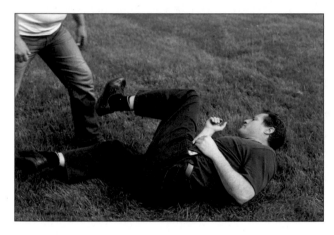

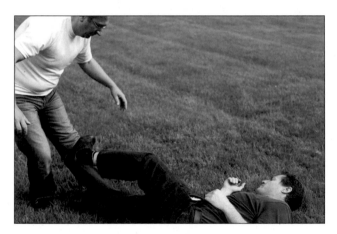

Note: Do not attempt to wrestle with your opponent's leg or bend it to a convenient angle so he would fall. Kick it like you are using your feet as scissors. The impact of the kick will make him fall at any angle and create a local trauma. For practice, tap it lightly and notice the sharp loss of your opponent's balance.

Break the Fall onto the Side

1. Cross your leg closer to the opponent behind the other, and squat on its heel, crossing your arms in front of your body and lifting the opposite leg.

2. Fall onto your side.
3. Kick from this position with your lower leg.

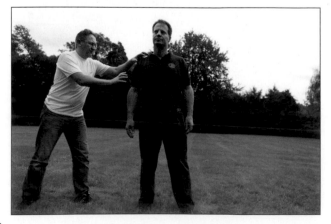

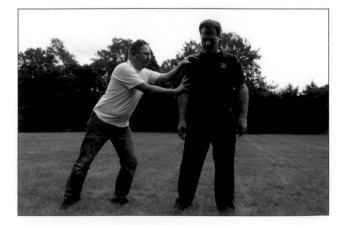

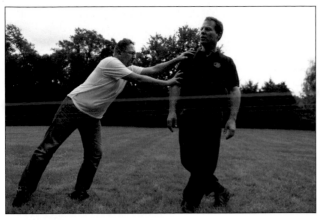

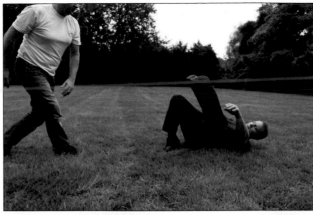

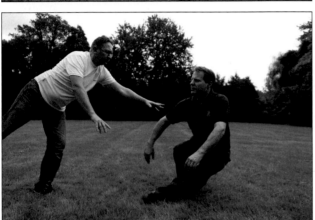

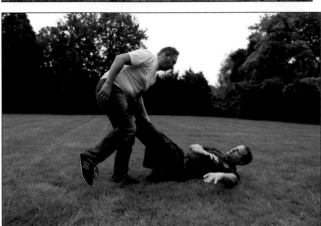

Breaking Your Fall Forward

Breaking your fall forward is done with your arms as shock absorbers, using a reversed pushup motion.

Keep your head turned to the side to prevent your face from getting smashed on the ground with a sharp fall.

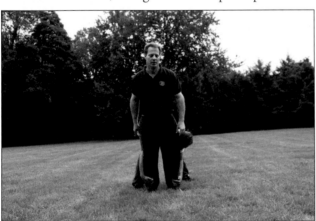

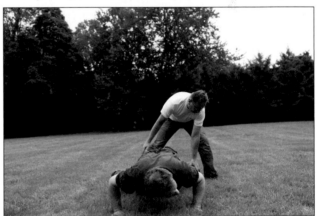

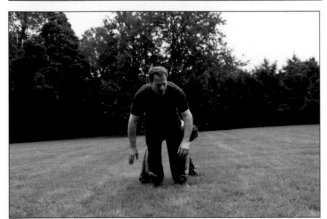

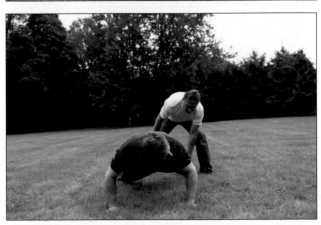

Forward Rollover (learning how to get up first)

Forward rollover can be used to break your fall from a horse, bicycle, motorcycle, and other such scenarios. In Krav Maga, it is used in attack scenarios and other various tactical situations. When encountering an attacker who is swinging a metal chain, or when part of a group held at gunpoint, a rollover would close the large gap between defender and attacker in a minimum amount of time and with the maximum amount of safety.

Krav Maga teaches you how to get up first. As you sit, you lean to one side, creating a forty-five degree angle with one leg folded on the ground at the hip and knee joints. Your other leg is crossed over where its knee is above your other knee. You then pivot your body as you get up, facing the direction your back was turned to.

1. Start with crossed legs.
2. Shift your weight and get up on one knee.
3. Pivot your body to the left and get up with a slight spring backward. If you keep control of your angles you are in a comfortable Krav Maga stance.
4. To practice the above steps with the force of the rollover, lie backward and lift your legs over your head. Throw your legs forward and land the side of your hip where the bottom leg is curled to a ninety-degree angle on the floor, while the other leg stays straight on top, foot facing the ground, knees on top of each other. With this momentum, you should be pivoting to the side and getting up with no assistance from your hands.

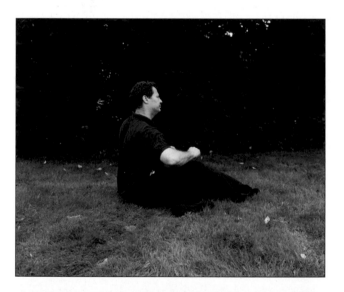

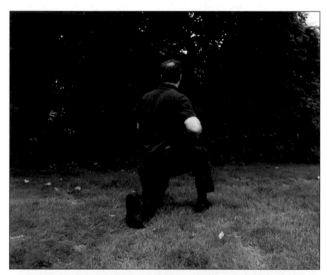

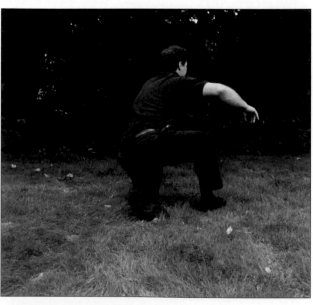

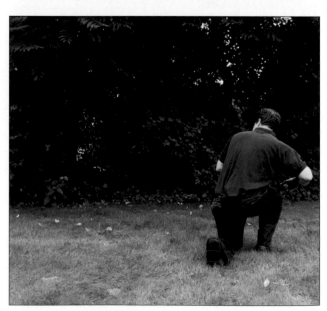

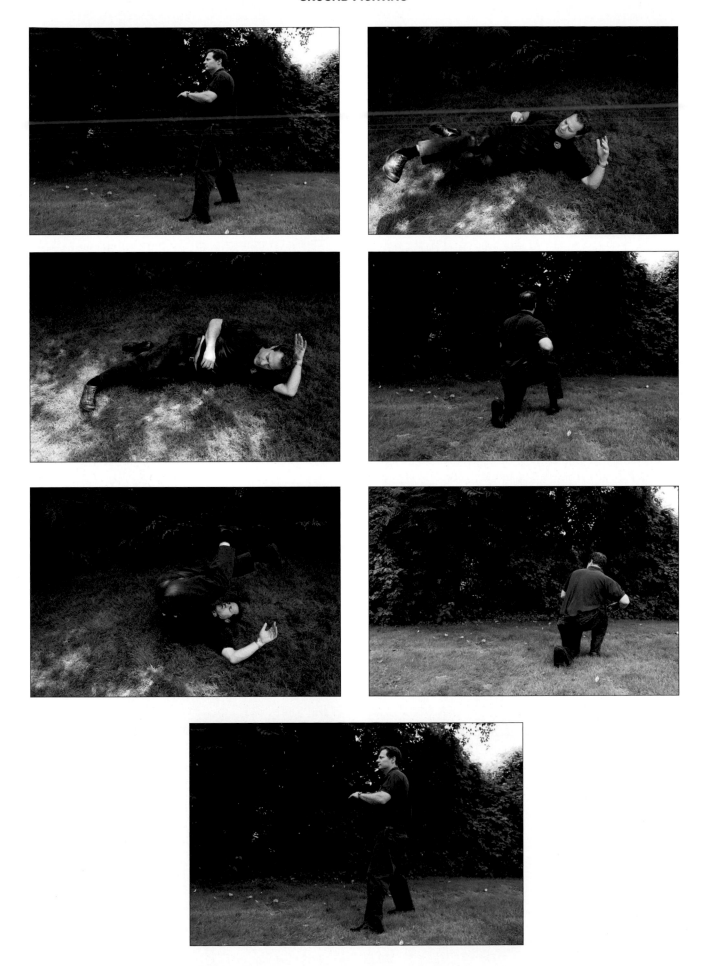

Forward Rollover (learning how to roll)

Your next step is to fall forward on your hands and then roll over. Your body should remember the getting up part by now.

1. Step forward and place your hands on the ground at shoulder level, where only the opposite hand points to that foot.
2. Shift your weight forward and slide your opposite arm toward your back foot, keeping the elbow locked. Imagine your arm is part of a wheel where the rest of it is part of your back and to the opposite end of your waist. If you are looking to your shoulder in the direction of your back leg, peeking at your potential opponent, and if your elbows are locked, your head will not touch the ground. You are rolling on your arched arm, one shoulder to the opposite side of the waist, and getting up the way you learned in the previous step. When comfortable, practice on a concrete floor.
3. As your legs roll over your head, keep pivoting your body. This causes you to land on the side of your leg as its knee is bent at ninety degrees. The ball of the foot close to the ground is being pointed, so it will help you spring yourself and get up quickly. Your other leg is positioned over your knee with the foot touching the ground.

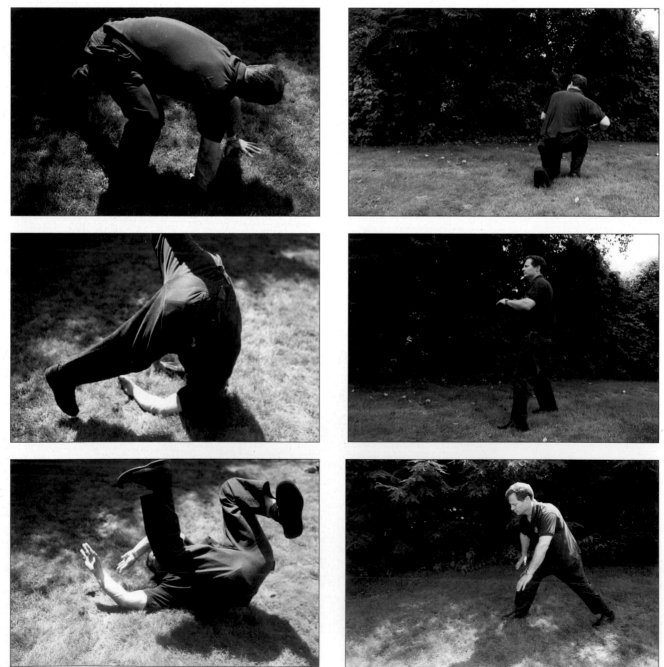

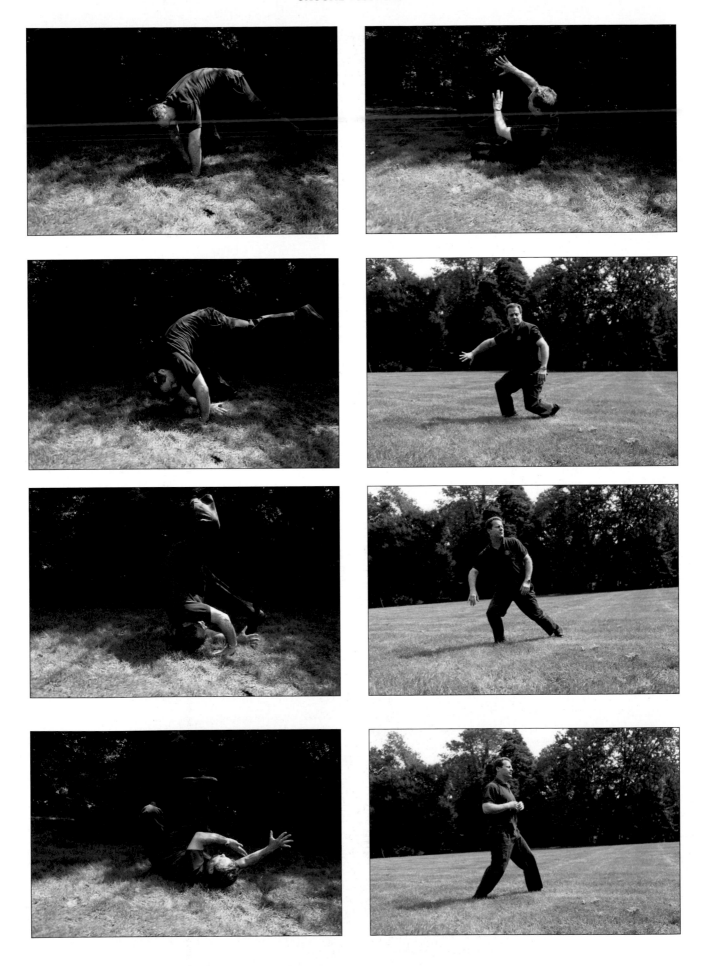

Note: This rollover can be finished with a few variations as you will see in this chapter and a few other chapters throughout the book.

Side Rollover

1. Place your hands on the floor with your left hand supporting your weight, your right hand sliding toward your back foot. Keep your elbows locked.

2. Rollover to the side.
3. Get up, standing on the side.

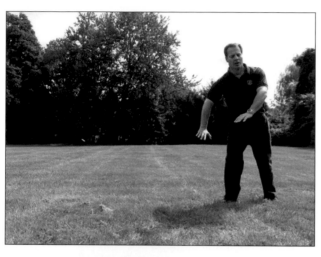

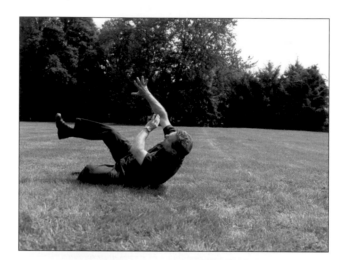

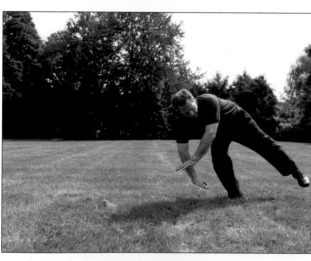

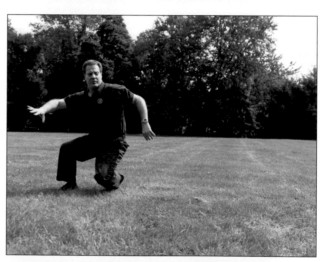

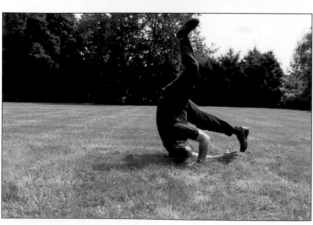

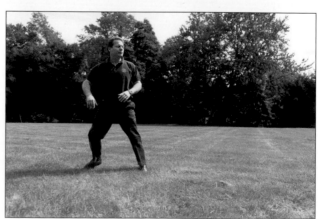

Tactical Use for Forward Rollover

If you sense danger behind you and it is too late to realize exactly what is going on, you can fall forward, roll over and get up in the reverse direction, ready to respond with a kick.

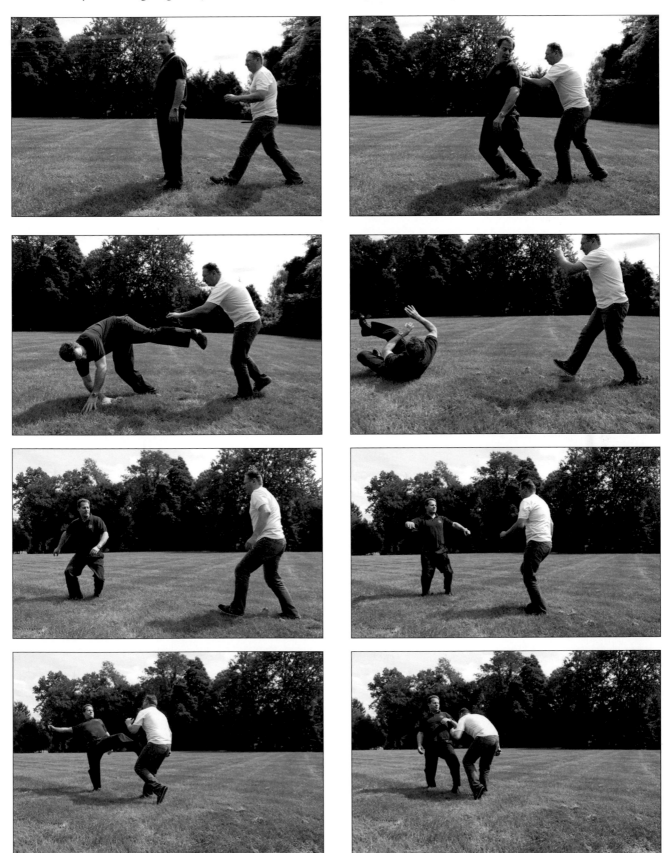

Backward Rollover

You can start by lying down on your back, rolling backwards on one shoulder using your hand to prevent your head from scraping the floor. This motion can help with quick movement in certain scenarios.

1. Sitting on the ground, roll backwards and stretch your legs straight over your head. Place your hands behind your shoulders on the ground and roll on one shoulder, twisting your head away from the ground.

2. Stand up on your feet.

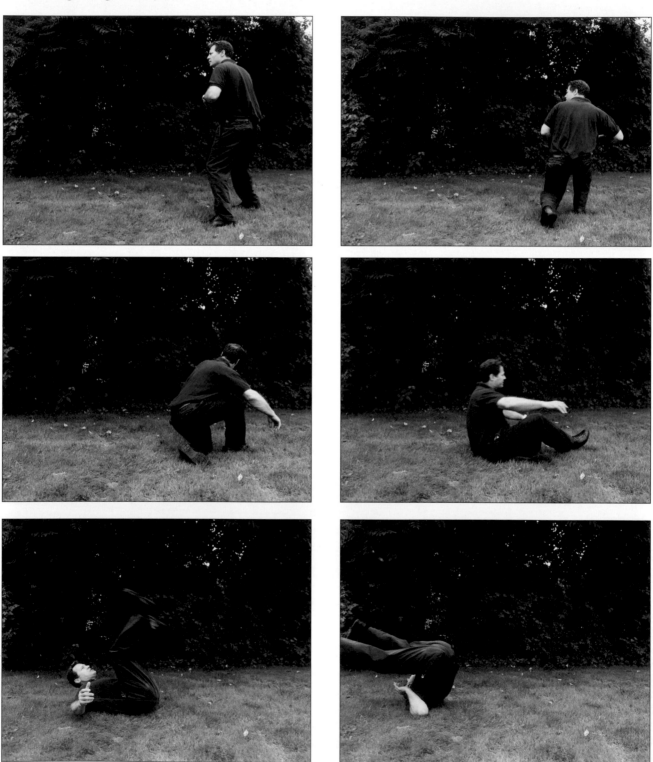

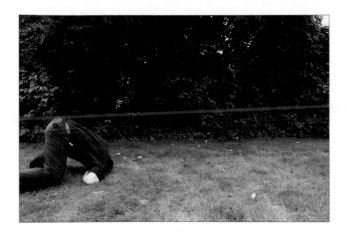
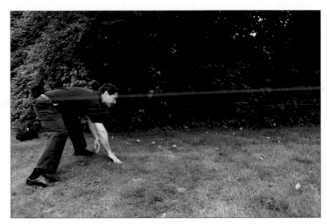

Ground Techniques

In jujitsu and wrestling, trained opponents manipulate each other's joints to inflict pain, hoping they'll surrender. Krav Maga does not intend to cover every aspect of joint manipulation, but instead teaches principles and shows students ways out of these situations. Many sports attacks are at a disadvantage in front of a Krav Maga expert—true experts do not sweat the small stuff and do not hesitate in putting their opponents out of commission.

In Greco-Roman wrestling, wrestlers can take a few seconds to try to manipulate their opponent's wrist or ankle as they do not fear an attack to the groin. If the result would be that swift, wrestlers would not have the time to surrender, and their careers would have been cut short. The Krav Maga expert attempts to knock the attacker unconscious before he has a chance to scream or surrender.

Defense when attacker is sitting on top of defender, striking defender's face and punching him

1. The attacker is sitting on top attempting to strike the defender.
2. The defender is blocking the attacker, simultaneously executing a bridge move, throwing the attacker on to his face while the defender parallels his forearm to his face to block him. He uses his other arm to punch the attacker in the groin. The punch should come immediately after the bridge, before the opponent has the opportunity to fall back down.
3. The defender keeps striking the attacker's groin as he turns out and gets up ready to kick and walk away.

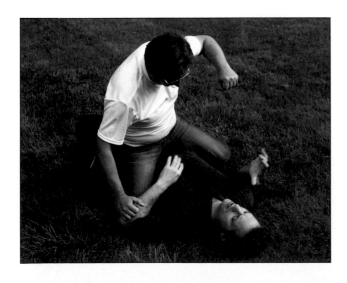
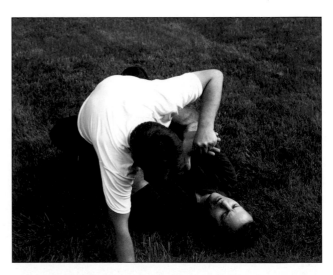

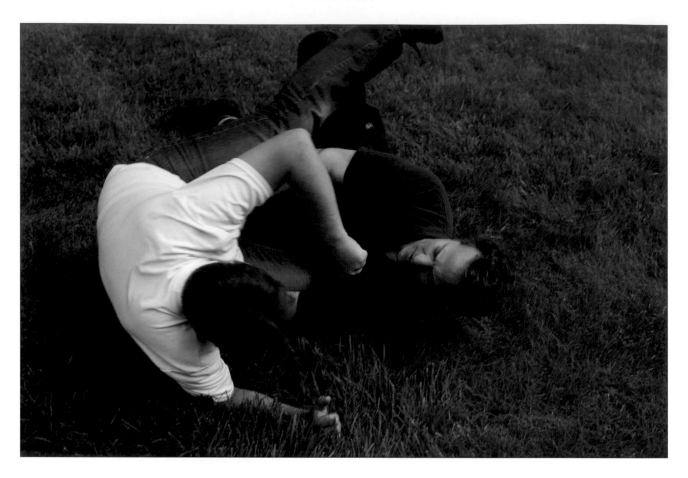

Note: In this technique, throwing the attacker out of balance diverts his first attempted strike while forcing him to use his hands for balance and prepare for his fall. Therefore, he cannot think about striking again. In addition, the defender delivers a series of blows to the attacker's groin, forcing him to roll over due to a combination of pain and force directed toward his center of gravity.

Defense against an attacker sitting on top of defender, choking him

1. The attacker sits on top of the defender and chokes him.
2. The defender releases himself from the opponent's chokehold by using a spoon grip with all five fingers on the same side of the opponent's wrist. At the same time, the defender creates a bridge by lifting his waist up, keeping heels close to the butt, throwing the opponent off his stomach. The defender extends his forearm parallel to his face to block the opponent's fall, punching the opponent's groin with his other hand.
3. The defender keeps striking the attacker's groin as he turns to the side, getting up ready to kick and walk away.

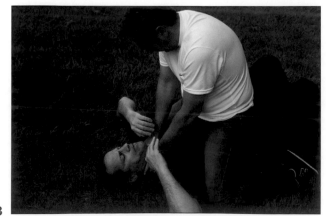

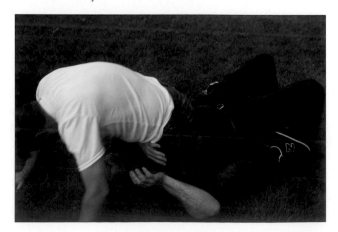

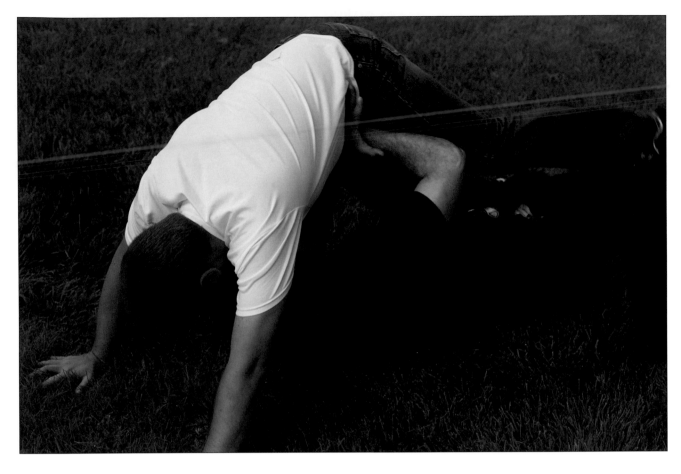

Note: Follow the steps in the previous drill for escape and counter attack!

Attacker is positioned to the side of the defender while choking or striking him

1. The attacker stands on his knees, next to defender, choking or striking him. The defender pushes off the attacker's thumbs away from his throat.
2. The defender uses his right knee to push the attacker away from his ribs, enabling him to smash the attacker's head to the ground with his left leg. The defender keeps holding the attacker's right arm to prevent him from escaping his fate.
3. Alas. The attacker meets his fate.

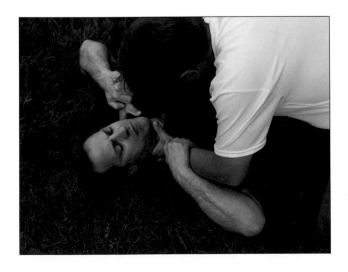

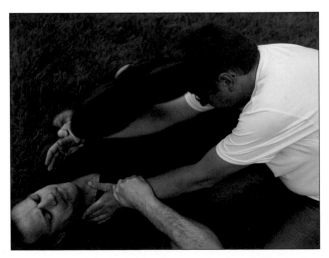

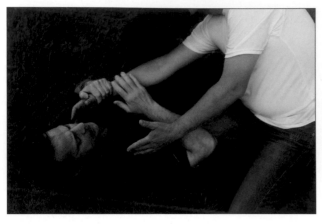
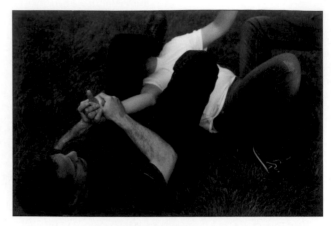

Note: If the attacker had his face close to the defender's, the defender would have used leverage on attacker's neck instead of using the above technique.

Release from hands pinned to the ground by rolling to the side

If the attacker pins your hands straight over your head, his weight will not be on your stomach, so making a bridge would not completely get him off your body.

1. The defender rolls as slightly as he can to one side to grab the attacker's wrist.
2. The defender rolls to the other side by pushing the attacker's elbow.
3. The defender is on top of the attacker's elbow.
4. The defender keeps crawling and rolling his body above the attacker's head to inflict greater pain on the attacker's arm.
5. The defender swings his legs as he leans on his arms, stepping with one leg on the attacker's forearm. This way he controls the attacker as he gets up and he now can kick the attacker in his head.

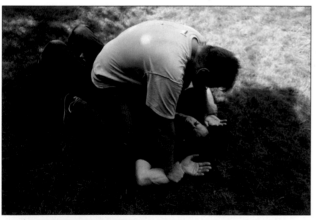
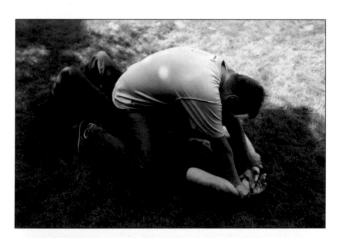

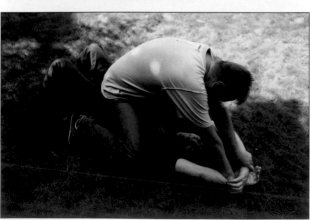
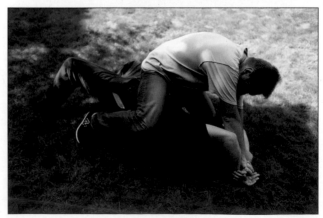

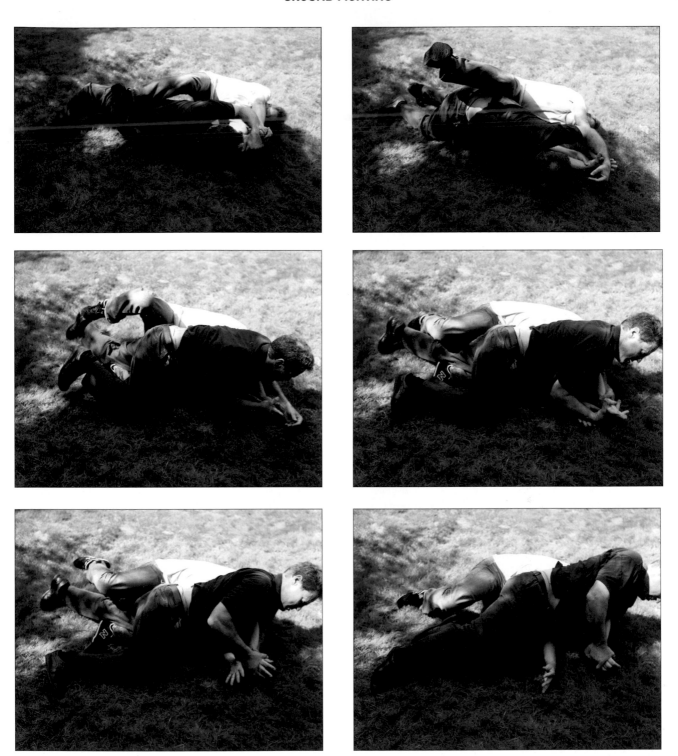

Release from hands pinned on the ground by bringing both hands to the belt

If your hands are pinned to the sides of your head, or you have managed to get into this position, the attacker's weight will be mostly distributed on your stomach.

1. The attacker pins the defender's wrists near the sides of his head.

2. The defender performs a bridge simultaneously bringing his hands down to his waist and turning his head to the side.
3. The defender counterattacks by striking the attacker's face or groin. The defender continues with escape and counterattack as required.

141

Defense against the attacker sitting on top with his torso leaning forward and choking

1. The attacker is sitting on top of the defender with his head close to the defender's head.

2. The defender rolls the attacker's head and body to the side by using both hands.

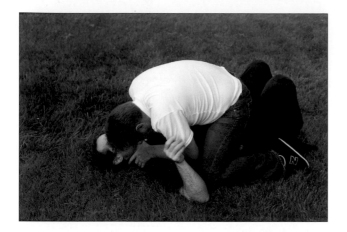

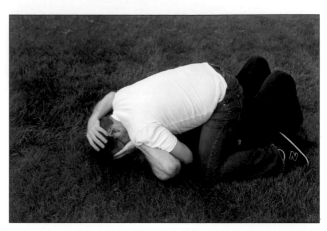

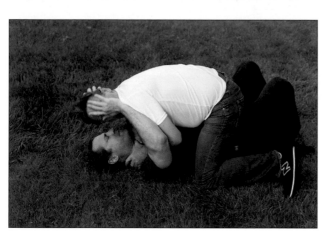

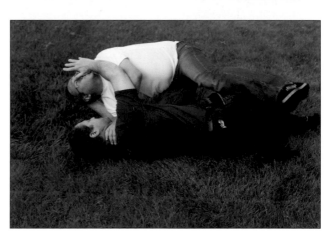

Release from a judo head lock

1. The attacker is holding the defender in a judo head lock.

2. The defender either pulls the attacker's hair, pushes in a nerve in their neck, or presses in the bridge of the attacker's nose.

3. The defender finishes with a throat pluck with his right hand.

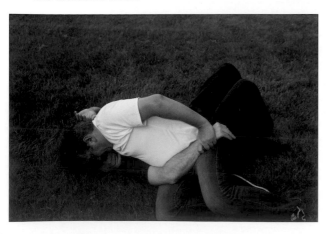

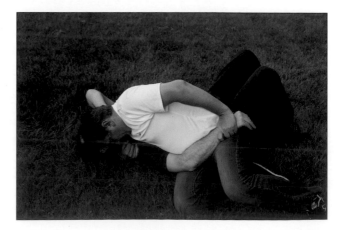

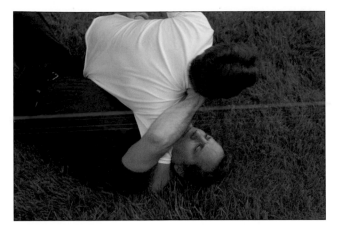
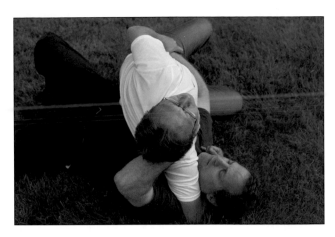

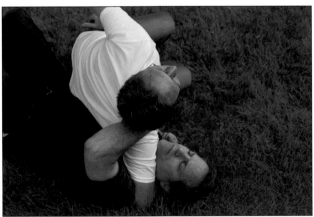
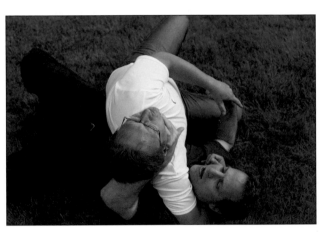

Note: Think about how you got into this position and how you could have prevented this by responding more quickly.

Release from a head-hold while sitting

The opponent can generate a great amount of force by pulling his hands toward himself, but generates much lesser force keeping his elbow down.

1. The attacker holds the defender in a head lock while sitting on the ground. The defender cuffs his hands on the attacker's wrists pulling down, lean-ing his head backwards to help him breathe easier. The defender twists his chin toward the attacker's hands to let the head slip out easier.

2. The defender uses one hand to lift the attacker's elbow up and get out.

3. The defender counterattacks.

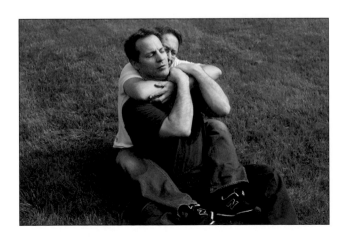
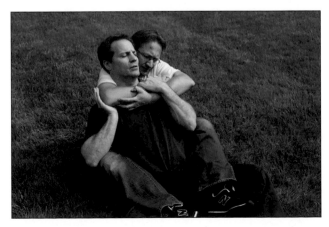

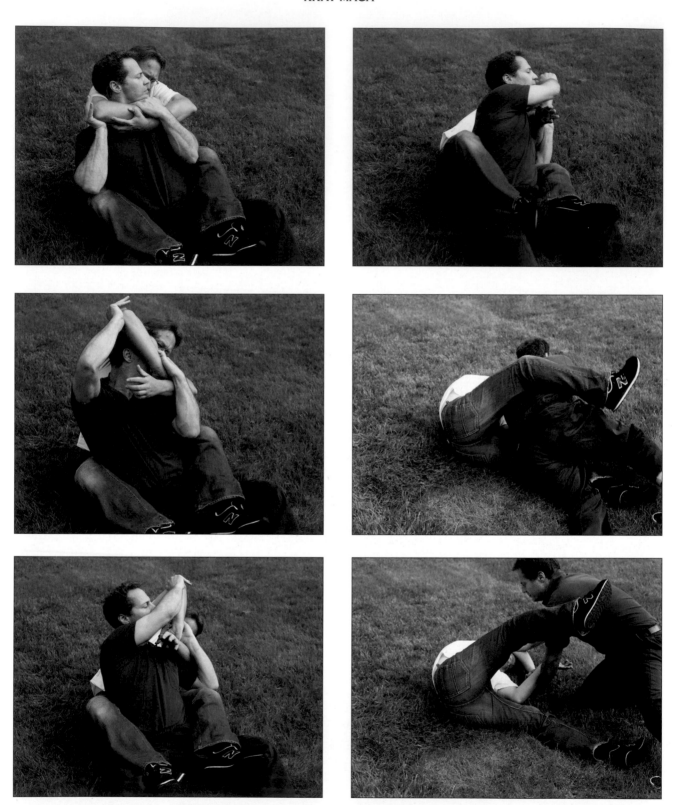

Release from rear-choke while sitting

When sitting, you are more limited than you are when standing, and it is hard to get a good pressure point on your attacker. Therefore, use his wrist to pull his body to a more convenient position. By throwing him to the ground, you would buy time to get up and kick him. Break his finger first if you need to, or go ahead and immediately grab a pressure point in his head.

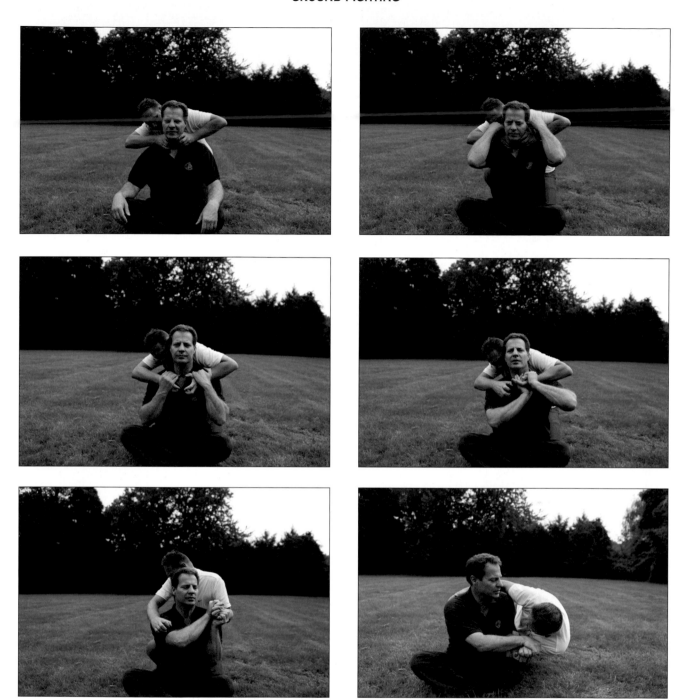

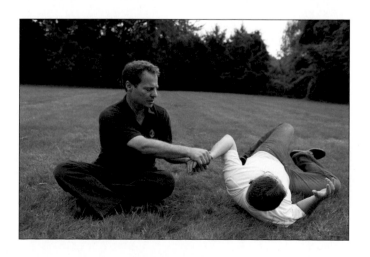

Summary

When fighting on the ground, one should consider striking the face area or the groin—whichever comes first. If the opponent attempts to grab your limbs with both hands, do not let him. You should immediately draw your limb back out of his hands and hit him. This will inflict pain and buy you time to inflict more severe damage to his body. If you hesitate, you are essentially letting him tie you down or virtually lock you behind bars. Hesitation could subject you to his mercy.

At this point, with the few techniques taught, you are ready for ground fighting drills. Fighting drills should be utilized where training partners try to hold each other in various other martial art techniques, while the aggressor attempts to control or strike as the defender attempts to escape and counterattack. The principles learned above can now be applied in dynamic motion.

In my years as the head instructor at the IDF, I have found this training method sufficient and have had the opportunity to see newly trained students overcome sports wrestlers and grappling martial arts fighters.

7

CLUB AND CHAIN

Attacking with a Club

In Krav Maga, club striking is taught as a rather quick and unpredictable move, as opposed to in other martial arts such as aikido where the attack is continuous. Students are taught to use a swing motion with a medium-sized stick, and with each strike they retract to the initial position to prepare for another attack. This makes it hard to defend and a gives a good challenge to your training partners. In reality, it is possible you would be attacked with a heavy pipe or a chair, requiring the use of the whole body to lift and strike, making it cumbersome to quickly retract and attack again. However, this only makes the attack more predictable and easier to defend. When using a stick or a club, use the tip of the object for contact, making the object less fragile and at the same time using its full momentum.

The following attacks are designed to get students familiar with the many possibilities of weapon use. The quicker and more effective method should be considered at all times. You could throw an object at the opponent, distracting him and buying yourself more time. You must assess each situation and see how to use the time you have. Think about the advantages and disadvantages of each decision.

If the club is short, hold it with one hand. Use two hands if it is longer.

Attack Techniques with a Club

1. Holding a club with the front hand in attack mode.
2. Front club swing.
3. Right side club swing.
4. Left side club swing.
5. Side stab with the butt of the club.
6. Straight stab with a long object (two-hand hold).
7. Uppercut strike to the groin.

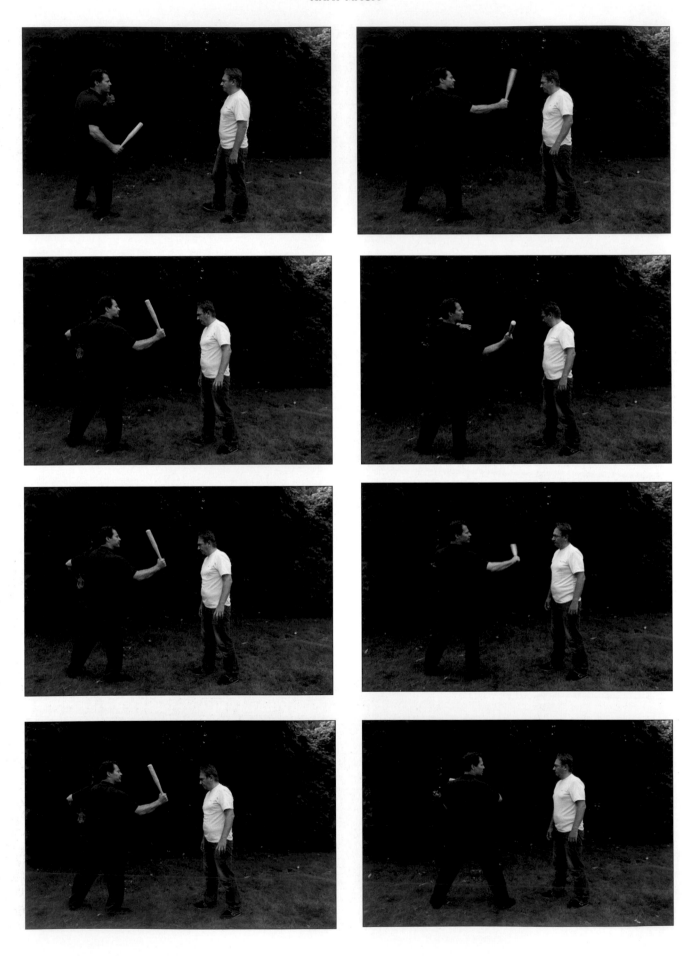

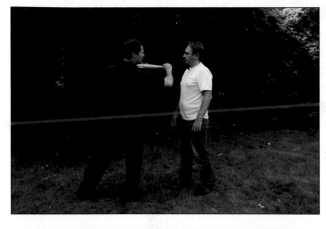

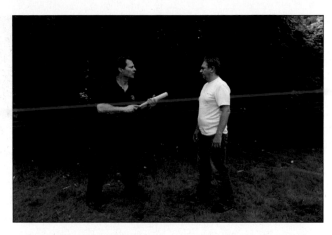

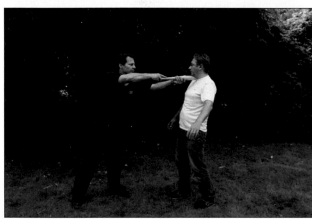

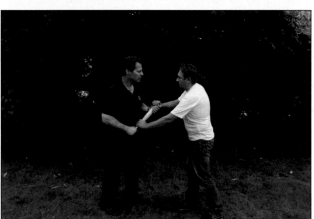

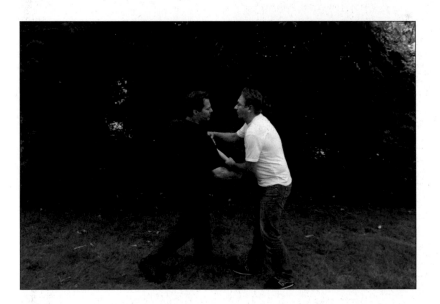

Training advice: After each one of the striking techniques is demonstrated, training partners should pair up and attack each other from each angle, moving back and forth and around each other. Punching pads should be used. This method keeps up the feel of continuous attack, providing the instructor and the training partner an opportunity to correct the student's attacks. Students often need to be reminded time and again to strike only with the tip of the club, and that they need to retract immediately afterward to maintain maximum speed during contact with the target.

Make sure the pad is placed close to the training partner's body and not directly in front of him. This helps train for a more realistic range. You may need to move backward to keep using the tip of the club as a contact point with the opponent's body if the attacker is advancing toward you. You will have the advantage of him being at a far enough distance from you that he cannot attack you with his arms or legs, or with a shorter weapon.

Defense against a Club Using Another Club or a Handy Object

1. The attacker strikes on top of the defender's head and the defender blocks with a club lifted diagonally up. The tip of the club is pointed downward, facilitating a slide out of the defender's reach. Sliding protects the defender's stick from breaking, and also helps with a faster counterattack.
2. The defender swings his club for a counterattack.
3. The attacker swings his club to the left of the defender's face while the defender is holding a club with his right hand.
4. The defender blocks the attack by striking diagonally down, close to the opponent's wrist.
5. The defender counterattacks.
6. The attacker swings his club to the right side of the defender's head. The defender is holding his club in his right hand.
7. The defender extends his hand to the right, blocking the attacker's club.
8. The defender counterattacks with the club.
9. The attacker swings his club over his head.
10. The defender blocks it with two hands while holding the club.
11. The defender counterattacks, using the handle of his club.
12. The attacker stabs the defender in the throat or face with the tip of his club.
13. The defender blocks it with two hands while holding the club, diverting the attacker's club with the tip of his own.
14. The defender continues to execute a counterattack, stabbing the opponent's club with the tip of the club.

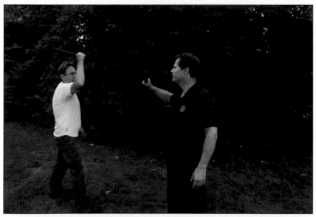

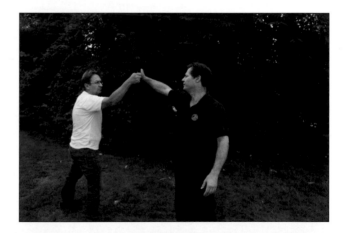

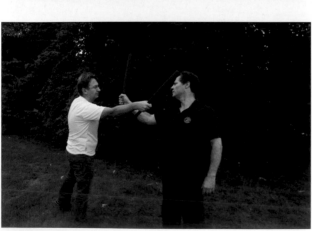

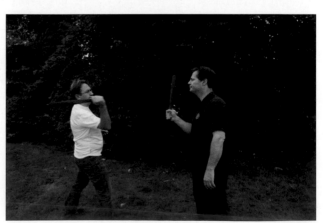

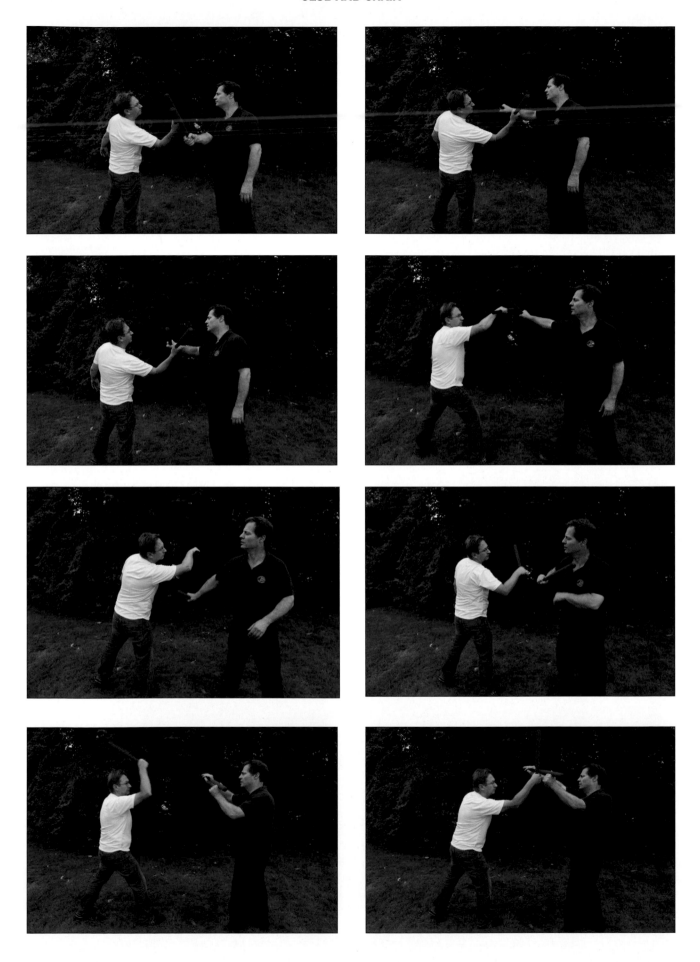

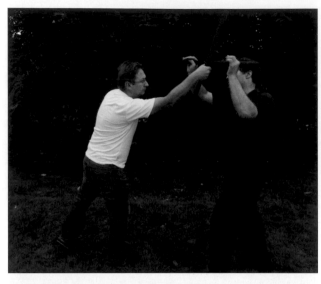
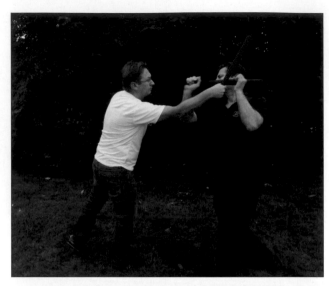
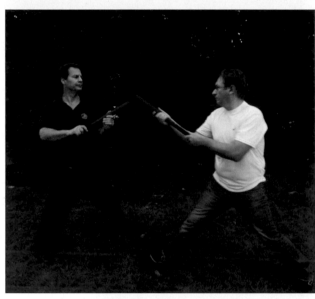
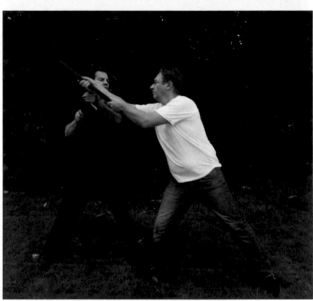
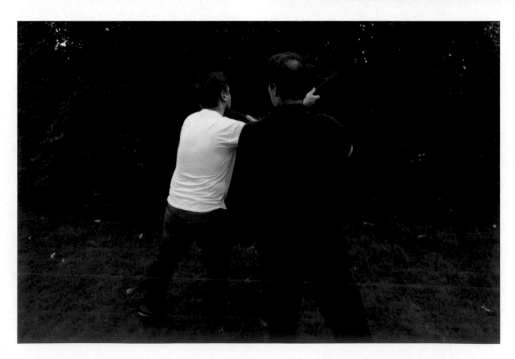

Attacking an Armed Opponent with a Club

Instead of waiting for your attacker to make the first move, use your club to strike him in the face or to block a potential strike while you are kicking him in the groin.

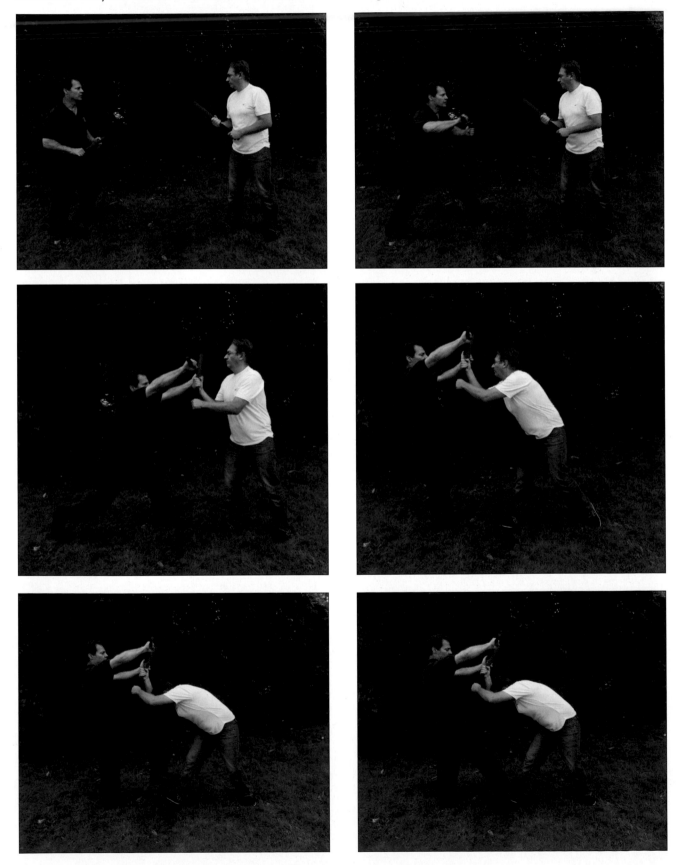

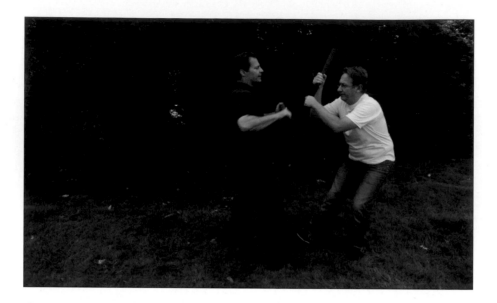

Note: If the attacker is trying to hit your legs with a long pipe, you can use a defensive kick to stop it with the bottom of your sole.

Defense against a Club with Bare Hands (head shot)

1. The attacker attempts to swing his club on top of the defender's head. The defender jumps forward, closing the gap before the attacker reaches his striking distance. The defender uses the outside of his forearm, letting it slide onto the attacker's wrist. If missed, the club would slide to the defender's forearm. The angle of contact will create more of a slide than a direct impact.

2. The defender lets the club slide down to the side of his body, and uses the opponent's momentum to strike him and grab the club.
3. The attacker falls to the ground as a result of the counterattack.
4. The defender follows with a knee kick or a stomp according to the situation.
5. The defender extracts the club from the attacker's hands.

Note: The defense is shown from two directions.

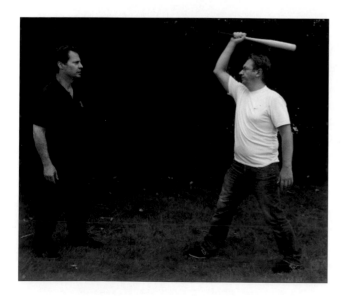

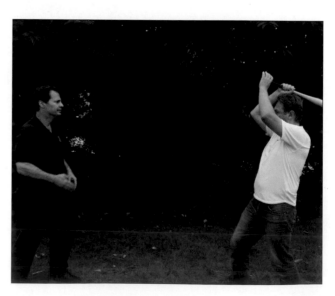

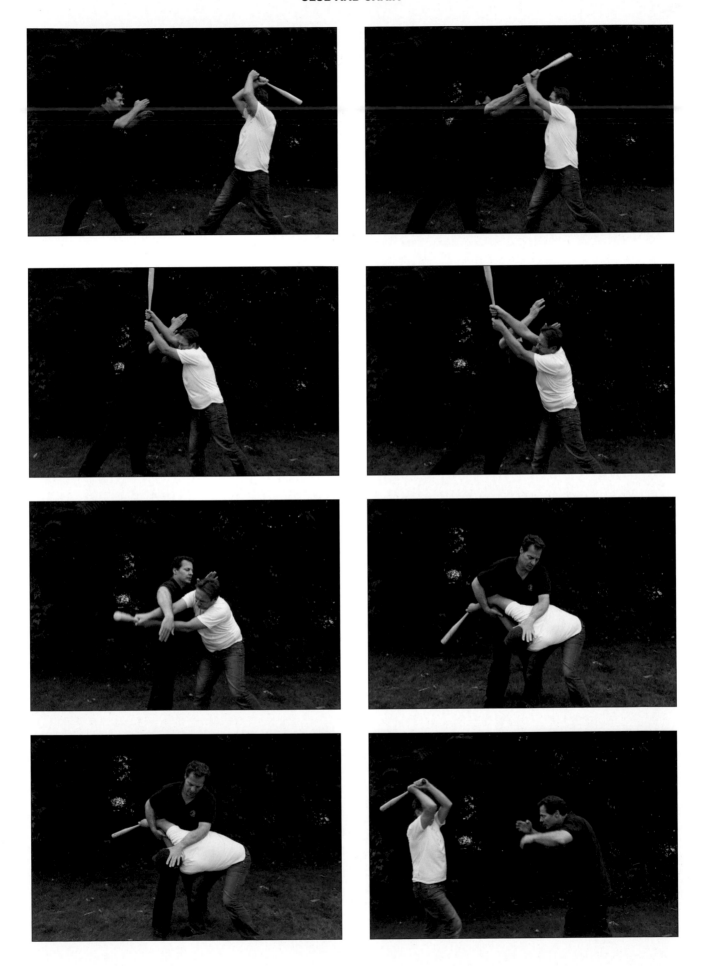

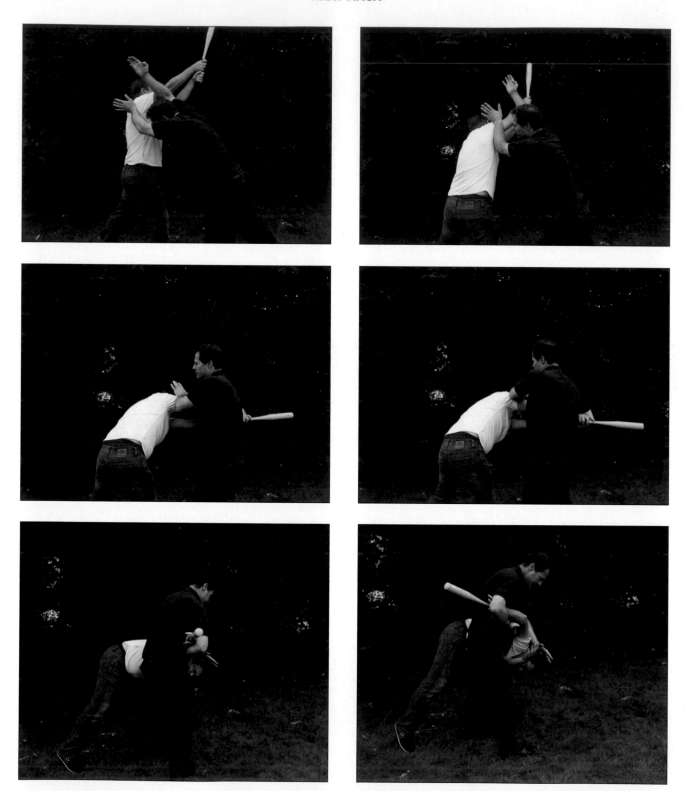

Defense against a Club with Bare Hands (side body shot)

1. The attacker swings his club forward with a horizontal shot to the defender's body.
2. The defender lunges forward, attempting to butt into his opponent's shoulder, while using his front arm to block the opponent's wrist or club keeping as close as possible to him.
3. The defender follows by locking his opponent's arms, executing a roundhouse elbow strike to his opponent's face.

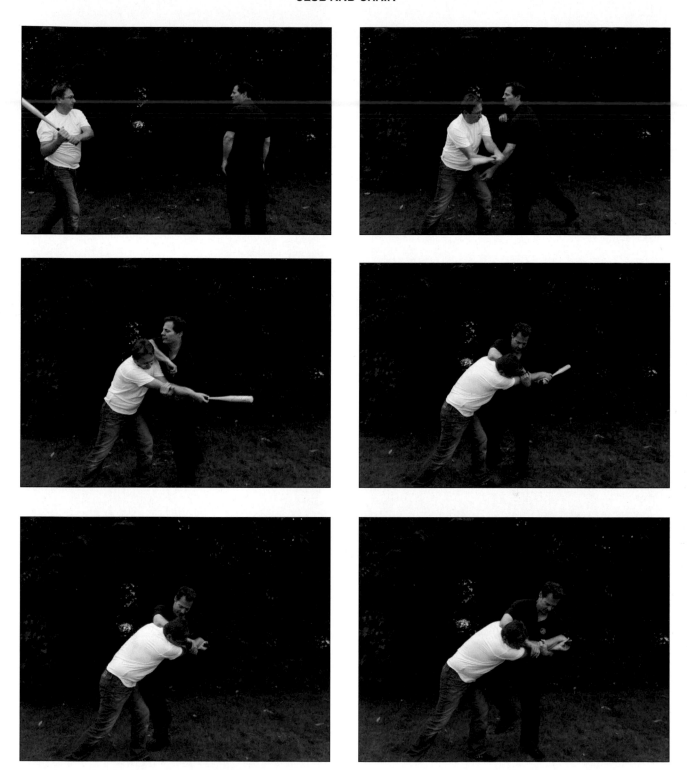

Preemptive Defense against an Attacker Armed with a Club

1. Rather than waiting for the attacker to choose which direction he will swing his club, the defender lunges forward and deflects any possible move from the attacker by blocking his wrist. The defender punches the attacker's face simultaneously, deflecting a possible attack.

2. The defender locks his arm onto the attacker's arm or club, pulling the attacker's body with his other hand. The defender delivers a knee kick to his opponent and continues to counterattack if necessary.

Note: In the following a frontal approach is demonstrated as well.

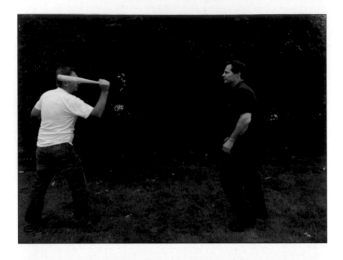 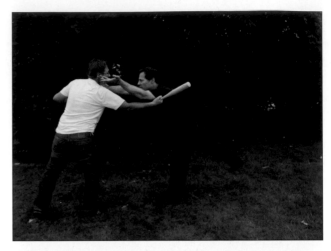

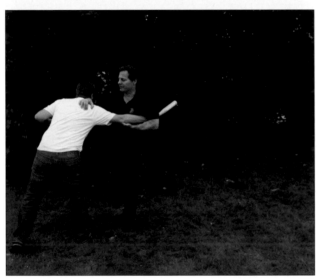 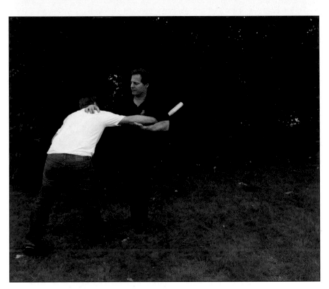

A Note on Sword Dueling

While most blade techniques are presented, Krav Maga does not practice sword fighting. Instead, sticks are used. In the IDF, when knife defenses are taught, a real knife is used at the final stage of the practice. However, soldiers rarely carry swords, and therefore they are not introduced to them in training. Civilians do not normally carry swords either. Instead, training sticks with techniques derived from sword fighting.

Chain Attack

Objects such as a motorcycle chain, nunchakos, or a ball and chain can be used as weapons. In this type of attack, the motion usually starts at shoulder level and ends on the opposite side away from the attacker. It can also end on a horizontal level. A good ending would be rolling over forward under the line of the attack and then kicking the opponent's center of gravity. Surprise is the key in this technique. Since the chain may cross your line of advance you need to start your move when it has just left the line.

1. The attacker is ready to swing his chain.
2. The attacker is swinging a chain or nunchakos as the defender begins to roll over.
3. The attacker's weapon is at the end of its motion, and the defender's leg is kicking the attacker from the ground up. In this case, you roll over without getting up, break fall on the ground and kick up as you learned in the ground techniques chapter.

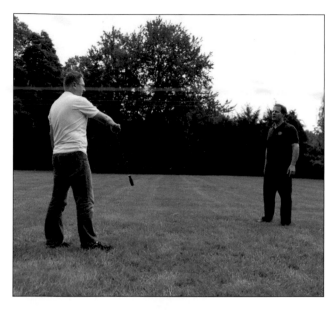

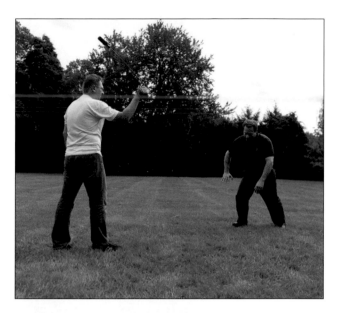

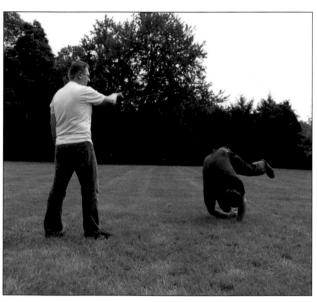

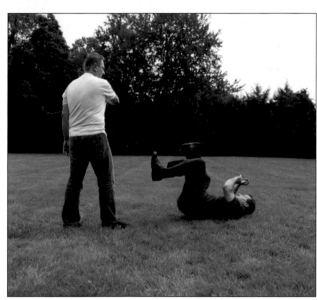

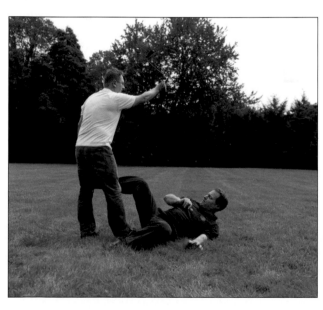

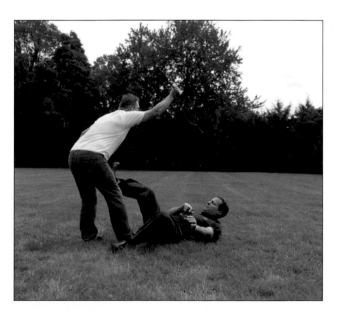

KNIFE TECHNIQUES AND DEFENSES

Small and sharp objects can be used for tearing the skin and arteries, and larger, pointed knives can poke and stab at one's flesh and vital organs from a greater distance. Poking the skin near the carotid artery and pulling the tip of the blade causes the artery to tear apart. The difference between slashing and tearing has no bearing on the result. Slashing pertains to a smooth cut inflicted by a sharp object. Tearing is a not-so-smooth cut done by a rather dull pointy object. The longer, sharp-tipped objects should pose more of a danger to the vital organs, the heart, lungs, or even the throat when held with the sharp point in front.

When your opponent is holding them top down, you should worry about a poke to your clavicle with a cut of the carotid artery, or your heart where a stab is through the ribs from the side. If the knife is held low with the tip pointed up, worry about your gut. A top-down stab hold, or a bottom-up stab hold require the opponent to get closer to you than if he was holding the knife in a straight hold trying to poke your throat or heart.

If you are wearing a heavily padded winter coat, your wrist, may be more protected against a small and sharp object. However, a large knife swung against your wrist, while not able to cut through your arteries, would stun you due to a painful hit on your wrist. You need to also watch out for your fingers. A knife can extend the user's range of attack or defense with less effort. An easy circular motion of the wrist, a medium speed poke, or a fairly fast slash, if aimed at your arteries or vital organs can swiftly leave you stunned and with the last breaths of life. This is just a small piece of advice to make you feel a little better. Now we get to the core techniques.

First, you need to learn an effective attack, and then you need to learn an effective defense. In the section on knife attacks, look at the attacker in each picture, and determine how you would predict the direction of the forthcoming attack. As you remember from an earlier discussion on reaction time, if the attacker changes his hold in the last second, you should already have planned your counterattack. Any last minute change will cause a delay in the attack. Once you have identified his initial possible attack, you should have moved in as if your attacker has started to close in.

If you can reach him quickly, you may move in, knowing it might prompt him to execute an attack defensively. As you move in, leave your hands down to the sides of your body; this will tempt him to stab you, and you can hence be almost certain what direction you should execute your defense in.

Generally, remember to try to look like an innocent lamb. Do not change to a defensive or offensive stance. You do not want your opponent to even think you are going to block or counterattack. That will end the fight faster, with no complications for you.

Using a Knife
Top-down hold

1. The attacker holds the knife in a top-down grip.
2. The attacker closes the gap, grabbing his opponent's clothes and raising his knife.

3. The attacker stabs diagonally into the clavicle, reaching the carotid artery.
4. The attacker stabs horizontally into the rib area.

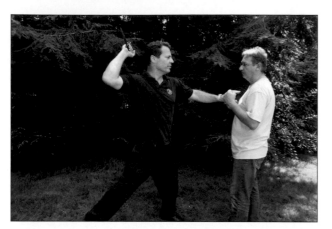
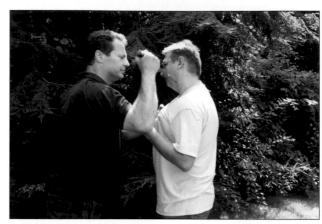

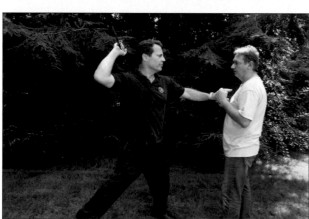
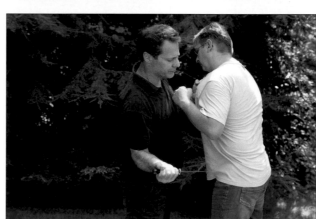

Under hold knife stab

1. The attacker holds the knife with his back hand, keeping his arm to the side of his body.
2. The attacker closes the gap, grabbing the opponent's clothes.

3. The attacker thrusts his knife into the opponent's abdomen, lifting it up to tear at his intestines.
4. The attacker stabs the ribs diagonally.

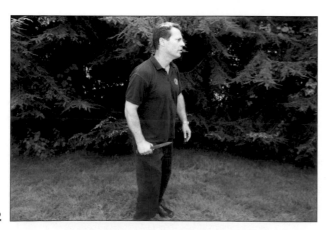
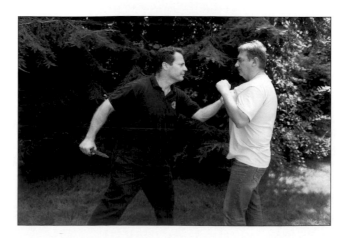

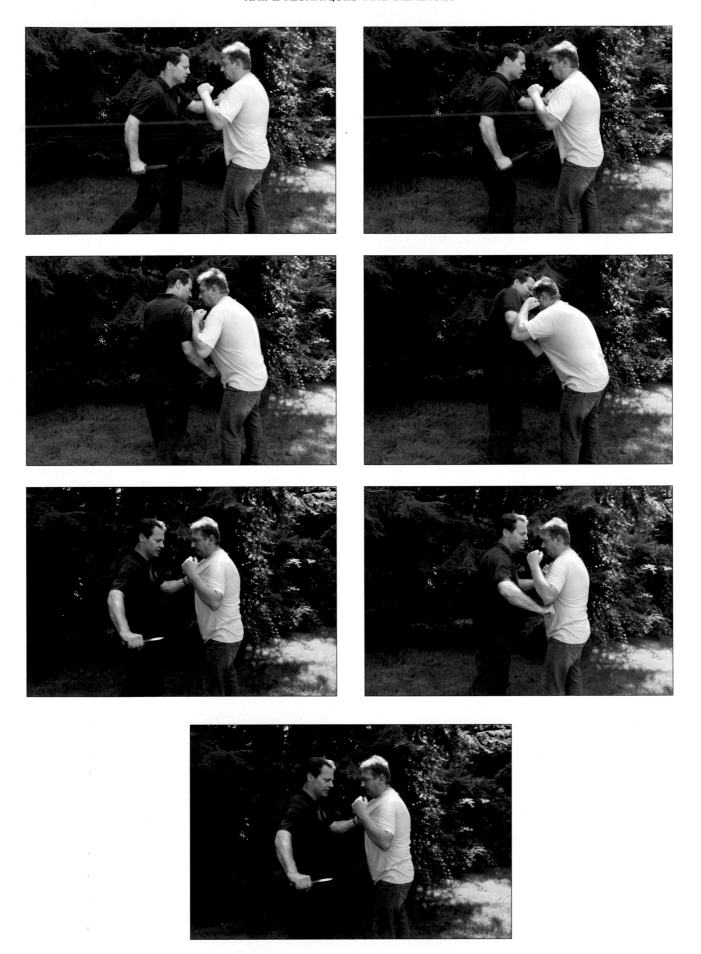

Straight stab hold

1. The attacker is holding his knife with hand in front, ready to stab the defender.
2. The attacker is closing the gap, about to lunge in, pushing his toes and landing on the front foot while the rear foot is raised straight to balance his tilted torso.
3. The attacker stabs the opponent's throat, chest, or abdomen area.

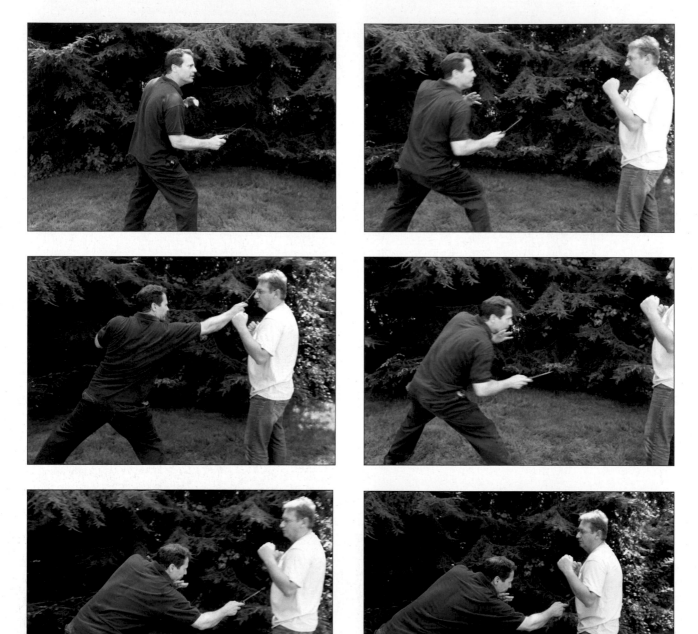

Note: The blade is held parallel to the ground to help it pass between the ribs.

The butt of the knife is sunk inside the palm, helping deepen the thrust. After the initial lunge, the gap is closed, and the attacker can repeatedly keep stabbing his opponent. Only the hand is retracted with each stab; there is no need to retract the torso when using a sharp knife in a straight stab.

Inside slashing attack

1. The attacker holds his knife with his front hand at shoulder level ready to slash the defender. The knife is held with his thumb and two fingers. Slashing has two components. The first component is the diagonal downward accelerating motion. The second component is pivoting the wrist clockwise. The purpose is to reach the arteries with the tip of a sharp object. A slashing move can be used defensively as well.
2. The attacker lunges forward.

3. The attacker throws his wrist from his shoulder to the direction of his opposite hip. Upon contact with the target's neck or wrist, the attacker flips his wrist clockwise, increasing his grip from three to five fingers. This is quicker when it's a stationary hold, when the knife is held in front, and is useful for defensive motions. In addition, the same wrist flip is useful when aimed at the carotid artery as it reaches with the tip of the blade even if the defender executed a last second block.

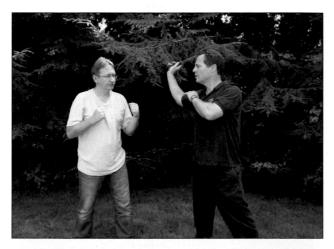
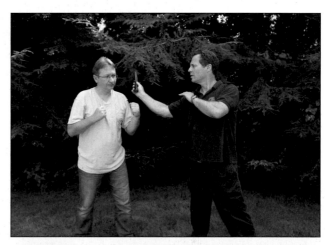

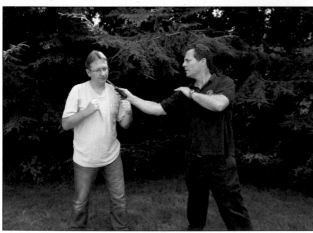
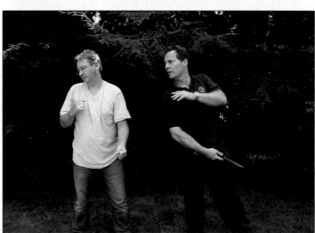

Outside slash in reversed motion

In an outside slash, even if the knife has only one sharp side, the thumb should stay on top for greater speed. Even if the edge of the knife is dull, the motion will facilitate a tear of the artery with the tip of the knife. The wrist, however, should start with a full grip, go on to a tossing motion, and end with a three-finger hold. Sufficient speed is the key.

1. The attacker holds the knife on his opposite hip with five fingers.
2. The attacker throws his wrist diagonally up to the direction of his shoulder, slashing the opponent's throat. Prior to contact, the attacker immediately changes his grip from five fingers to three, which helps increase force.

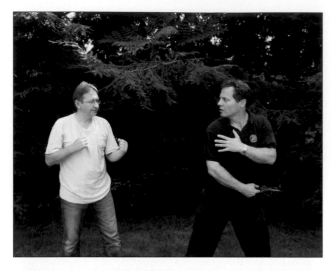
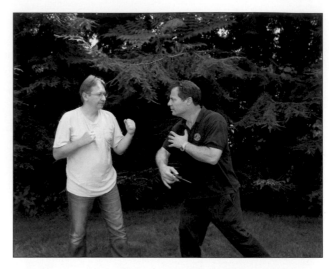
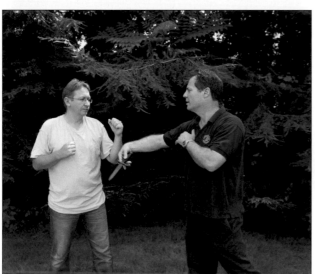
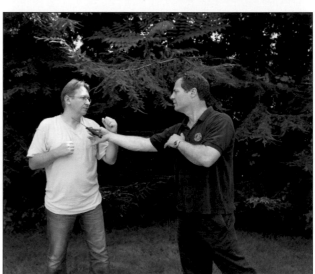

Defense against Knives Using Your Legs

We would use kicks if we had enough time to identify the danger of an armed opponent ahead of time. We may, however, prefer to use our hands instead, depending on our proficiency, and the moment's convenience.

Top-Down Hold Defense with Front Kick to the Groin

1. The attacker is holding the knife with his right hand, tip pointed down. The attacker moves his left foot forward preparing his right hand for a stab. The defender initiates his move by leaning his weight forward. The defender is lunging by pushing his toes forward, landing on his left foot with toes pointed out. Pivoting his body helps for a better reach. The idea is to land comfortably balanced, at least at the same time the kick is executed. If landing on the base foot occurs in diagonal angle prior to kicking, it eliminates a possible friction that will cause you to wobble should you try to extend your reach as you go. This ensures that all the kicking transforms instantly into the desired direction.

2. The defender pivots his body, landing diagonally on his left foot as he kicks the opponent in the groin.

3. The defender retracts his body and leg to a ninety-degree angle ready for a repeated kick if necessary.

4. The defender is closing the short gap rising up, and then landing down with a hammer blow to the back of his opponent's neck.

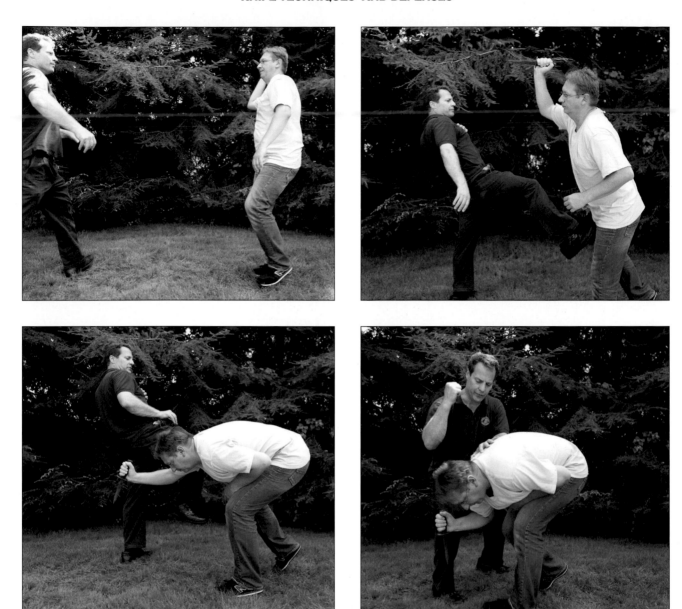

Note: This is a planned reaction to an attacker preparing to stab from the top down. You should take into account that he would need to close the gap and use a little extra momentum while preparing for the stab. While you are expected to kick the attacker as his hand is going backwards, you should take extra precaution by using the opposite leg. This positions your body slightly outside the direction of the stab.

Straight Hold Defense with Roundhouse Kick to the Groin

1. The defender spots an attacker holding a knife in a straight stab position.
2. The defender executes a low roundhouse kick to the groin with the opposite foot to the attacker's front leg. The motion is driven by throwing the opposite shoulder down to the floor, lifting the base foot accordingly, and kicking the opponent's groin with your other foot. The shoulder throw to

the ground is taken from an instinctive body sneak. A complete body sneak could be used as a last resort, but should be cut short and used to initiate the kick only, providing a counterattack before the attack is initiated.
3. The defender follows with a side kick to the opponent's knee.

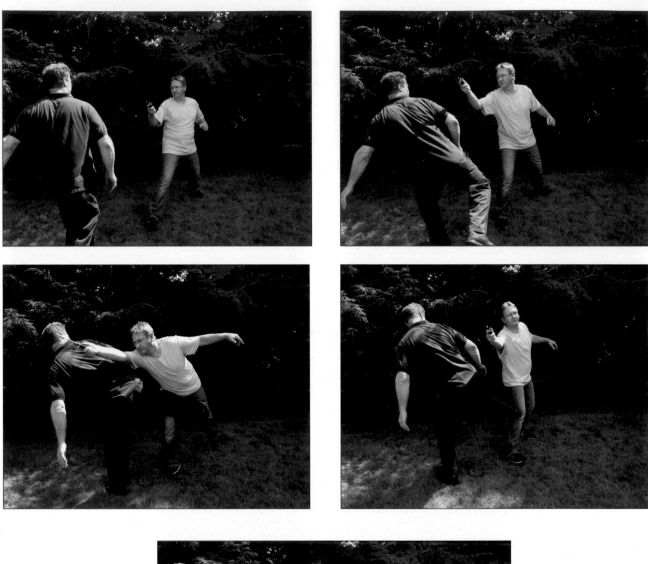

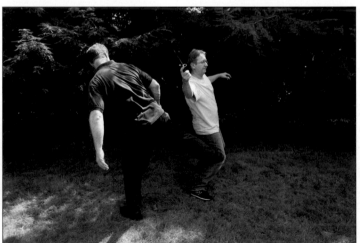

Straight Hold Defense with Armpit Kick

1. The attacker advances forward, holding his knife ready for a straight stab to the throat.
2. The defender lifts his front leg from the spot and kicks the attacker under his elbow. Note that the aim is toward the armpit, and the contact is on the outside of the foot to facilitate a greater catch.

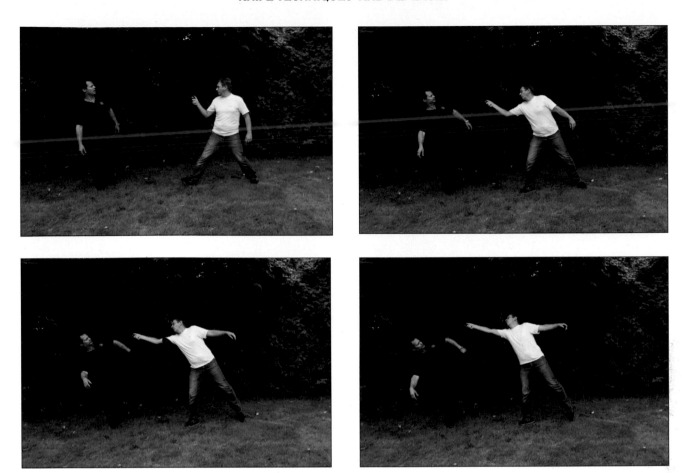

Note: This technique, although not preferred, has great potential if the distance and angle call for it. It's not a circular kick; an attacker's arm can have quicker reach than a defender shifting his weight and then lifting his foot for a kick. That is why this technique does not hold preference.

Under Hold Defense with Scissors Jump Kick

1. The attacker comes forward, holding a knife to the side of his body with the tip pointed up for an upward thrust to the gut or diagonally to the ribs. He holds his knife in his back (left) hand, or is walking and you move when his opposite foot is getting closer.
2. As the attacker steps forward with his right leg to close the gap, the defender lifts his right foot and jumps on his left foot as he drops the right foot down slightly pivoting his torso clockwise. The right leg is lifted slightly prior to the kick with the left foot, which facilitates immense and surprising high kick power. The kick hits the opponent in his sternum or chin. In this scenario, the foot opposite to the knife is used, preferably with a slight torso pivot to extend the kicking range and position the torso away from the direction of the stab.

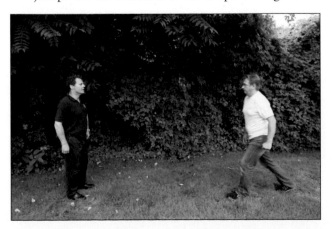

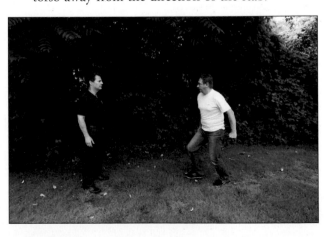

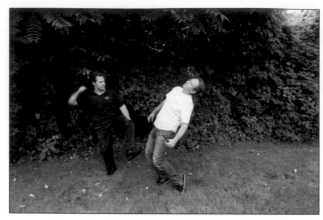 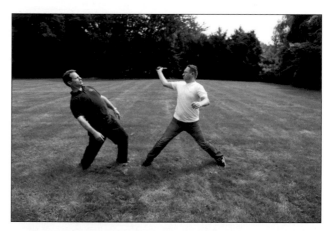

Note: Once you decide to execute this kick, you should concentrate on the timing. It may not be your best choice, but it could be the only choice you have as time runs out.

Inner Slash Defense with Front Defensive Kick

This motion is similar to a top-down hold in the direction of the slash.

1. The attacker is holding a knife in the initial position of an inside body slash.

2. The attacker advances, and the defender leans backward with his torso to evade the knife.
3. The defender continues with a defensive kick to the attacker's arm. The defender continues with hand strikes.

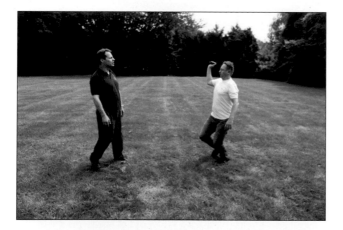 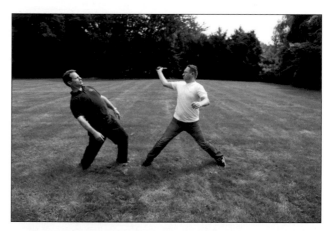

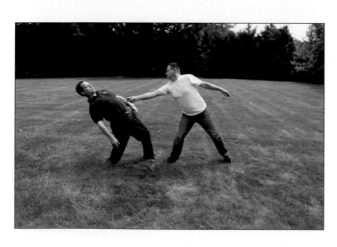 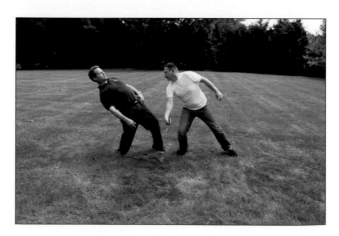

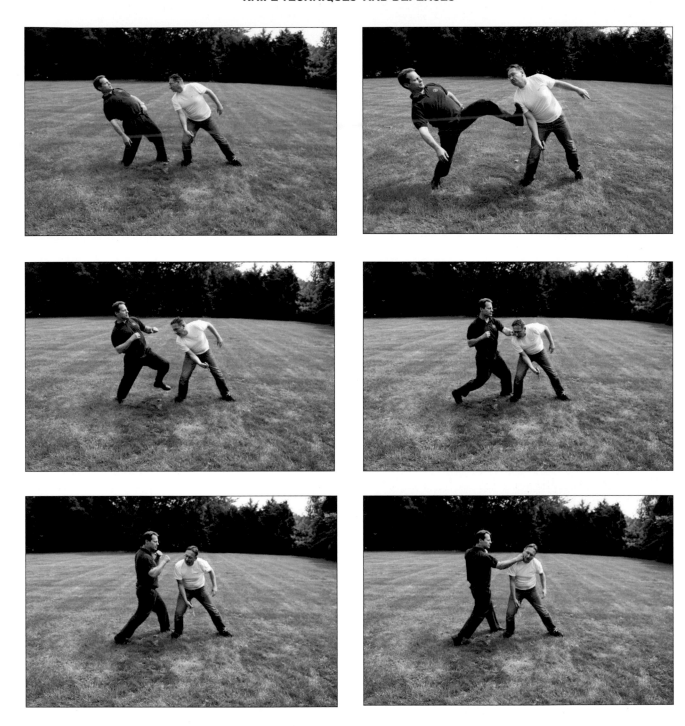

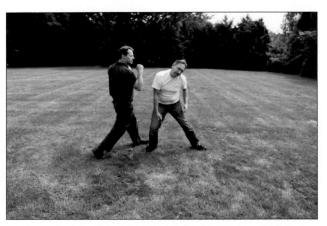

Outer Slash Defense with a Front Defensive Kick

1. The attacker approaches, holding his knife crossed over his body.
2. As the attacker begins to slash, the defender leans with his body backward to avoid the blade.
3. The defender continues with lifting his front leg to kick the opponent's groin or abdomen.

4. The defender continues to use his fists to counter-attack his opponent. The knife will probably be tossed to the ground so it might not be possible to grab it from the attacker's hand.

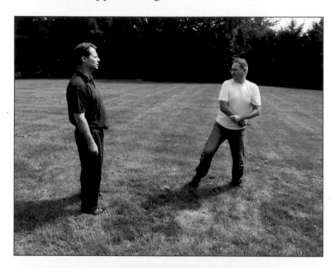
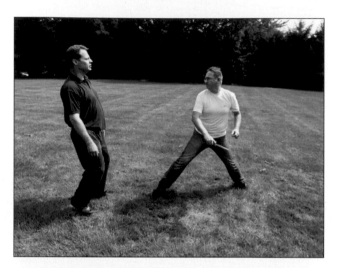

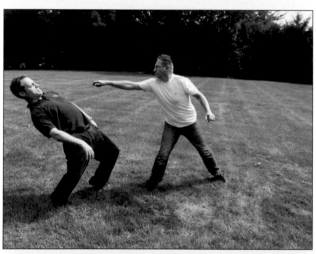
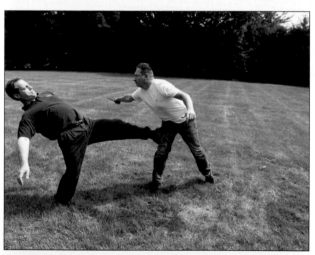

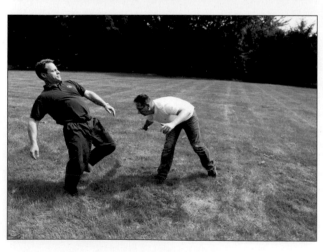
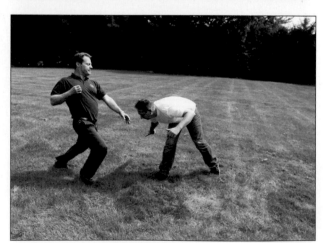

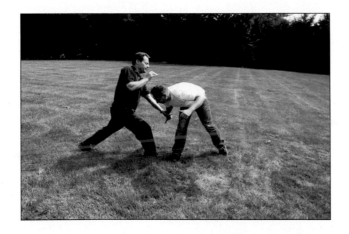
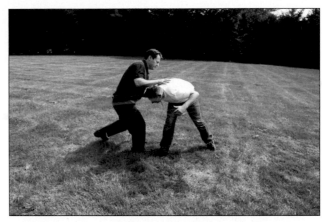
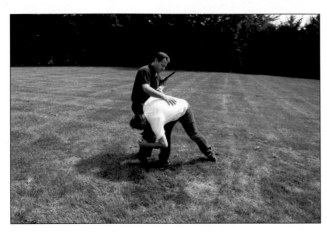
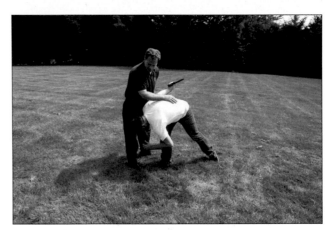

Note: If the attacker is closing the gap with the intent to slash and his knife is in front of his body, his stance is similar to a straight stab, and the defense techniques would be chosen accordingly.

Bear in mind that attackers put all their energy in the first attack. For that reason, for each of the knife holds presented above, the best anatomical stance is chosen by maximum related momentum.

A few variations of directions, body angles, and direction of attack are possible. Training partners are encouraged to try this. Deciding what direction to move in should generally be based on your opponent's capabilities, judging from his stance and how he holds his knife. Then, consider if it is faster for him to reach you with a kick, a punch, or a knife, and then react. An attacker leaning forward will most likely use his knife. Most of the time, use of the appropriate response demonstrated above will work.

Defense vs. Top-Down Knife Hold in the Attacker's Front Hand

1. The attacker is holding the knife top down, ready for a swing from the opposite direction of his knife-holding arm. The attacker is actually standing with his side to you. While the attacker's motion could be slower, he will probably attempt to close the gap slowly, perhaps expecting an attack from you and hoping to stab your leg or arm. You should act like an innocent sheep and wait for the window of opportunity to kick him in the center of his body. You may immediately follow with a hand strike while attempting to block his knife with your arm if needed. If possible according to the angle he is standing, kick him in the groin.

2. The defender kicks to the center, or the groin if possible.

Defense against a Knife with a Low Side Kick to the Knee

1. The attacker approaches from the defender's side with a straight stab hold.

2. The defender executes a low side kick to the attacker's front leg.

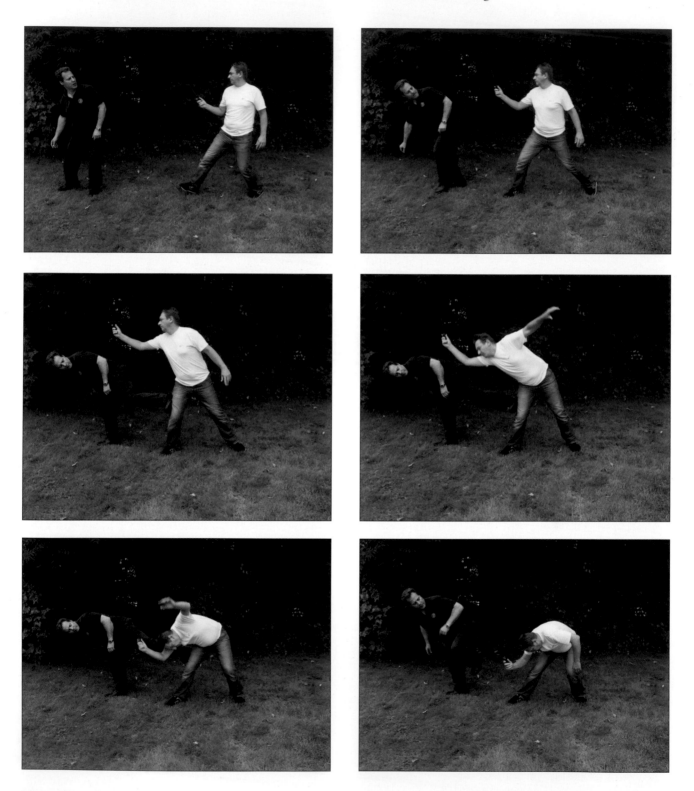

Note: We only provided one example of approaching from the side. In all other scenarios, the defense and counterattack should be the same: side kick to the opponent's front leg.

Defense against a Knife with Distraction and a Kick

1. The attacker holds a knife in a straight hold.

2. The defender throws an object into the attacker's eyes and follows with a low roundhouse kick.

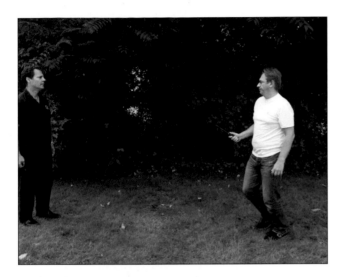

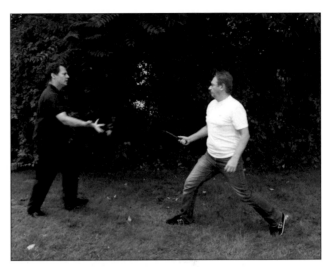

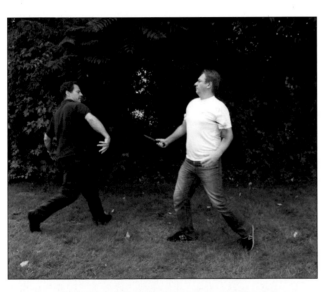

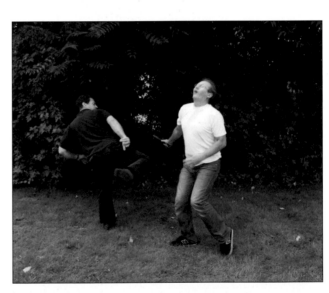

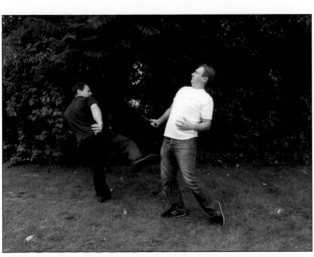

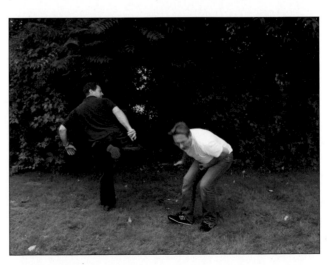

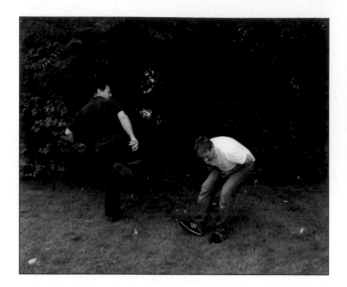
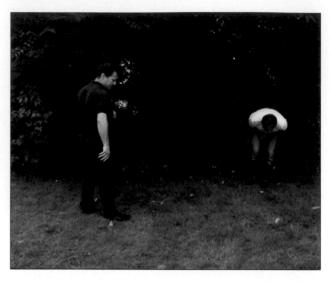

Note: Hope you have figured out by now that any distraction can be helpful. You can create a distraction by throwing an object as you're getting on the defensive. You can use your watch, your keys, or anything that you hold to throw at the opponent's eyes and buy you a few seconds. Move in immediately and kick the attacker. The sooner you try this distraction technique, the better the chance that it will give you the upper hand. When you do not have anything in your hand, spit. Make sure not to distract yourself. You need to attack immediately after your distractive maneuver. You should use your judgment regarding the type of kick you will use. Kicking an armed attacker is risky, but less so if you do it before he attacks you. It is less risky to position your body away from the predicted direction of the knife.

In Krav Maga if you are using kicks vs. a knife, always use a side kick to the knee when the attacker approaches the defender from the side.

If the attacker approaches the defender from the front, then kick him either in the groin, or on his chest or chin. You could also roundhouse kick his groin and follow it with a side kick to the knee after the initial advance and reposition to the side of the opponent.

The most dangerous knife attack is the straight stab with the front hand. The second most dangerous is the slash, which has almost the same reach.

The straight stab provides an immediate contact with the tip of the blade. The slash would involve whipping the blade into the side of the throat. We can see the intention of the attacker by the type of hold. The range of the slash is almost as much as the range of the straight stab.

The third most dangerous is the circular attack from the bottom up, and the fourth is from the top down.

A straight stab with the rear hand can be countered with a roundhouse kick to the opposite direction, or a jumping scissors kick to the chin like a bottom-up stab.

If you notice the attacker on time, position your body in neutral position so you can have a peripheral view and also be able to control the timing. If you do not have the time, you will probably have to resort to defending with your hands.

There are three considerations to identifying and choosing the best option using these three methods of preemptive attacks with kicks.

First, look at your opponent's knife grip. Second, which hand is he holding it in? Third, your options are either kicking the head or the groin area—whichever is farther from the knife in order to avoid a counterattack and a stab in the leg. Straight stabs are generally at the center but you should only kick below it and not above, as it would take longer for you to kick than for the opponent to stab.

Remember also that a direct kick to the center of the body, be it chest or crossed arms, stops the opponent with its initial impact.

Remember: the three frontal maneuvers are a front kick to the groin, a scissors kick to the chest or chin, and a defensive front roundhouse kick. Each one has a tactical component. For example, the front kick is tactically executed with the defender's leg across the hand holding the knife and not the one in front. This forces the defender to move his body slightly to the opponent's side, away from the slightly angular top-down direction of the knife. If the attacker chooses a top-down stab with the knife in his front hand, you could use the time the attacker takes to stab, executing a roundhouse kick to his groin with the leg opposite his front leg. You might also choose to do the second part of the roundhouse kick and not a straight stab, and execute only a side kick to the opponent's knee. You need to practice all aforementioned options until you are comfortable with them.

Another tactical component involves the response to the straight stab. The counter-kick would be a roundhouse kick to the groin, followed by a side kick to the knee. Execute the roundhouse kick as a continuation of the tactical maneuver that is triggered by the instinctive throw of the shoulder opposite to the attacker's front hand to the ground, and the shifting of your body weight to the side and out of the stabbing range.

But the initial instinct motion is honed more to promote the timing and force of the counter-kick than a complete evasion. At least you are in the right direction to escape if you are running out of time.

The scissors kick involves abruptly lifting the defender's leg below knee height and in front of the attacker's knife-holding hand, and then dropping that leg back to the ground to lift the opposite leg while pivoting the torso.

This brings you to a jump kick to the chest or chin. Make sure to correctly reposition your body, keeping it slightly away from the direction of the blade.

So for the straight front hand stab, you will use a roundhouse kick to the groin, followed by a side kick. If it is a low straight stab, you might skip the groin but instead complete that same tactical evasion and move on to kick the knee from the side instead. For circular top-down or horizontal top-side, you should kick the groin.

Remember that with circular moves, the opponent first has to close the gap and then go on to the circular stab. So when he starts to close the gap, move in and kick him.

As for a bottom-up or a bottom-to-the-side motion, respond with a scissor kick to the chest or chin, depending on the height of the opponent. You do not want to waste too much time going to a higher altitude. Rather, you want to accelerate forward. If the attacker is holding a bottom-up hold in his front hand, go for a roundhouse kick to the groin followed with a side kick to the knee. Consider delaying your kick after you start the evasive motion to ensure your kicking leg will not be in the path of the tip of the knife.

You should execute the same last response if the attacker is going for a rear hand straight stab because he has to first close the gap before moving on to the circular stab, but by throwing your shoulder in the direction of his front hand and not to the knife-holding hand.

Now what if the attacker is standing in forty-five degrees with his hands crossed over his chest and a blade pointed with a top-down hold?

He could be waiting to see you move and aim for your leg or arm. He could either be calculated, trying to ensure a series of attacks, or lunge forward with his body and knife in opposite directions. This can be a little confusing.

From his position, he cannot lunge with the same range as a front stab, but if you try to kick him he could stab your leg. He could also just be advancing slowly, hoping to execute a fast figure-eight attack.

The key in choosing your move is identifying the most efficient capacity from the initial stance. The direction of the blade, and the size and type of knife might give you an idea about your attacker's intention and tactical inclination. Do you think he is planning a defensive poke, or a preemptive attack? In addition, you need to be aware of his lunging capacity.

A preemptive kick to the chest might also be useful against someone holding two knives in a top-down hold. You never want to project your intention or ability to defend yourself. Instead, you want to surprise your opponent. However, let's say someone approaches you with the intention of countering your defense. It would probably be best to wait and kick him as he enters your range and follow up with your hands, or wait a split second more and use your body and forearm for defenses. Let's talk about kicking an opponent who is about to slash you. Well if he is standing ready for a front hand straight stab, he might use a slashing motion to deflect your wrist first, but his initial motion would be the same as a straight stab so you would react and execute a defense vs. a straight stab as discussed above.

But if he is standing with his hand like a barber using a razor, hand in front of his shoulder thumb down, what do you think the preferred kick would be if you are standing in front of him? The blade is pointed forward and not downward, and the damage to your arteries is done with the top of the blade. This gives the attack a greater range and a faster reach forward than it would with a circular top-down motion. Since the slash occurs when the attacker is in punching range, the attacker could reach your body faster with his hand even if you try to move out of the way. This is why I would prefer you delay kicking if you choose to use that option. You would execute it after throwing your upper torso backward, evading a quick slash and trying to kick his arm afterward. But generally, I would prefer you didn't kick at all at any point.

Defense with Bare Hands against an Attacker Armed with a Knife

In the following demonstrations, the attacker will use his right hand to hold the knife, and each picture will have precise explanations. If the attacker uses his left hand, reverse the instructions.

Defense against a Top-Down Knife Hold

1. The attacker aims his knife at the clavicle, holding it with his right hand. The defender blocks it with the middle of his forearm with his thumb pointing down. The defender strikes the attacker's face simultaneously with his free hand.

2. The defender swings the attacker's hand with a half circle, pushing the the attacker's wrist away with the defender's forearm before the defender grabs his wrist with his hand. This prevents the blade from hooking on to the defender's wrist. This move is almost as if you are letting the attacker stab you in the torso. Pushing his wrist forward ends the stab in front of your body. With this motion, you can follow the opponent's wrist if he is attempting to stab you in the ribs with the same hold.

3. Defender switches hands in order to grab attacker's hand with defender's right hand. He then delivers a hand strike with his left hand. If the first counter strike was sufficient, the defender uses his right hand to extract the knife after the swing.

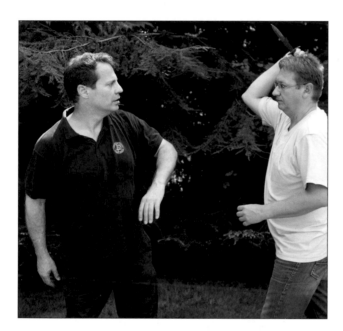

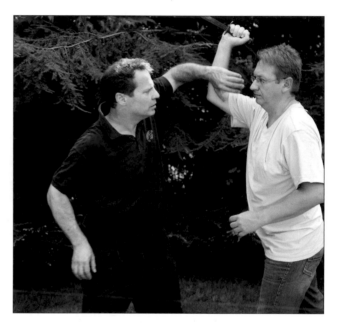

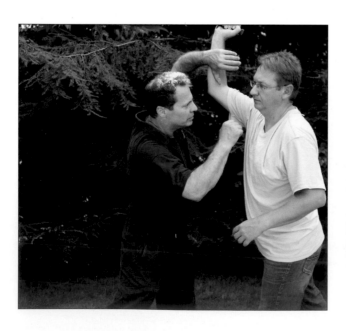

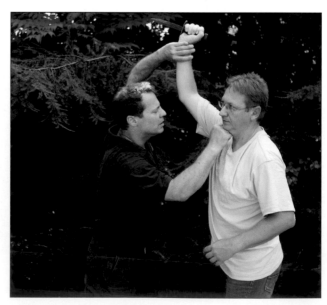

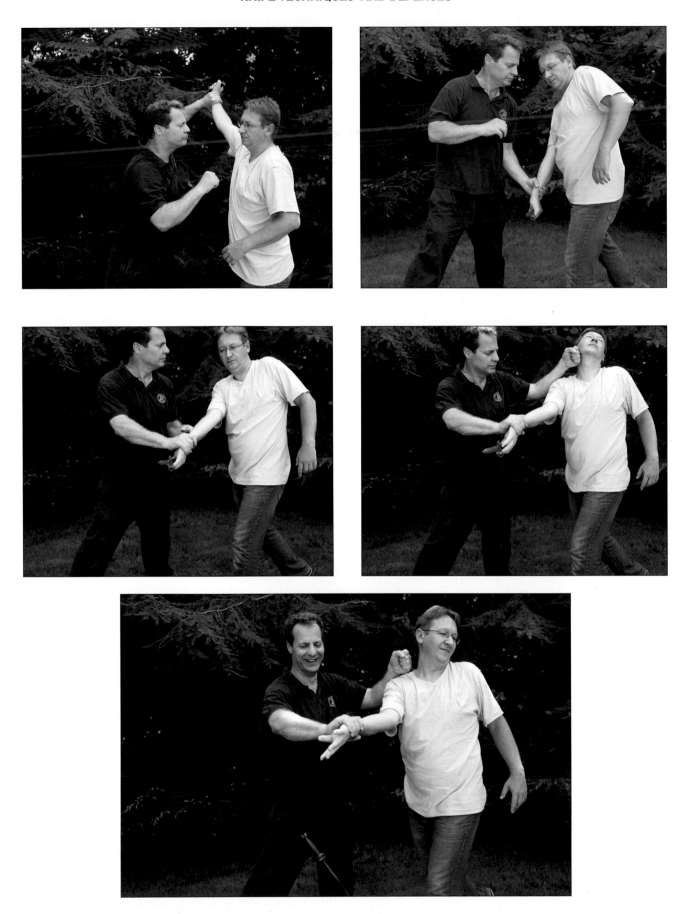

Note: You can continue to pull your opponent's head backward and knee his tailbone.

Instinctive Defense vs. Attacker Holding a Knife in an Underhand Hold

1. Attacker stabs with an underhand hold and defender slides his feet moving his torso backwards, blocking the knife with his left forearm. Defender is counterattacking simultaneously to the attacker's face. Note that defender has moved his torso away from the knife.
2. Defender follows with a second attack after he has got a hold of the hand holding the weapon.

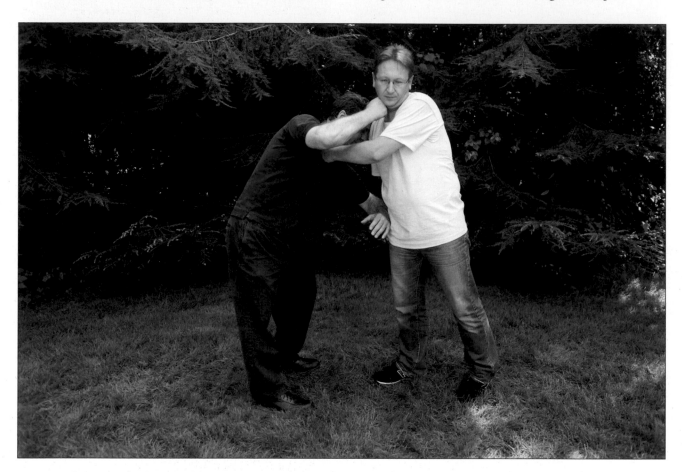

Defense with Forward Move vs. Attacker Holding a Knife in an Underhand Hold

1. As you see the opponent running toward you, meet him halfway. As you lean forward you pivot your torso to the right and your upper body leans down so that your forearm can catch the opponent's wrist as he moves it back gaining momentum for the stab. You strike him with your right hand to his face.
2. Since you have moved close to him, even if he retracts his hand, you have it. You limit his hand's motion by keeping your elbow slightly lower than your wrist, and you slide your hand to grab his wrist immediately after the block and counterattack.
3. As you grab his wrist, strike his face again if needed, and move your right hand to join your left hand holding his wrist. You create leverage on his wrist.
4. The leverage on his wrist is executed by keeping both hands in front of your belt. You roll your left wrist towards you like a motorcycle handle, and you push his small knuckles down with your right hand, delivering a kick to his groin with your right foot.
5. When his hand resistance loosens, peel the knife out.

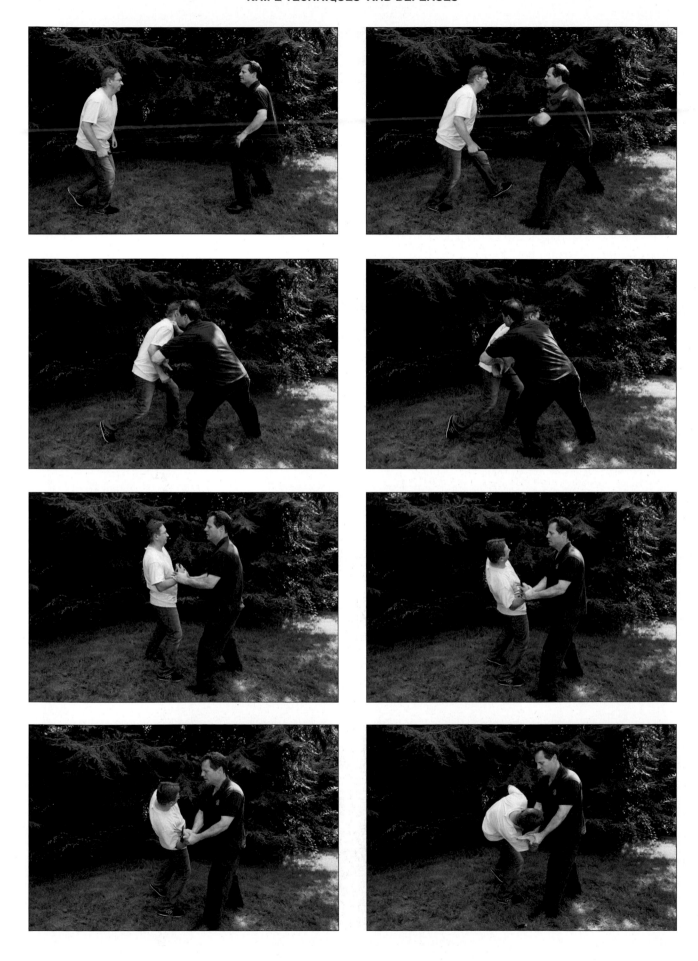

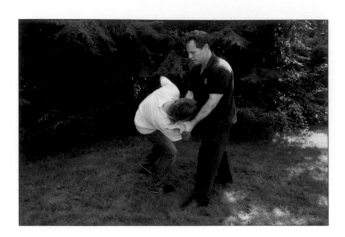

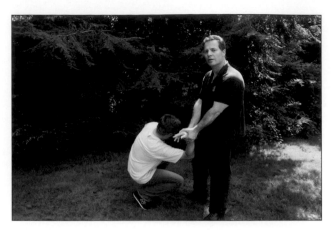

Opponent Approaching from the Side with Low Stab to the Ribs

If an attacker approaches you from your side holding a knife to the side of his body with the blade pointed up, it is likely that he will try to stab your ribs diagonally upwards since in this position, your abdomen is not in front of his knife.

1. Attacker approaches from the side holding a knife with the blade pointing up.

2. Defender pivots his torso toward the opponent blocking the opponent's forearm with his left hand, delivering a hand strike with his right hand.
3. Defender executes another punch, and grabs the opponent's wrist if possible.

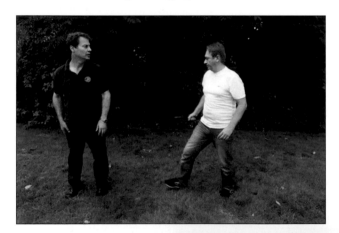

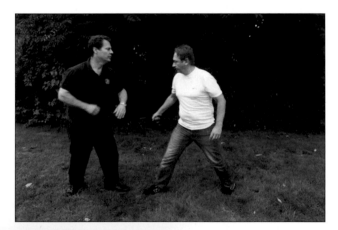

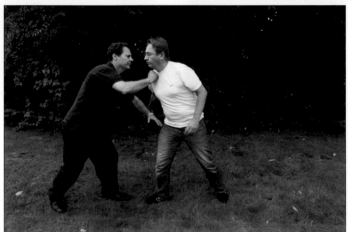

Note: the following variation of this technique is not recommended since an attacker retracting the knife will cause your arm to get cut!

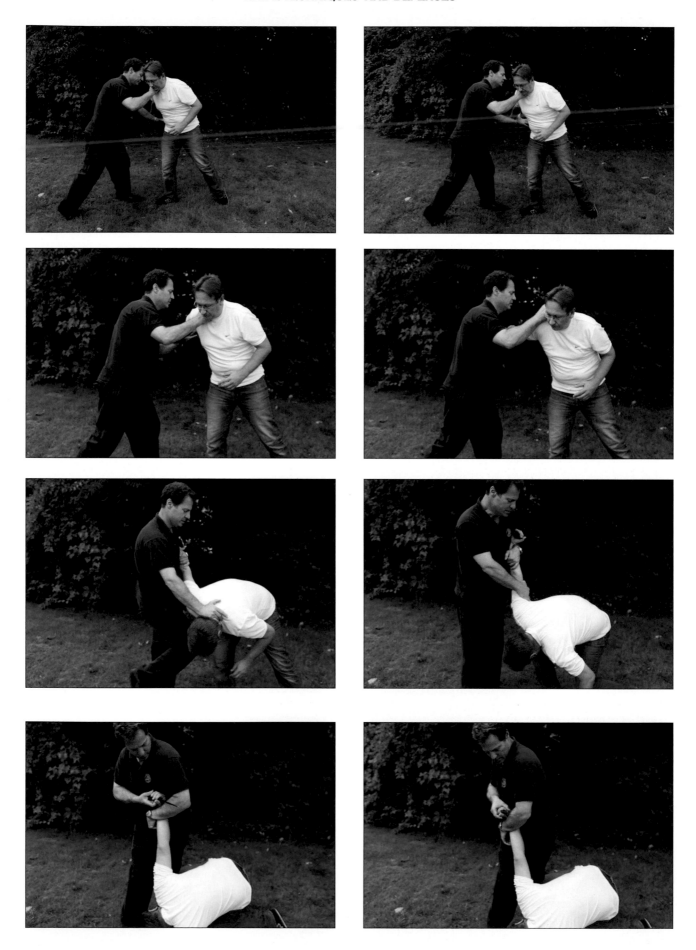

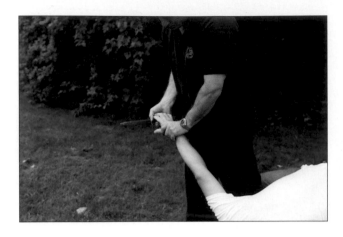
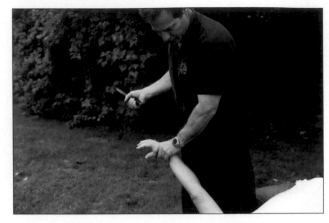

Defense vs. Underhand Knife Hold with Center Approach

1. Attacker is holding a knife in an underhand hold. Defender is standing with his right hand closer to the center of his opponent's body facilitating faster reach facing the opponent from the front.
2. Defender blocks the attacker's underhand stab with his right hand and simultaneously punches him with his left hand.
3. Defender switches his hand to grip the attacker's wrist and delivers an outside knife hand strike to the attacker's throat.
4. Defender proceeds to disarm the attacker as needed.

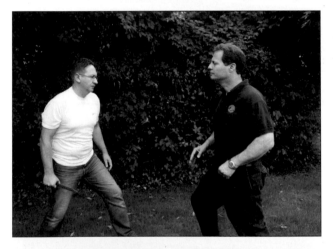
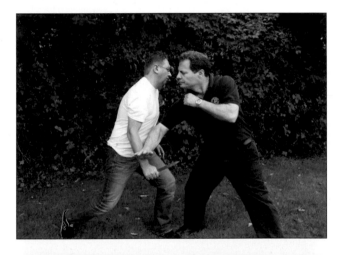

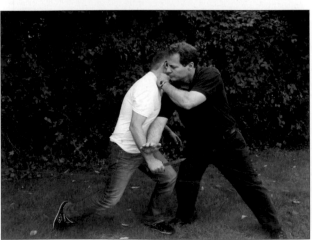
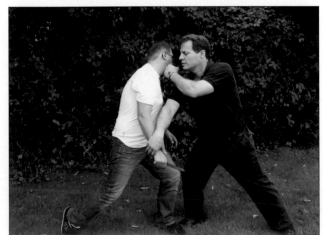

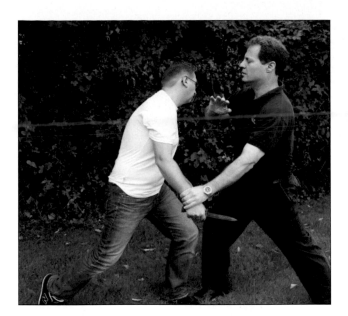
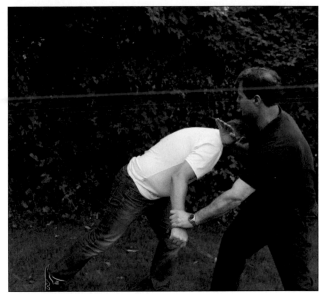

Defense vs. Front Inverted Grip Stab

1. Attacker is holding a knife using inverted right hand grip stabbing backwards diagonally to the defender's abdomen.
2. Defender is executing an outside forward block with his left hand, with simultaneous counter strike to the opponent's face with his right hand.

3. Defender follows to grab attacker's knife hand with his right hand and continues to execute a kick if possible, or a cavalier takedown to get the opponent off balance and to the ground.

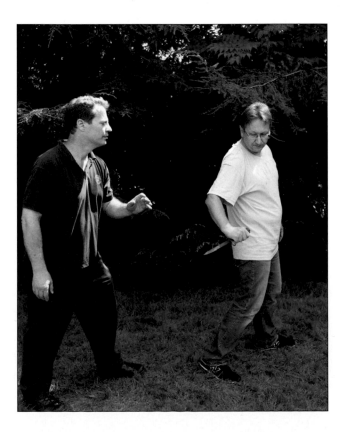
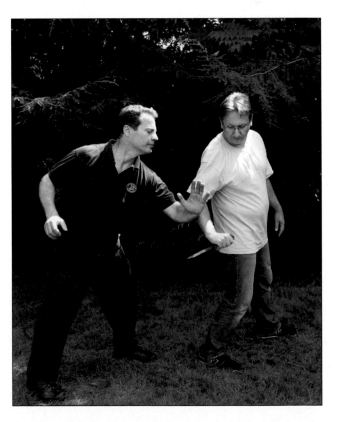

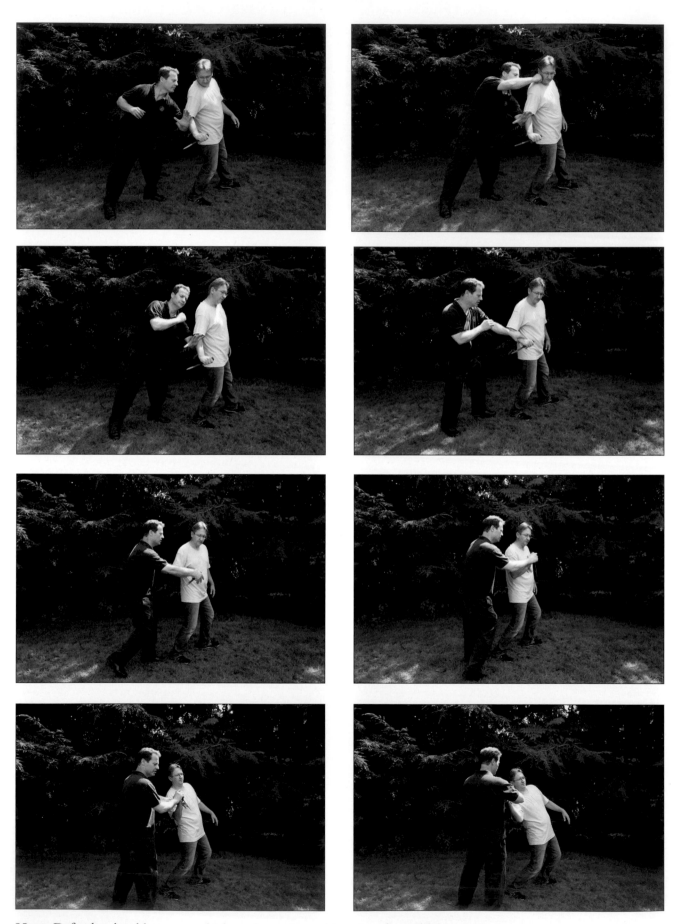

Note: Defender should execute a kick to the groin at this point if possible!

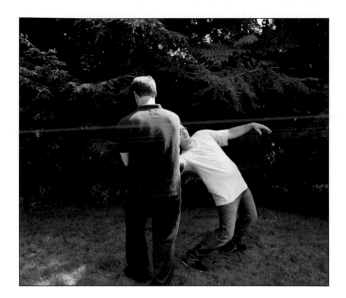 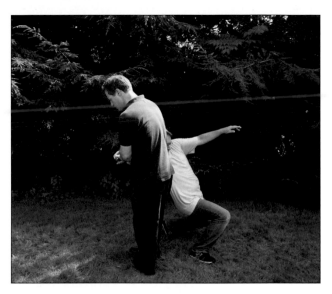

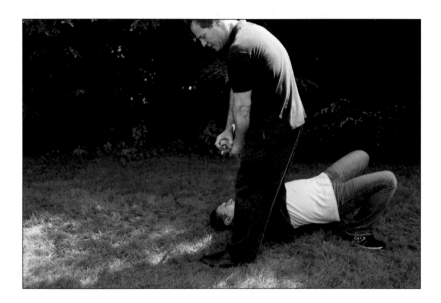

Defense vs. Front Straight Stab

1. The attacker holds his knife in front, ready to stab the defender in the heart or throat. The defender stands with his hands down without projecting his defensive plan.
2. The attacker stabs, and the defender places his forearm in front of him to meet the attacker's wrist with the center of the forearm. The initial contact is with the defender's inside soft part of the forearm.
3. When defender feels the contact with the attacker's wrist, he pivots his forearm clockwise, pushing his thumb forward. This motion propels the attacker's hand out of the defender's body range.

4. The defender simultaneously delivers a right-handed punch to the attacker's ribs as he lunges forward with his left leg. The forward body move limits the attacker's hand from repeated stabbing.
5. The defender catches the retracting opponent's hand delivering another strike to the opponent's face.
6. The defender joins his right hand to grab the opponent's hand with a cavalier.
7. The defender pulls the attacker's forearm, bringing his front leg backwards so he can kick with the other leg. He then executes a kick to the attacker's groin and peels the knife out of the attacker's hand.

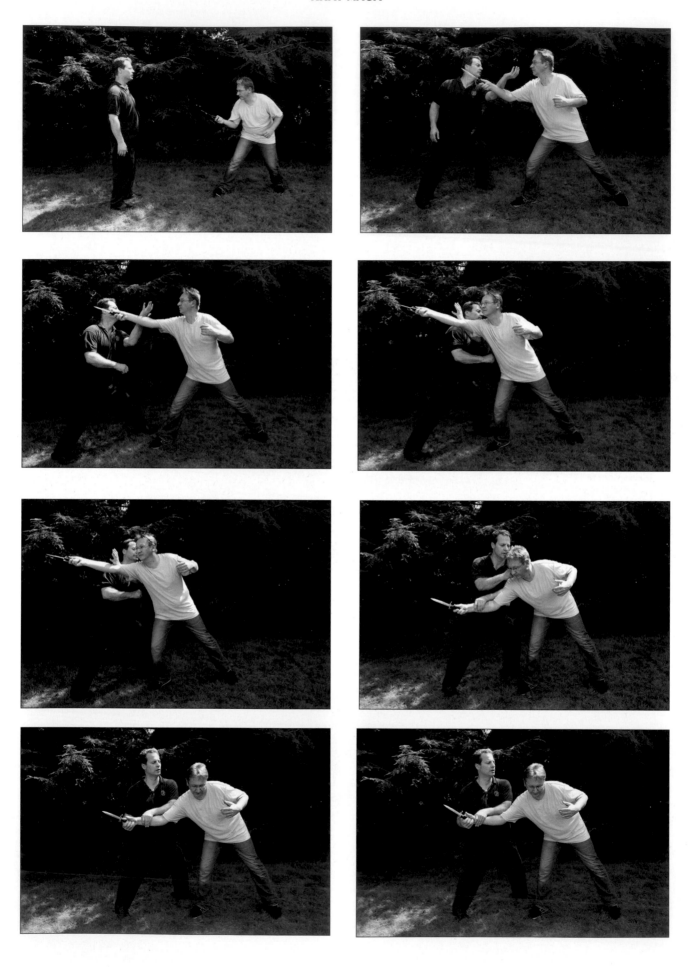

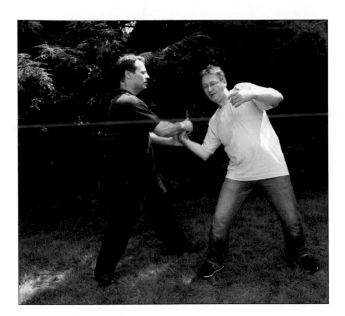

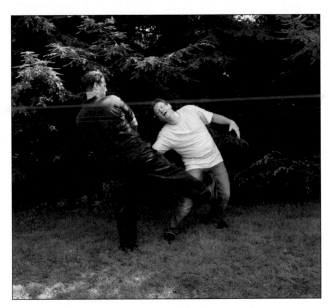

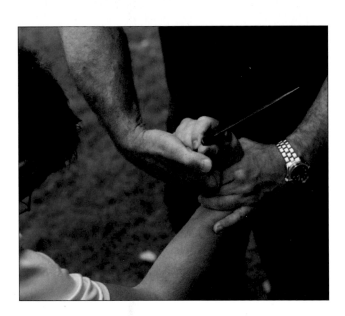

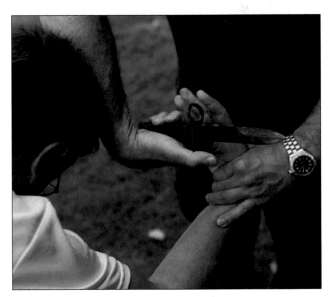

Defense vs. Attacker Holding a Knife in a Straight Low Hold

1. Attacker holds his knife in front ready to stab defender in the heart or throat. Defender stands with his hand down without projecting his defensive plan.
2. Attacker leans low forward as he aims to defender's abdomen. Defender adjusts his height by bending his knees and places his forearm in front of him to meet the attacker's wrist with the center of the forearm. The initial contact is with the defender's inside soft part of the forearm.
3. When the defender feels the contact with the attacker's wrist, he pivots his left forearm clock-

wise, pushing his thumb forward. This motion propels the attacker's hand out of the defender's body range.
4. Defender moves forward to catch the retracting opponent's hand delivering a punch to the opponent's face.
5. Defender joins his right hand to grab opponent's hand with a cavalier. The defender switches his front leg, pulling the attacker's arm, pivoting it to unbalance the attacker.
6. Defender executes a kick to the attacker's groin and peels the knife out of the attacker's hand.

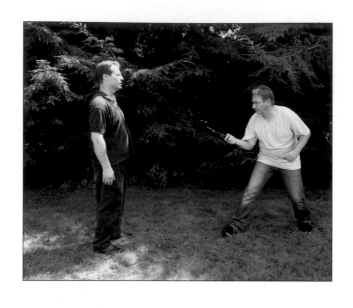

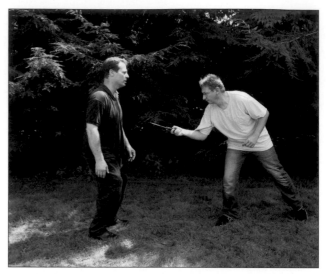

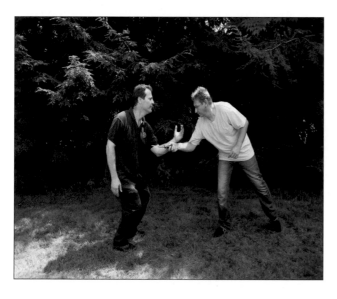

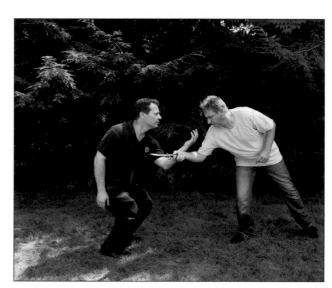

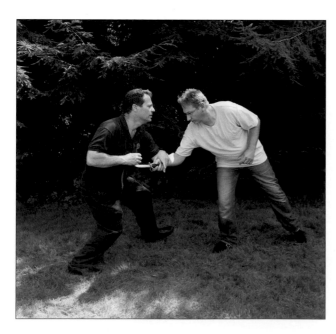

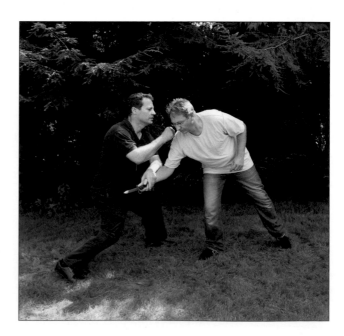

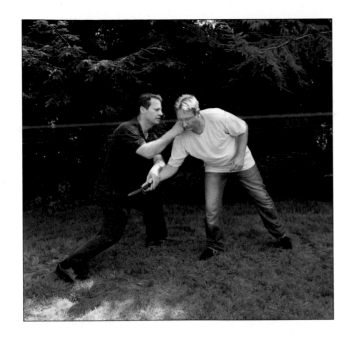

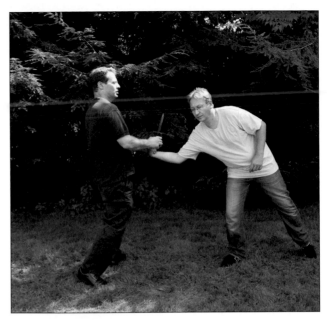

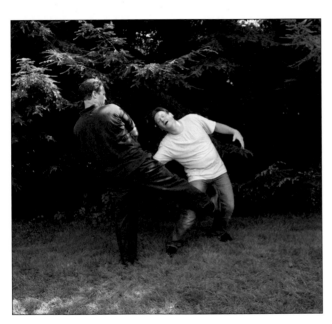

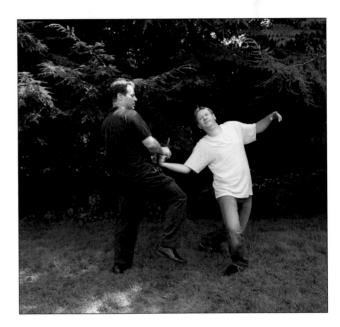

Defense vs. a Straight Knife Hold with a Center Approach

1. The attacker holds his knife in front, ready to stab the defender in his heart or throat. The defender stands with his hand down without projecting his defensive plan. The defender's right leg is closer to the attacker.
2. Defender blocks with his right arm, bending his knees to meet the attacker's wrist with the center of the defender's inner forearm.
3. As the defender feels the attacker's wrist, he pushes his thumb forward counterclockwise and the back of his hand forward. That moves the opponent's hand out of the defender's body range.
4. Defender moves forward, switching hands to grab the opponent's hand with his left hand, delivering a knife hand strike to the attacker's carotid artery.
5. Defender grabs the attacker's shirt with his right hand and executes a knee kick.

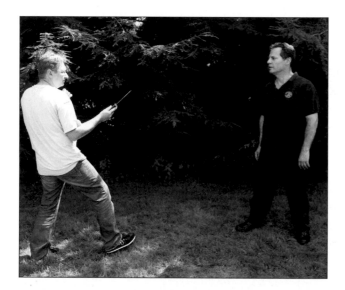
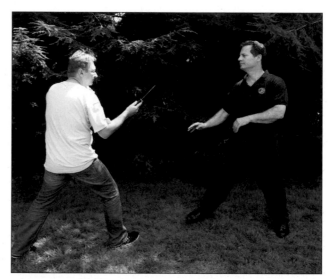
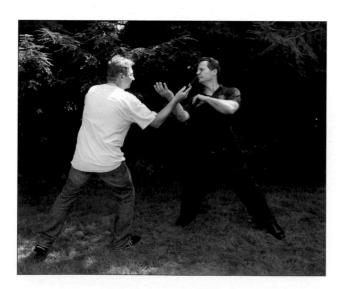
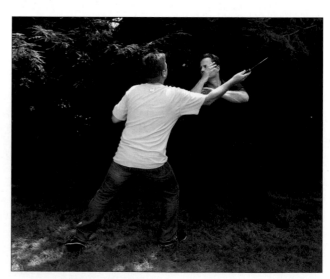

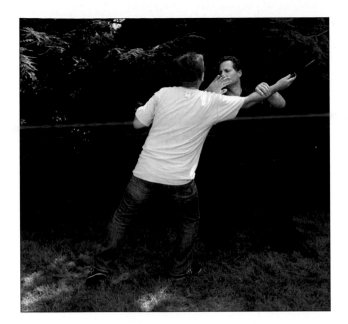

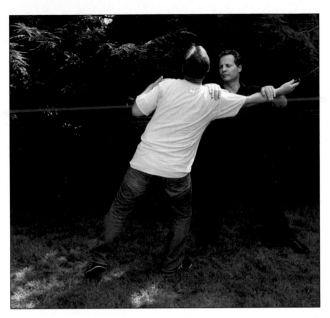

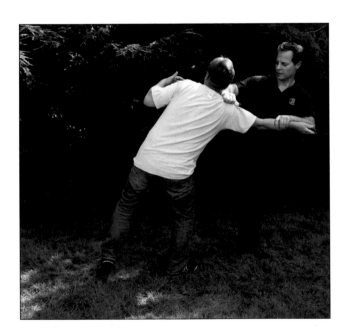

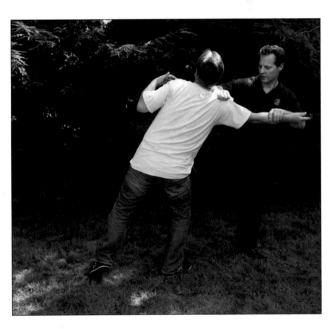

Note: While you need to align the middle of your forearm with the opponent's wrist, if the opponent attempts to stab you as low as your groin area, you can use an instinctive defense vs. underhand hold moving your torso backward, or an inside defense vs. kick. These scenarios however, would not give the opponent the advantage of maximum speed to reach you.

Instinctive Defense vs. Knife Slash from Close Distance

1. Attacker is standing close with a knife hidden behind his back.
2. Attacker slashes immediately and defender executes an outside defense and counterattacks with a

strike to the opponent's face (note that the defender initially cannot see the knife and performs an instinctive defense).

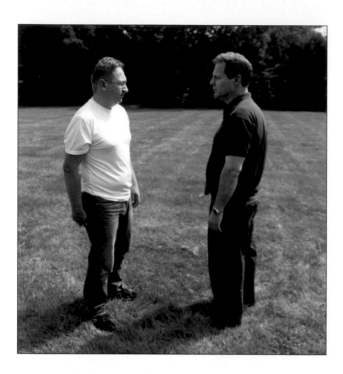 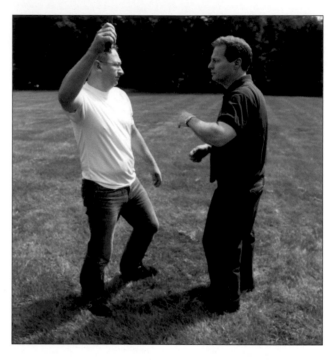

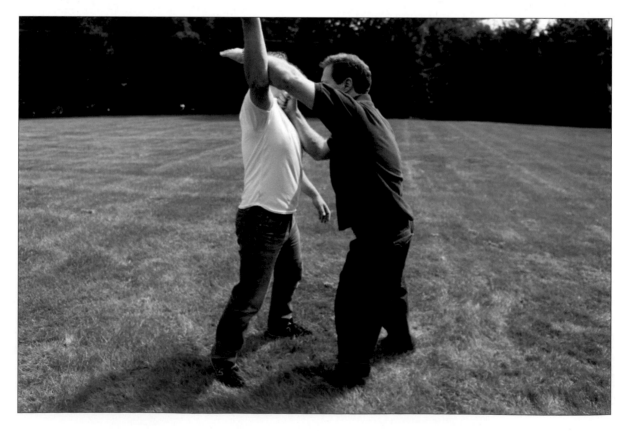

Defense vs. Attacker Holding a Knife in a Slashing Hold

1. Attacker holds his knife in a slashing position.
2. Defender chooses to forgo the first slash and lean backwards with his body.

3. Defender retracts his body forward, meeting the attacker's arms with defender's forearms sliding forward, and strikes the attacker in the face.
4. Defender grabs attacker's neck and hand in order to knee his tailbone.

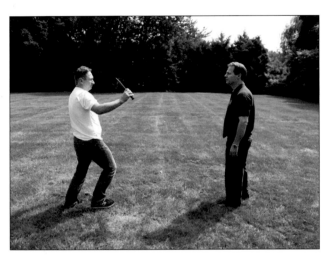

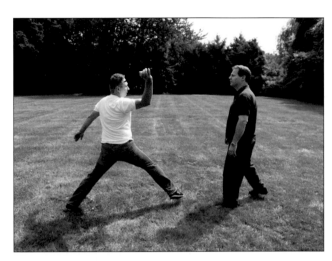

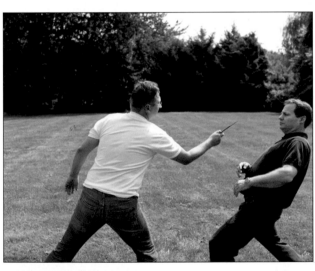

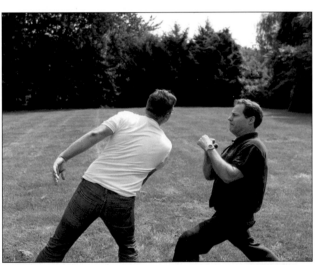

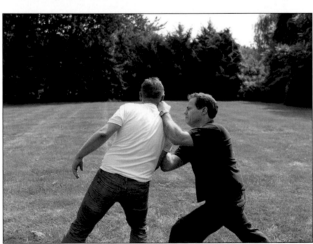

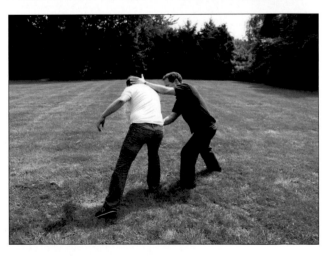

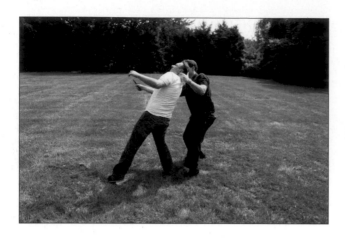
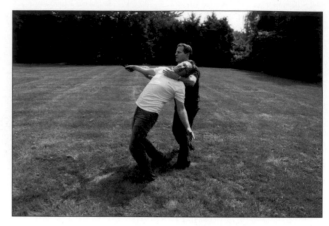

Note: This method of repositioning yourself behind the attacker has proved to be the best for controlling unexpected repeated attempts to reach you with the blade.

Defense with a Knife or Handy Objects
Defense with a knife vs. top-down knife hold

1. Attacker holds a knife in a top-down grip while defender hides his knife to the side of his body slightly behind his back.
2. Attacker moves forward closing the gap, raising his knife to stab downward.
3. Defender pivots his torso and stabs the attacker's throat.

During practice, tap the attacking training partner on the sternum with a bare hand to avoid endangering his body. The defense can be demonstrated with a handy object such as a rolled-up magazine, which is a safer method of training, especially when the attacker's training partner is holding a real knife.

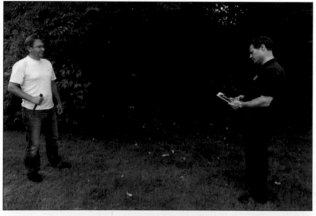
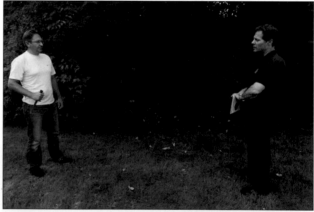

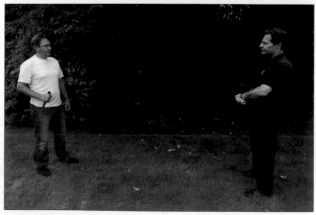
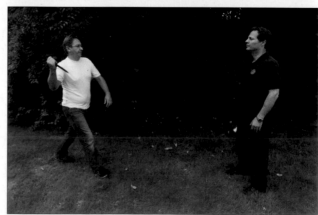

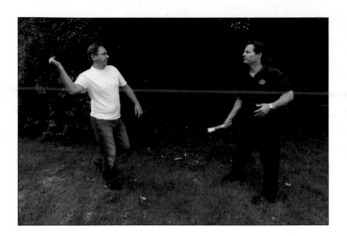
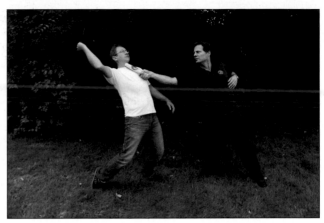

Defense with a knife against an attacker holding a knife in an underhand hold

1. The attacker holds a knife with his backhand, his arm to the side of his body.
2. The defender hides his knife behind his body with his right hand.

3. As the attacker closes the gap, the defender pivots his torso and reaches with his knife to strike at the attacker's knife-holding wrist.
4. The defender then continues to slash or stab the attacker's throat in a continuous motion.

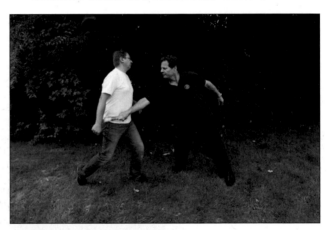

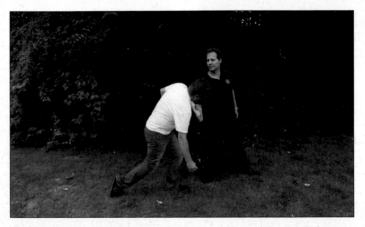

Note: Using a folded magazine against an opponent's neck can stun the opponent. It is a great weapon for practice with low risk to the training partner, but in a real situation it could also strike the opponent's vagus nerve and lower his pulse. This could buy you time for an additional knee kick. The folded magazine is more than enough to stop the train of thought of your opponent, delivering a stunning effect. Remember, however, that in reality you would need to continue hitting your opponent with one of your limbs, and then disarm the knife.

Defense with a handy object against an attacker holding a knife in a straight stab hold

1. The attacker is holding his knife with his right hand in front, ready to stab the defender. The defender is holding his folded magazine in his right hand, hiding it behind his back.
2. The attacker is closing the gap with a stab, as the defender blocks it with a perpendicular slash to the attacker's wrist. The defender pivots his body, reaching forward as far as possible.

3. The defender continues to slash attacker's wrist, blocking the hand holding the knife.
4. The defender counter-stabs the attacker's throat.

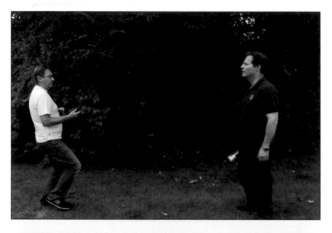
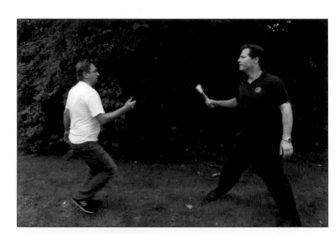

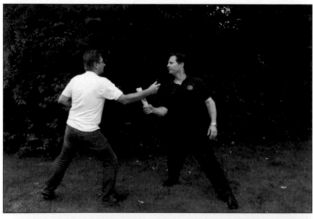
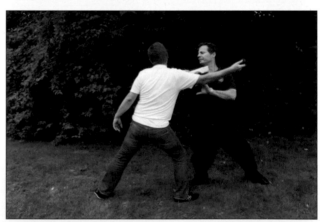

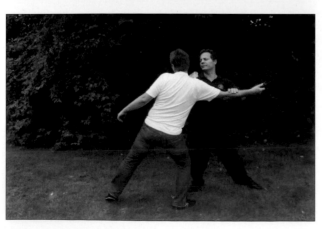
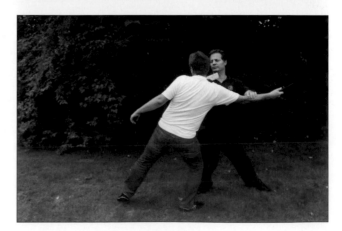

Defense with a knife against an attacker
holding his knife in a straight stab hold

1. The attacker is holding his knife with his right hand in front, ready to stab the defender. The defender is holding his knife in his right hand, hiding it behind his back.

2. The attacker is closing the gap with a stab, as the defender blocks it with a perpendicular slash to the attacker's wrist. The defender pivots his body,

reaching forward as far as possible pivoting his wrist in a counterclockwise motion to deflect the stab.

3. The defender continues to stab the attacker's throat with the same motion.

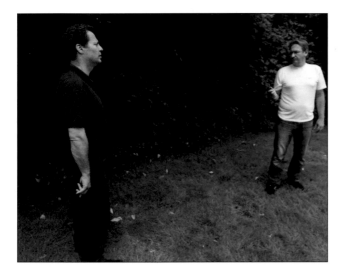

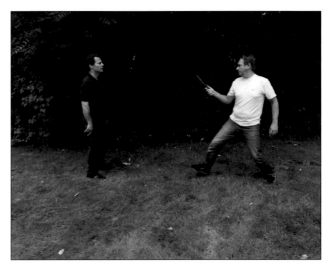

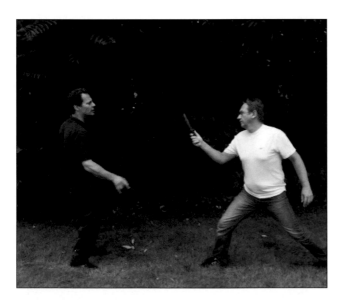

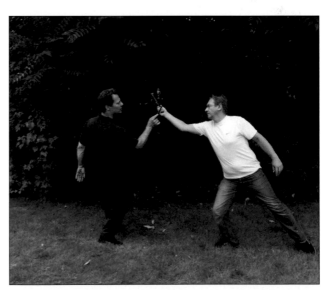

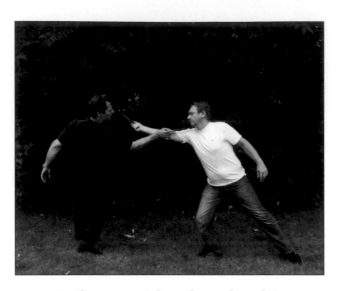
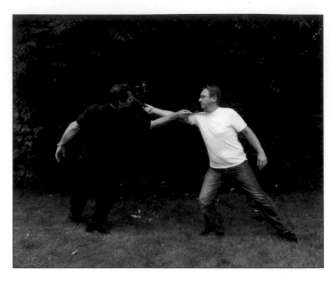

Defense with a handy object vs. an attacker slashing with a knife

1. The attacker slashes and the defender's torso leans backwards.

2. The defender retracts his body, pointing and sliding both hands forward and stabbing the attacker.

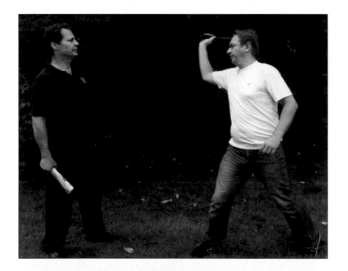
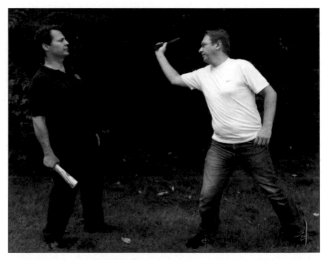

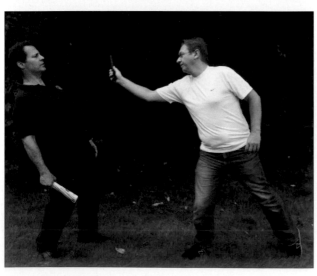
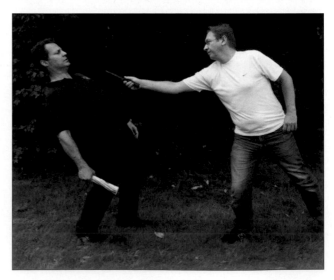

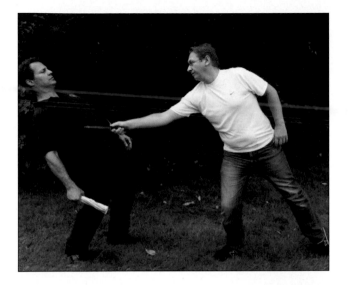
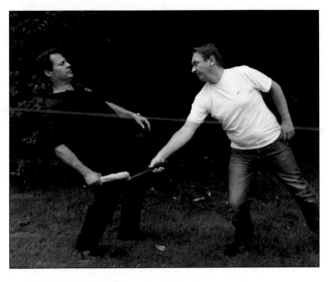
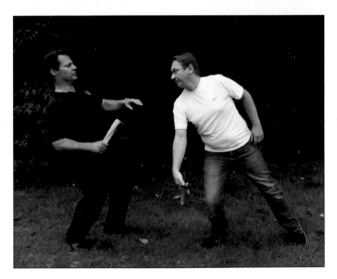
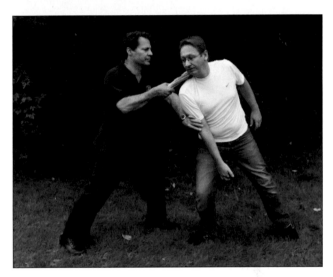

Note: Of all defenses vs. knife slashes, you need to know that the attacker is moving in for a reverse slash and knows how his body contortion propels him in such a way that it is hard to make him stop. Escaping the first slash, with his torso leaning backwards, will stop the first step, but moving in and counterattacking can be risky if you miss his throat with your stab. Go over all the above defense techniques and sort them out so you will have a backup plan if the first one fails. After all, even with weapons you still may need to resort to hand-to-hand fighting.

Knife Fighting

Besides the various defenses mentioned above, there are a few other hints to succeed in a knife fight where two opponents have a weapon and are ready to fight.

During defensive moves against a knife-armed attacker, I would recommend standing normally and not projecting your defense or attack. If you hold your knife in front of your body, you have more time to wait for your attacker, as your knife is closer to where you want to use it. However, by holding the knife to the side of your body, you are not projecting your potential and should only bring it up when the opponent closes in. When you bring it up, you need to immediately use it, otherwise your wrist becomes a target for your opponent's blade.

Try to stab the opponent's hand since it is the hardest to defend.

1. Both opponents stand in front of each other with a knife in their front hand.
2. Aim at the attacker's knife-holding hand.

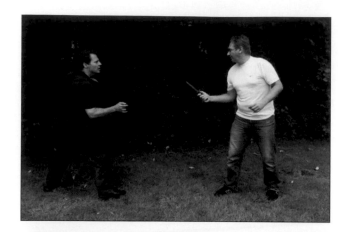
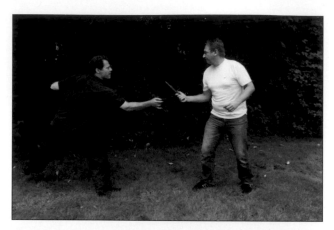

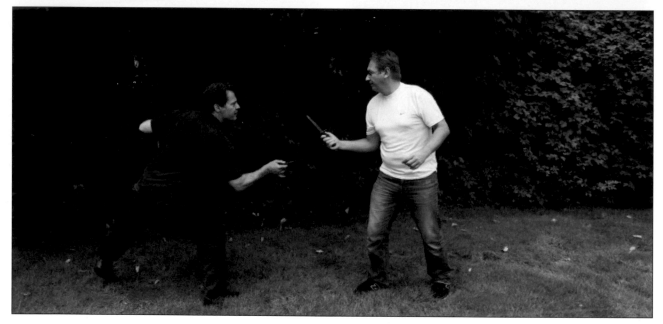

If he tries that on you, you may have to drop your weapon-holding hand down, while blocking his weapon-holding hand. Then stab him with your knife.

1. The attacker attempts to slash the defender's wrist that's holding the knife.

2. The defender drops the knife-holding hand lower to avoid being cut.
3. The defender blocks the attacker's hand with his free hand.
4. The defender lifts his hand, holding the knife back, and stabs the opponent in the throat.

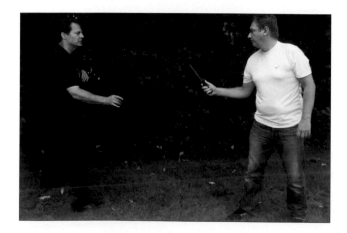
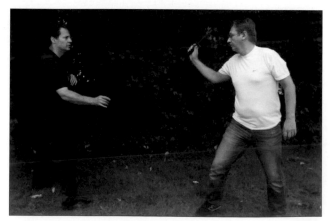

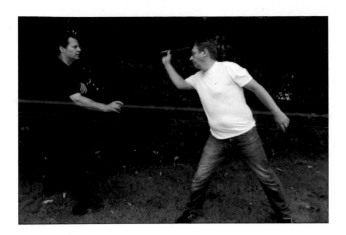 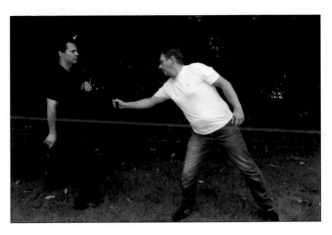

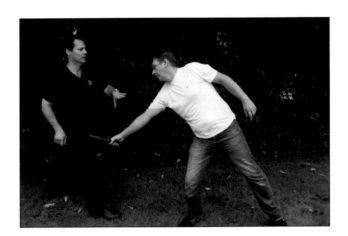 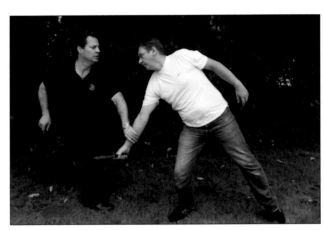

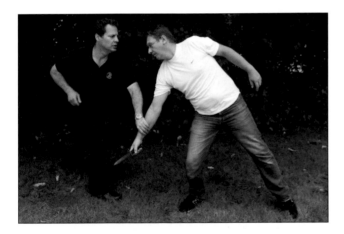 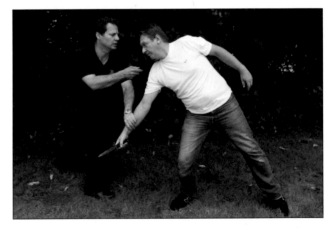

Note: There are double-edged practice knives made out of rubber that you can chalk-dye for fun practice. Use an old T-shirt, and use caution on your partner's eyes and throat. You could add protective eye, head, and neck gear.

Do not forget you have a second hand and a front leg for attack and defense. Use them as necessary. In practicing a knife fight, you basically practice your static defenses that you learned before in a dynamic movement. Try to keep it realistic.

As you practice "fighting," remember that you need a two-second reaction to any scenario, designed to end your opponent's mobility or life. The more time passes, the greater the risk to your life.

If Your Opponent Is Trained in Continuous Attacks

Obviously, all your leg counterattacks are intended to destroy. Kicking has the advantage of greater distance than a knife, providing greater reach. Timing is the second crucial factor in leg techniques. Since the attacker needs to close the gap before using his knife, defend yourself about halfway before he attacks.

Hand defenses against knives are based on timing as well. In some cases, you may need a second strike, where it is easier to reach a less vital point, or you may put all your energy in blocking a stab. Your hand defenses take into account that the attacker will try to stab again and again. The fact that you strike him at the same time prevents him from successfully passing the knife to his other hand after you have grabbed his wrist. You are trained to move in and grab his wrist as it retracts, but if it doesn't, position your body and hands in the same way to make it difficult for him to continue attacking you.

This reinforces the need to identify the first possible attack according to the attacker's body position and type of knife-hold. Once you have identified the swiftest motion your opponent can make, you only need to put your energy into your first defense. While your attacker is trained to perform a continuous attack, and is probably going to try and execute such, you will foil it all. You will therefore immediately cause a reversal of fortunes.

Knife Throw

Modern bayonets are well balanced and almost guarantee a kill when thrown by a sufficiently trained commando soldier. However, they are rarely expected to be used for that purpose. Instead, anyone who needs to know how to throw a knife gets intensive instructions and practice in this special need. As an IDF Krav Maga instructor, I've learned that modern bayonets can easily penetrate metal oil barrels I've used for practice.

However, when sitting in a dining room, it was the fork that got stuck to the wooden door rather than the butter knife. While almost any object thrown can provide a distraction, the killing power should be practiced to perfection if someone intends to make a habit of it. The quality of the knife should be considered as well. Some knives were well made for throwing and are easy to throw with very little training!

Principles of the Knife Defense

Mastering the principles of Krav Maga brings you to a state where you can better rely on your body and make split-second decisions that help you survive fights. Above all, remember that you do not fight with the techniques you practiced, but instead by applying the principles you have learned from the techniques. Realistic scenarios will require immediate solutions and with Krav Maga your mind and body would be ready with the appropriate response.

It is important to be a step ahead of your opponent, seeing as he has the same capabilities you do but as an aggressor. You need to learn to identify the danger and move fast, taking advantage of the short window of opportunity. Note that you have to do it while training your body in quick chain reactions.

Consider your opponent's capability in using straight attacks from a greater distance and circular attacks from a shorter distance.

If the starting point is from a greater distance, and your opponent has paused for a moment, you might have time to move your whole body and meet him halfway either with a kick or a hand defense.

If the attacker is lunging forward with a straight stab, start with throwing your forearm toward his wrist and pulling the rest of your body away. Land forward as you counterattack and then try to grab his wrist for further control and safety. At this point, you control his arm and he cannot use the blade against you. If your opponent is attacking with a straight stab, it would be faster for him to lunge with the blade forward than for you to move your body out of the way. Yet remember that with a straight stab stance, he can lunge and stab you from two to three steps away in a split second.

Stand still and just deflect his knife-holding wrist with the inside of your forearm by spinning it inward. Your arm motion will pull your torso at a horizontal forty-five degree pivot. Immediately after, deflect your opponent's wrist, and fall forward as you can plan your landing position while in motion. You can also grab his retracting hand at its exit point, not giving him the freedom of movement.

Remember that you are looking to strike him with your free hand at the same time. If, during training, your opponent or training partner knows what to expect from you, he will pull his arm behind his back so you cannot grab his wrist. Punching his face will foil any attempts to bring his arm back and try to poke you anywhere in your body. Obviously you can hit him lightly to buy yourself a second or two and then grab his arm. Or, you can hit him lightly again until you get control over the knife.

If you are caught by surprise from a short distance and you manage to see the motion of a hand, but you don't have time to determine whether the hand has a blade or not, your blocks should be instinctively directed to your opponent's wrists. You should counterattack with your free hand immediately after. If you see that your opponent is or might be holding a knife, you can kick and stop him before he plans to stab. For a straight stab, you should preferably go for a roundhouse kick to the groin. If he is lunging low, he would have to stand low a second before and would not have much of an option to continue after the one lunge since his body will land low. Still, it would be too dangerous to execute a roundhouse kick to his groin if the knife is at the height of your abdomen, as you can get stabbed in your thighs as you try to kick. You can use the same evasive body motion, skip the roundhouse kick and go for a side kick to his knee after he lands. This is also the follow-up step of the roundhouse kick if he is stabbing your throat.

Finally, you should plan your action if you see him holding the knife with his body ready to lunge. He could be shifting his weight from leg to leg and tossing the knife from one hand to another to baffle you, but if you attack him first, you will break his train of thought.

If your attacker is switching hands as he gets closer to you, make your move when you think you can reach him. If the knife hold is for a straight stab, wait for him to get to a range within reach. If his hold is for a circular stab, you can make your move earlier.

If you manage to see your opponent approaching from the side, give his knee a side kick while diving with your torso to under his extended arm. This is a good response to any kind of knife hold.

If he is holding his knife top down for a circular attack, go for a front kick to the groin, and if he is holding the knife bottom up to the side of his body then give his chin a front scissors kick. A final consideration is to pay more attention to where his knife is positioned in relationship to his body. If it is more to the side, it would be a circular attack, and if it is more in front of him then it would be a straight attack.

Although slashing is a circular motion, its advantage is use of the tip of the blade to give an extended length to the point of cutting away from the attacker's wrist. The motion of the wrist facilitates a looser, faster movement than the regular circular stabbing motion does. If the blade is hidden behind the attacker's back, just instinctively block his wrist if he swings his hand at you.

You just have no time to know what he has in his hand when you initiate your reaction and you are trying to aim your outer forearm to his wrist, in the same fashion as in a circular top-down hold attack. If he is holding the knife loose, expect a slash aimed at your throat and not your body.

You can lean your torso back and retract it landing on his forearm coming with the middle of your forearm on his arm continuing with a reversed slash while striking his face with your free arm. Blocking his immediate slash is not suggested as his loose grip can still send the blade into your throat as the force and speed of the slash will deflect your blocking hands. Direct kick to the knife-holding arm is possible in certain scenarios, but not suggested. However, never attempt a circular kick to the knife-holding hand, since you will never make it unless the attack is not challenging.

Remember that your opponent is using his hands to hold his knife. A hand is much faster than a leg. But from a longer distance, it is faster to reach with your leg as you use the leaping time to prepare your foot for an exact hit. At the same time your attacker can use his fast hand to damage your leg if he can see your intention before you close the gap. You need to time your kicks when he is not paying attention, or at the moment he starts to stab.

If the attacker is holding the knife top down in front, he needs to first get close to you and then stab you. You should plan your block and counterattack accordingly. Avoid exposing your body to the knife as you move to close the gap.

If the attacker is changing directions as you move in or as he moves in, keep in mind that it is important not to project your movement to ensure he is in an attack mode and not in defense mode.

If he is planning to change direction in the first stab, you could block it and counterattack. However, if he fakes the first stab, you block the air, and at the same time don't get stabbed. As your body follows your forearm while trying to grab his wrist, counterattack him with a punch. Your defensive position against a straight stab would not give him much opportunity for a follow-up stab.

If he starts with a fake circular stab to your clavicle, and then changes his aim to the side of your ribs, your kick to his groin should stop him on time. If you used your arm, you went to the top of his shoulder following his wrist and then pushed it in front of your body to help him complete the motion in front of you and not inside your ribs.

If he is lunging at you with a bottom-up hold and then changed course to a rib stab, get him before his hand leaves the side of his body. Your last resort is to execute an instinctive defense against the knife to the rib. But if you see his hand moving to a circular horizontal bottom-up hold, execute an instinctive defense against a rib stab. Be careful in the follow-up and avoid grabbing his whole arm, unless you manage to strike him first. His retracting hand might cut the inner side of your elbow.

If confronted with an opponent holding two knives, first you have to think about what options he has. Both of you can strike at each other, but he has not one blade, but two. This makes it easy for him to poke and cut you in the short range. However, in the long range, he would need to extend an arm and a shoulder to gain maximum reach, leaving his second hand behind and out of reach.

For the long range, if you are planning on kicking him, you need to consider only his front hand stab. If you use your arms, you need to consider a follow-up stab with your opponent's back hand that might need to be blocked if you don't manage to counterstrike him quick enough.

But your opponent, who might be trained with two knives, would rather wait for your kick or punch so he can respond poking your limbs . . . You need to try and catch him within a reasonable distance where it is not too early and definitely not too late.

If he is flailing his arms, it works to your advantage, taking into account the reaction time principles you have learned. In the end it is all about the timing. You need to break his train of thought immediately, not letting him stab with his second hand, by striking

one of his major pressure points—preferably in his face or head. Keep in mind that kicking will give him more time to try and stab your legs since it takes more time to shift the whole body than to extend a blade. If you kick ensure the direction of your kick is not in his immediate line of attack.

Combine the fight with a kick if you are in a two-step range and follow with a knife stab—straight or circular in the closer range—and then punch with your free hand and you have a challenging method for your training partner's practice.

So far, you have learned a few techniques and training methods. However, you need a little more training in a realistic setting in order to master knife defenses.

There are a few things you need to incorporate into your training. First, hone and distill Imrich's principles. You need to respond to your opponent's body positioning and apply the techniques selected according to the type of approach. For example, if an attacker stabs an under-hold with his knife in his front hand, then treat it like a front stab and execute the appropriate hand defensive technique.

If the attacker is stabbing straight and with his rear hand, then you have the time to treat it as a short range stab, and move your foot forward before your wrist. If the attacker is holding the knife in his front hand, then you need to treat it like a straight stab even if the tip of the knife is not pointed straight. Remember to approach the wrist from a more favorable side so as to not cut your forearm.

So if the opponent is holding his knife down to his body, and making advances in a slow or fast motion, and suddenly changes his grip , you need to go for his wrist. When you can reach it, hit his face or groin, whatever comes first. So, supposedly he feigned one attack, and you went for his wrist. If his wrist is not there anymore, then you have already punched him. As mentioned in the above techniques, you need to position your forearm after the defense motion in the best position to limit his next attack.

In your training, you need to reach the stage where your training partner is freely trying to continue and attack you, or fake an attack from any position possible. You need to follow the principles of identifying the most efficient approach your opponent has from his body positioning, which can change as he gets closer. Bottom line is, when he is close to you and he moves, you move in and deflect his last positioning and counterattack at the same time.

Remember, your training partner will probably try to cut you as he already knows where your hand is going, so you have to pay attention to the distance he keeps as he moves, and see if he is executing an actual attack or not. After a few trial and errors, you will be able to prioritize your motion according to the position of your wrist before he is in lunging range.

The direction of the blade, location of the knife-wielding hand, and distribution of your opponent's weight for a stab or cut should all be considered in judging his potential attack/defense capabilities and reaction time.

Knife Threat in a Vehicle

The following sequence of pictures is provided as extras with general instruction. There are scenarios in tight and limited spaces that may limit the motion of the defender and the attacker. Do the best you can. Prioritize according to your danger analysis.

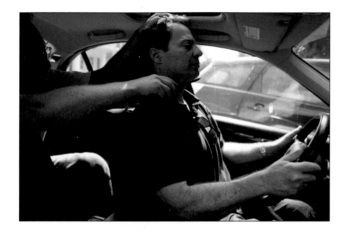
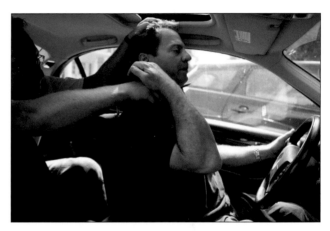

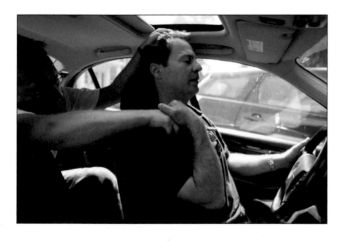
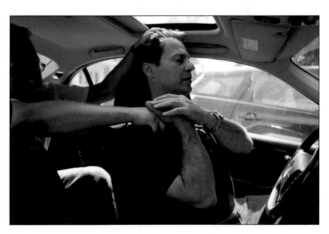

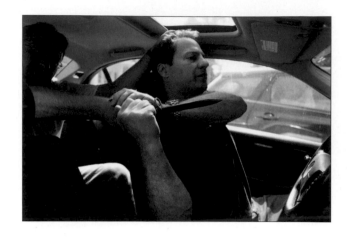
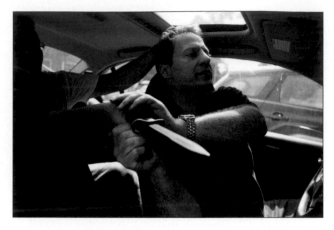
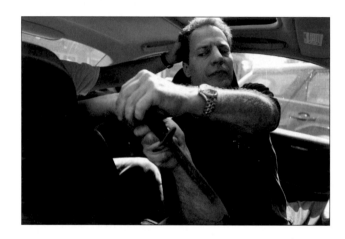
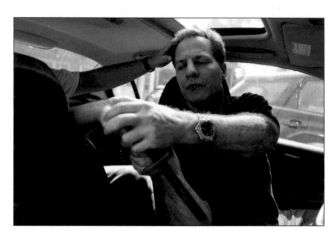
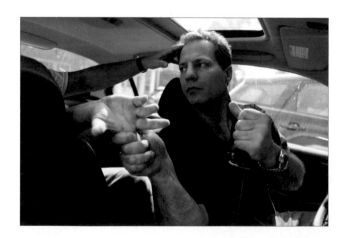
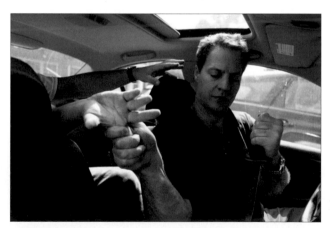

HANDLING PISTOL THREAT SCENARIOS

Your enemy's intent can range from robbery or execution to taking you hostage, but as long as your hands are free you must take your chance when you have it. Understanding reaction time is one of the major components of your defense. Your attacker's decision to shoot takes at least another split second. If he points a gun at you expecting you to do as he says, he is giving you a chance, which means you can initiate the next move. Even if he decides to execute you, he might hesitate for a second, perhaps to get a better aim, or perhaps to savor the moment.

Your job is to first move the barrel away from your body. You need to train your body to make the minimum movement with only your hand reaching the barrel and deflect it before you do anything else. You may swivel your body to point the barrel away from you if the gun is pointed at your back. You definitely do not want to stare at the gun, showing your intention to reach for it. That might make your attacker shoot you, being afraid that you will try to take it.

Take into account that your attacker is not going to give up his weapon. You will move in the direction of your attacker. If he tries to pull his hand back and aim again, you should have already gotten a grip on his weapon. Consider that he can use his free hand or his legs to strike or kick you as well. Once the barrel is not pointing at your body, follow immediately with a simultaneous counterattack. Finish by acquiring the weapon.

I will show you gunpoints at various angles with their respective defenses. However, if the angle and body position is slightly different, keep in mind the following advice where order of priority is concerned.

First, your mindset should be to use the short time you have without thinking too much about the dangers. If you do, you may be dead mid-thought. Second, you need to move the barrel away from your body without projecting your intention. If the barrel is poking your body, you may need to use your body to swivel away, or deflect the opponent's wrist instead. Third, you need to attack your opponent to buy time and gain control of the hand holding the weapon. I will show you a technique that will combine all your needs into continuous motions. You need to attack your opponent until you feel he loosens his grip and resistance. You can then extract the weapon out of his hand.

Fourth, you need to be conscious that the barrel is not pointed at any innocent bystanders if possible. And you need to be ready to use his weapon immediately, or use your body to handle additional attackers. If you do not, you may have wasted your time and your life.

And finally, after you have extracted the pistol, move away from the opponent so he will not be able to reverse your fortune again. Do not hesitate to shoot him if he tries to reach you. If his weapon does not function, you can still kick.

Your attacker may have other weapons in his possession. Be alert!

Defense against a Gunpoint from the Front with the Barrel Pointed at the Chest

1. Look forward at the attacker's face keeping as relaxed as possible, and raise your left hand, bringing your index finger underneath the barrel. Do not move the barrel. Practice this move until you are comfortable with the speed of execution.

2. From above, position your thumb and index as a cradle, and move your palm toward the opponent's line of the sternum, as if you were going to tap it. This quickly diverts the barrel away from your body, and makes it easier for you to close in and grab the pistol. Do not proceed and grab the barrel until the pistol hits your opponent's sternum. You do not want to slow down the barrel diversion by making a more complex move. Allow your body to pivot as you shift all your weight forward.

3. Grab the pistol. If you have lost your balance, shift forward and land on your front foot. Put all your weight on your front hand, keeping the attacker's hand down. Use your hand and weight to keep the barrel pointed to the ground away from your body. At the same time, strike your opponent in his face with your right fist.

4. Once your opponent does not resist or falls down, bring your right hand close to your body so you do not cross the line of the barrel. Put it as a tray under your left hand, grabbing the hammer of the pistol and pulling it toward you.

5. At the same time, your left elbow will be pushing his arm to extract the pistol out of his hand. Be careful not to break his finger, as this will reduce the possibility of another shot being fired.

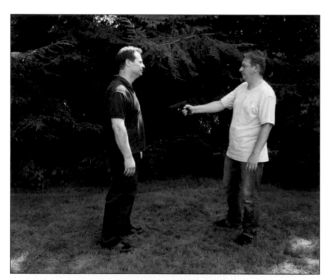 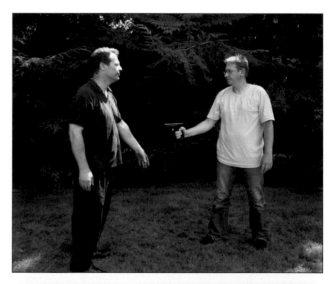

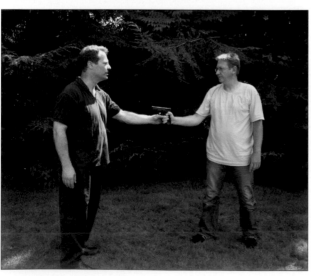 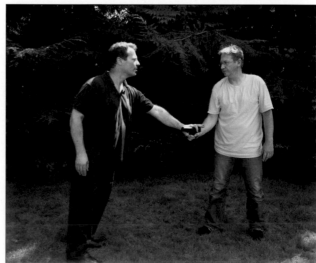

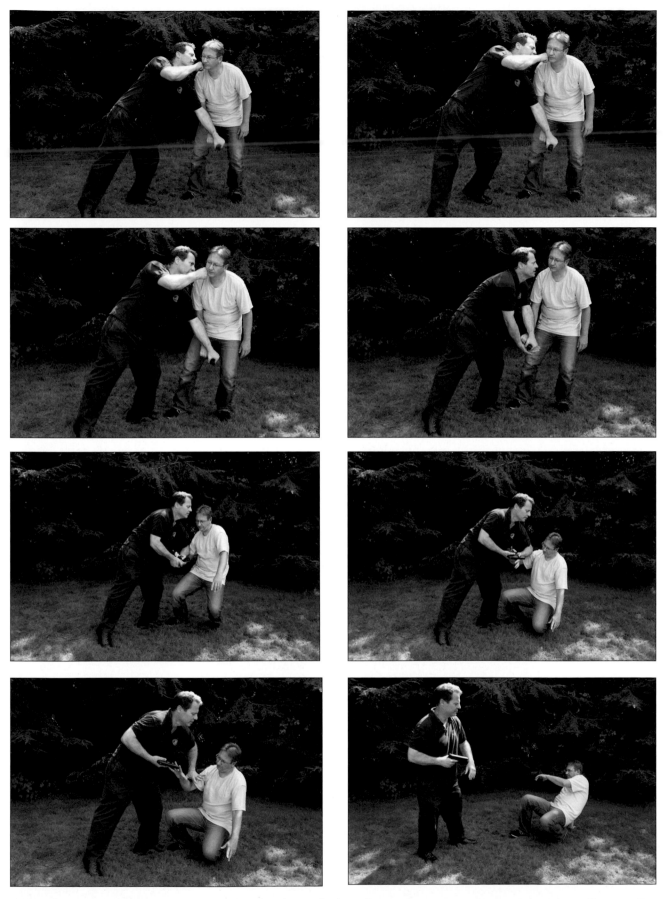

Note: Ask your training partner to pull and redirect the barrel toward you to make it more realistic for you. For training purposes you can hit his front shoulder a few times to loosen his concentration on his grip of the weapon.

Defense against Gunpoint from the Front with the Barrel Pushed into the Forehead

From this position, you should hope your opponent will tell you to raise your hands up, since it takes longer to bring them from your waist to the opponent's wrist. Do not complain if you are not asked to raise your hands up. Start your motion by violently tilting your neck away from the barrel. Never move both hands toward the barrel at once, since you are making your intentions obvious to your attacker, slowing down your motion and your ability to move your body away.

1. The attacker points a pistol at the defender's forehead.
2. The defender violently tilts his neck towards his left shoulder.
3. The defender raises his left hand and taps the attacker's wrist. At the same time, the defender's head leans to the left, followed by his body moving forward. (This is preferable and more comfortable than grabbing the barrel and having to lean backwards).

4. The defender slides his left hand along the attacker's wrist and forearm, moving his head with it. This will also ensure a less loud noise if a shot is dispensed. The defender is hooking the weapon with his right arm, by tapping the attacker's shoulder and then sliding his hand on the attacker's arm, until his wrist gets hooked to the defender's chest. Executing a simultaneous strike to the opponent's groin is a matter of judgment in this scenario. You want to buy time and ensure he would not attack you with his free hand, but at the same time you want to immediately hook the weapon.
5. The defender executes a counterattack with his left hand.
6. The defender's left arm, fingers pointed down, hand turned clockwise reaches for the weapon's barrel. The defender extracts the weapon by breaking the barrel down.
7. The defender proceeds to strike the opponent's temple with the barrel of the pistol.

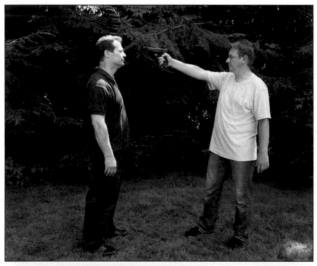

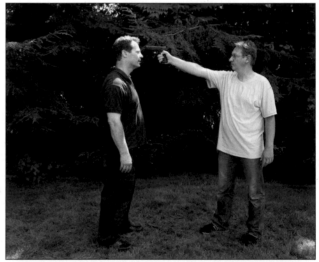

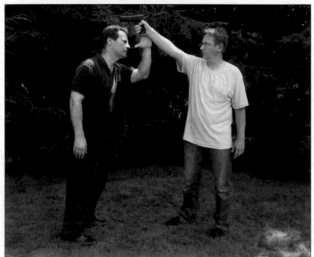

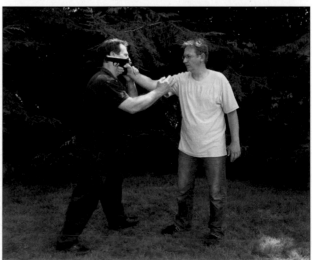

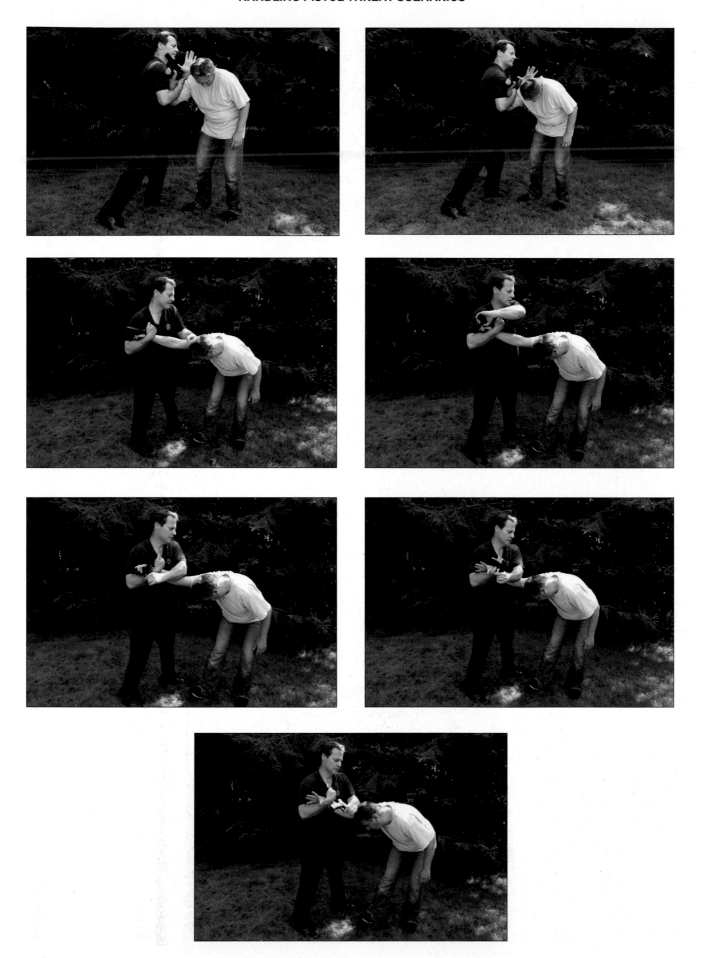

Defense against a Front Barrel Pushed into the Side of the Stomach

Note: In this scenario you will need to deflect the opponent's wrist instead of the barrel.

1. The attacker shoves his pistol barrel low into the defender's abdomen.
2. With the defender's palm, thumb and fingers down, deflect the attacker's wrist while the defender pivots his body to get away from a possible redirection of the barrel.
3. To secure the barrel and avoid a redirection, defender steps in diagonally forward, and joins his right hand palms forward and thumb and fingers down to grip the weapon.
4. The defender pivots his body forward, hitting the attacker's abdomen with the weapon's barrel.
5. The defender continues to turn his hands and body and peel the weapon out. However, there is a great possibility that the attacker has already been shot from the impact or been hit by the barrel and has loosened his grip, which makes extracting the pistol possible on the spot.

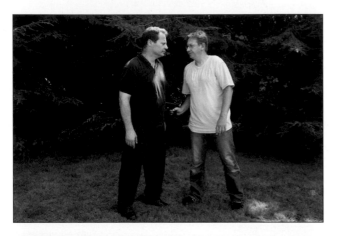

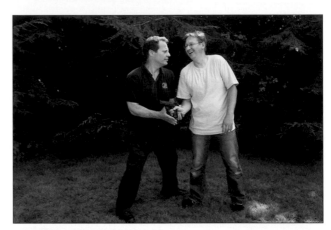

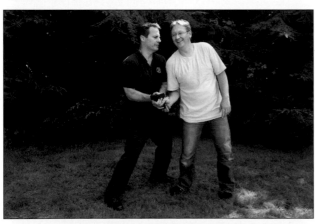

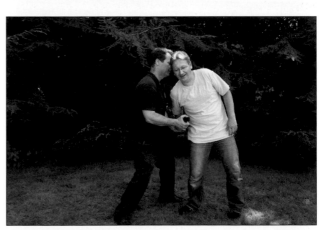

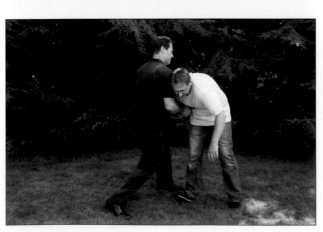

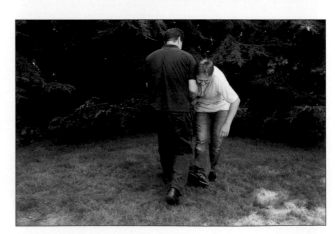

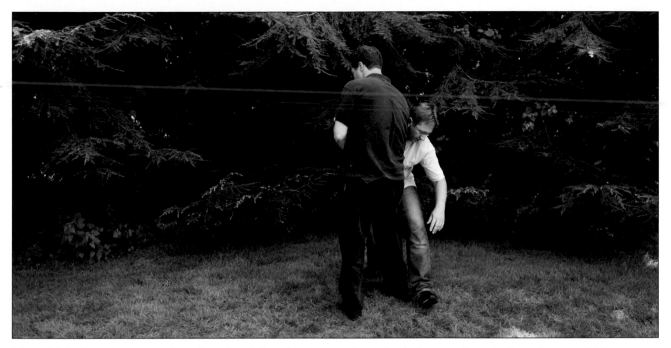

Note: If the barrel is pointed to the side of the ribs close to the defender's arm, the initial motion would be executed with the defender's forearm to push the gun away and grab the pistol with both hands.

Defense against Gunpoint from the Rear with the Barrel Pushed into the Back (inside turn)

The defensive reaction here must start with a body motion, since hands cannot reach. Moving the body takes more time than just moving the hand. To be safer, tell your mind that you will face your opponent with your body in a split second and just face him. This will tune your mind to control the complex pivoting motion. In fact, your feet will push off the ground just enough for a full turn jump and you will face your opponent while the barrel is left to the side of your body (do not try to contact the barrel with your forearm before you complete the turn).

1. The attacker points a pistol poking into the defender's back.
2. The defender pivots the barrel away, leaning toward the opponent.
3. The defender strikes the opponent in the face while his left arm makes a hook motion, reaching the opponent's armpit and ensuring the range of motion is covered entirely in case the opponent attempts to retract and redirect the weapon. The counterattack and hooking of the weapon are done simultaneously here.
4. The defender elbows the attacker's chin. (Note that if the attacker is not subdued, you can grab his shirt and knee him as well. The general rule is to continue attacking while the gun is under control until the attacker loosens his resistance.)
5. The defender's right arm, fingers pointed down, hand turned counterclockwise, reaches for the weapon's barrel.
6. The defender extracts the weapon by breaking the barrel down.
7. The defender proceeds to strike the opponent's temple with the barrel of the pistol.

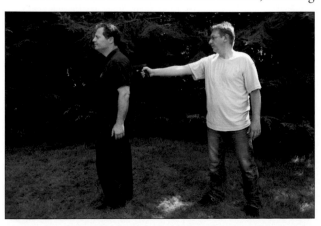

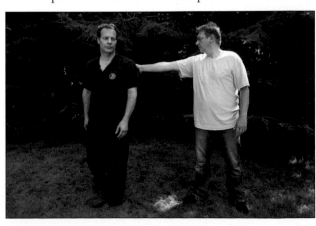

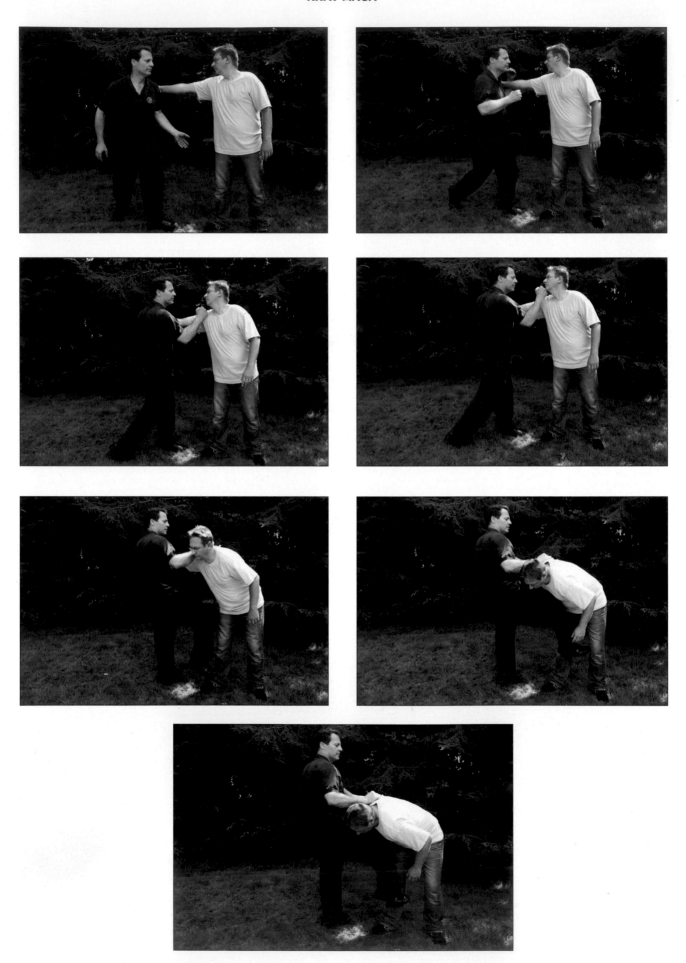

Defense against Gunpoint with the Barrel Pushed into the Back (outside turn)

Note: The defender should turn in the direction facilitating the shortest move. If the barrel is pushed closer to your right shoulder and you are standing with your left foot in front, you should turn right.

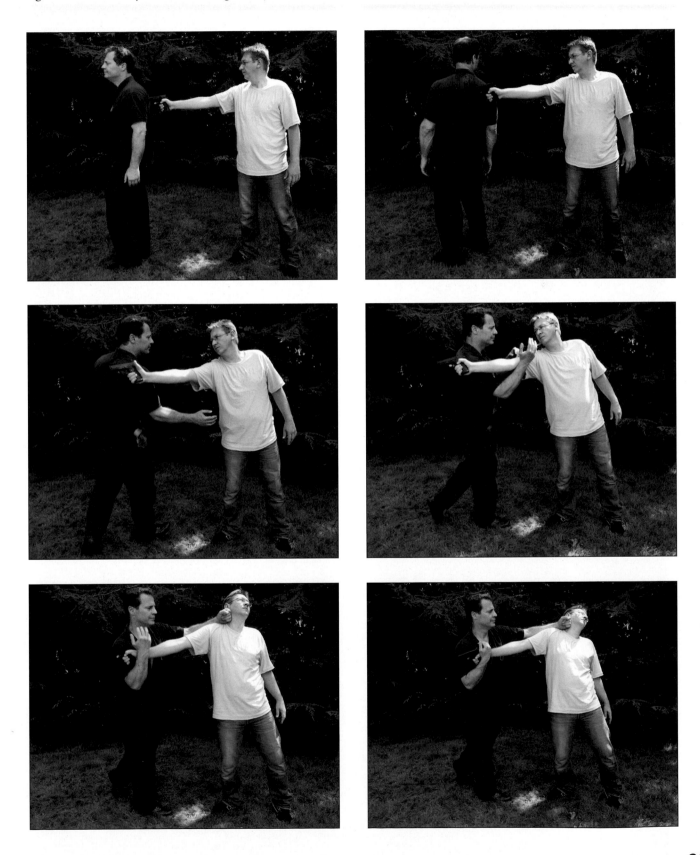

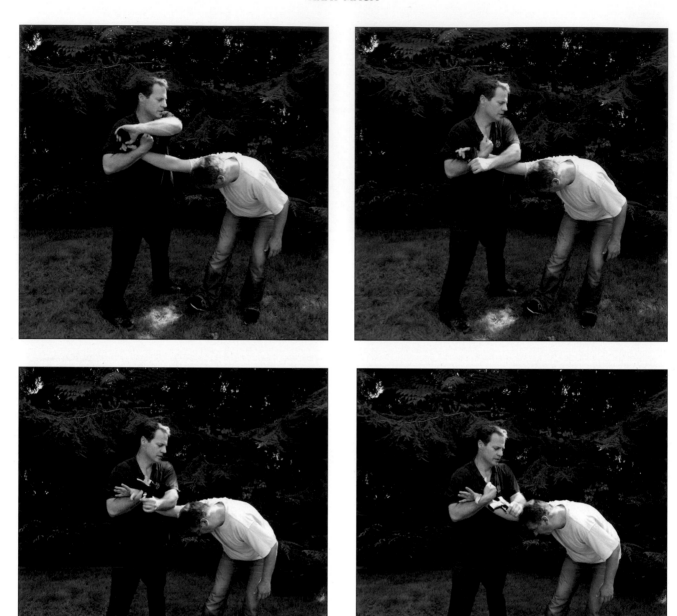

Defense against Gunpoint with the Barrel Pointed to the Back of the Head

1. The attacker points his pistol barrel into the back of the defender's neck. The defender's initial motion is to violently tilt his head toward his shoulder to ensure the barrel is not pointed at his head.
2. The defender slides his neck on the attacker's arm and falls on the attacker to get his ear away from the gun.
3. The defender executes an open hand strike to the opponent's groin.
4. The defender hooks the attacker's weapon-holding hand.
5. The defender strikes the attacker's head.
6. The defender moves to extract the pistol, grabbing it with his thumb pointed down, and extracting it by flipping his thumb up.

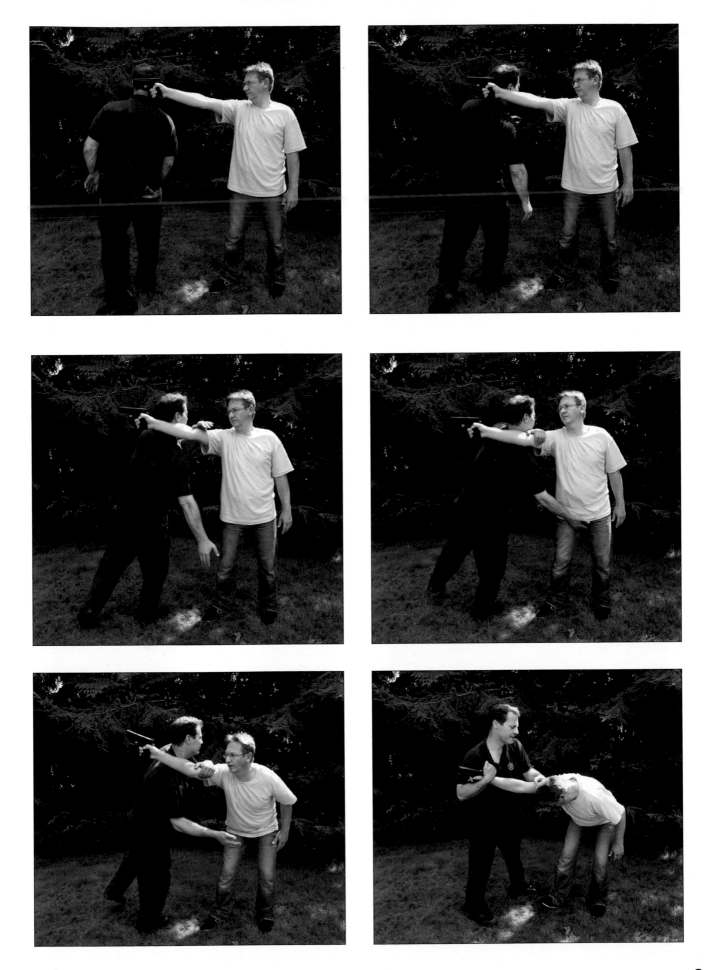

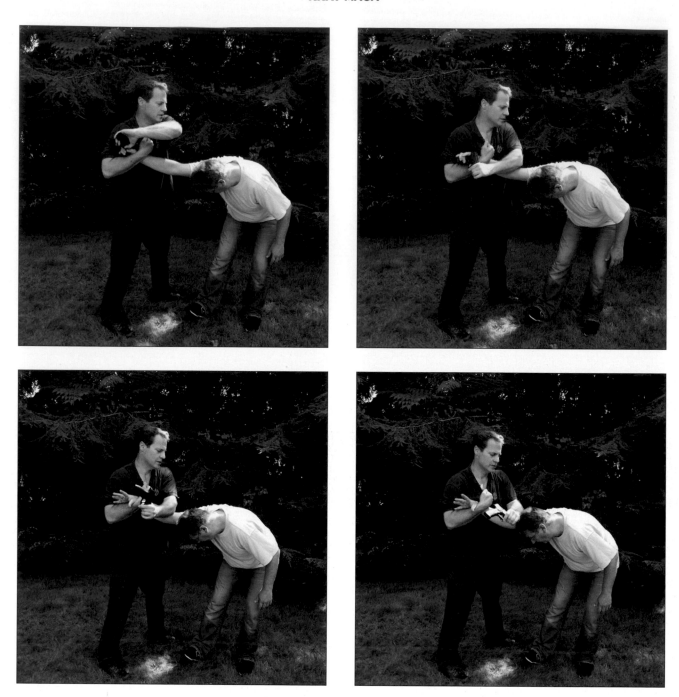

Note: In reality, you may decide on fewer counterattacks if they are not necessary.

Defense against Gunpoint with the Barrel Pushed to the Temple from the Side

There are two options to use according to your judgment.

1. The attacker points the pistol to the defender's left temple.
2. The defender ducks his head forward and lunges toward the attacker, hooking the pistol with his left hand and striking him in the groin with his right.

3. The defender elbows the attacker's chin.
4. The defender proceeds to extract the pistol with his thumb down. See "defense against pistol threat from the rear" for further steps.

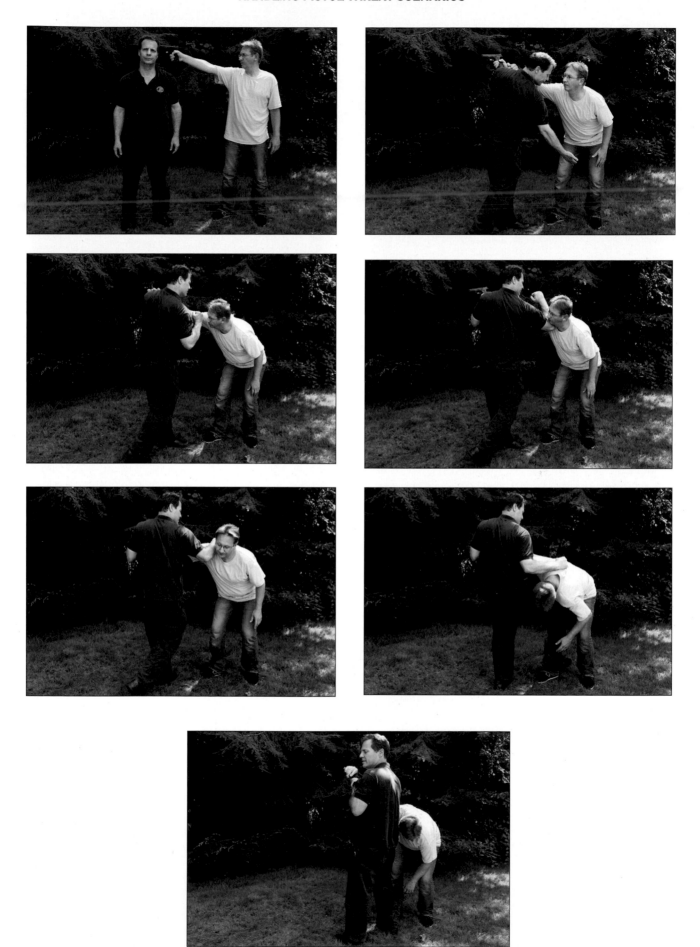

Second option

1. The attacker points a pistol to the defender's left temple.
2. The defender violently ducks his head down, pulling his upper body with it and looking upwards at the attacker's hand.
3. The defender executes an outside defense to the attacker's wrist, keeping his thumb down.
4. The defender turns left and grabs the attacker's forearm with the same hand.
5. The defender strikes the attacker in the face with his right hand.
6. The defender joins his right hand under the attacker's elbow, grabbing the hammer area of the pistol.
7. The defender extracts the pistol.

Defense against a Head Hold with the Left Hand Combined with a Pistol Threat to the Right Temple

The following scenario usually involves a loose head hold from the back and then a cold barrel on your temple.

Hopefully the attacker would be reluctant to shoot you since the bullet can exit your head and enter his arm. This may buy you another second.

1. The attacker grabs the defender's mouth and points the barrel to the defender's temple from the back.
2. The defender violently moves his head back, while turning it sideways away from the barrel, and hooking his right hand fingers and thumb onto the attacker's pistol-holding wrist and pulling it to his shoulder.
3. The defender joins his left hand to grab the opponent's pistol-gripping hand with both hands, palm facing the pistol.
4. The defender pivots to the right, reinforcing the leverage on the pistol-holding hand, pivoting both hands counterclockwise and forward to extract the pistol.

Note: You must first concentrate your efforts on moving your head away from the barrel and then hooking the barrel in front of your shoulder. Then you need to proceed to escape the hold and extract the weapon.

Defense against Gunpoint from Front in Sitting Position

1. The attacker points the barrel into the defender's forehead as the defender sits on the ground.
2. The defender hooks the barrel in an upward motion with his thumb and index fingers, ducking his head to the opposite side and leaning forward.
3. The defender brings his right hand to grab the pistol in the hammer area.
4. The defender is pulling on the right hand, keeping the barrel away from his body with his left hand.
5. The defender extracts the pistol with his body weight.
6. The defender is prepared to get the weapon in a shooting grip.

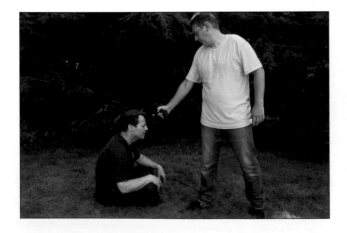 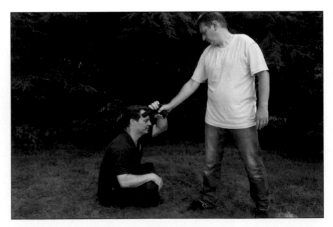

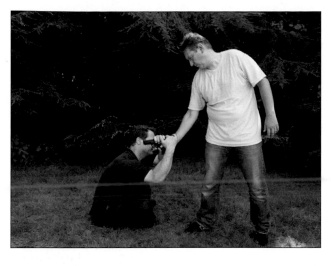

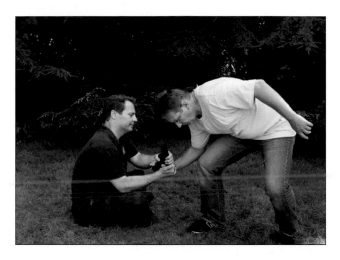

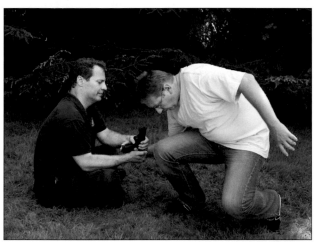

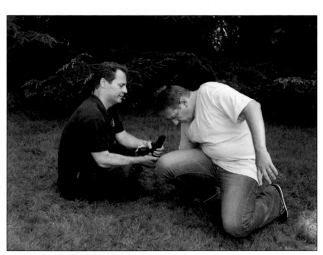

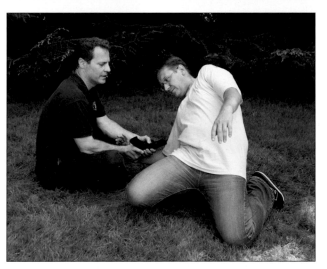

Note: If the attacker is much heavier than the defender and tries to retract the gun and pull the defender up, the defender may need to counterattack from a standing position. This is not a problem since the defender has enough weight to leverage the attacker's fingers and extract the pistol before being pulled. As a general rule of thumb, try to land on your back after grabbing the pistol if there are other armed attackers in the area. In hostage scenarios, you will be more protected on the ground this way. From this position, you can shoot in any direction. In addition, it is preferable to fall backwards after getting a grip on the pistol, keeping the barrel away from your body and pushing your legs forward to keep your opponent away from you.

Defense against Rear Gunpoint in a Sitting Position

1. The attacker points a pistol at the back of the defender's head while the defender is sitting on the ground.
2. The defender hooks up the barrel with his thumb and index fingers pointing up behind his neck, ducking his head underneath the gun and leaning back.
3. The defender hooks down the opponent's wrist with his free hand and uses both hands to point the barrel away from the direction of his body. His best option is to lean all his weight on the opponent's wrist and swivel his body, lying on the ground and facing him. If the pistol is extracted before the completion of the turn, there is still no harm done.
4. The defender extracts the pistol out of the attacker's hand (if you are sitting down, gravity gives you more force on your grip than if you are standing up).

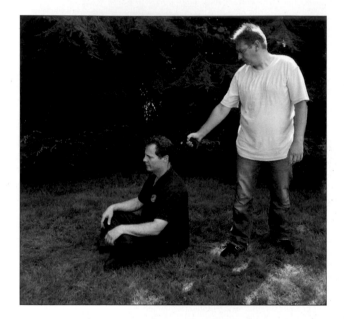

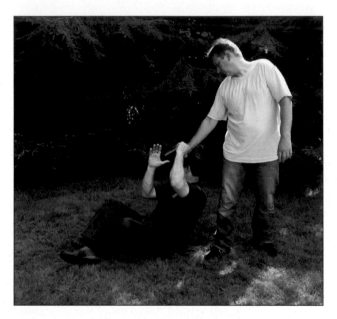

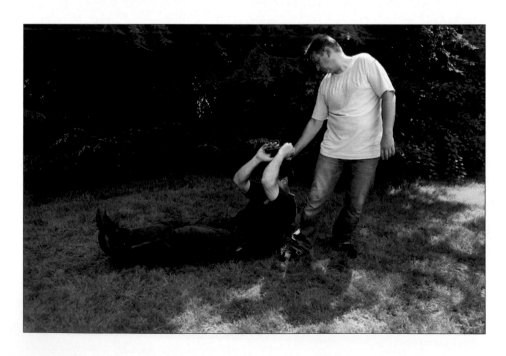

When the Opponent Is Not Near But It's Worth a Shot

If an attacker is a few feet away, you can drop to the ground with a front break fall, hoping he will miss. You can then roll over if you find cover nearby. If he is closer, you can just roll forward and kick him as in the defense vs. chain in Chapter 7. If he is still not close enough, you can continue with a second roll. Sounds crazy? Yes and no. If he needs another second to re-aim and if he is not the greatest shooter, you could save your life.

You can try throwing your keys at him and moving diagonally away from the line of fire, following with a roundhouse kick. The flying object may cause him to retract his hand in a defense move and you can shoot when the barrel is not pointed at you.

You can also roll over and lift him for a throw. He would need his hands for balance and would not be able to re-point the weapon at you. See the chapter on military applications against assault rifles pointed at a group taken hostage. You can of course gamble and wait for him to get closer.

If you turn your head over your shoulder and the attacker points a gun at your back, try to deflect his wrist and move back toward him. Grab his body for a lift off the ground, then throw him on his face.

On a final note, the technique might not be always exactly the same due to differences in height and positioning. But you must strive to respond with the most efficient and effective manner and appropriate counterattack to control your opponent.

Tight Scenarios in Vehicles

The following series of pictures were intended to demonstrate how to use your judgment in tight spaces that limit your movements. Use your knowledge from prior chapters, analyze the dangers and put your priorities in the correct order.

Attacker is in the passenger seat

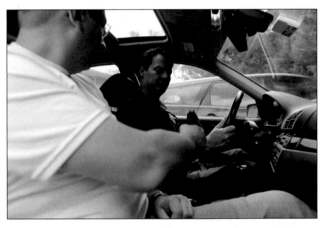
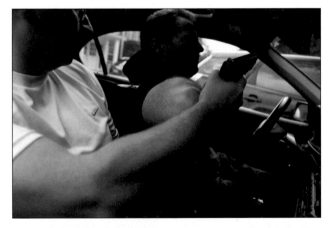

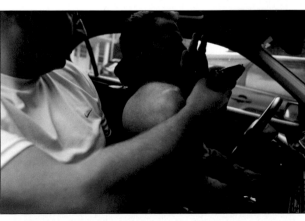
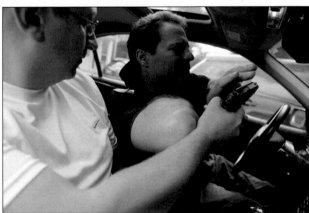

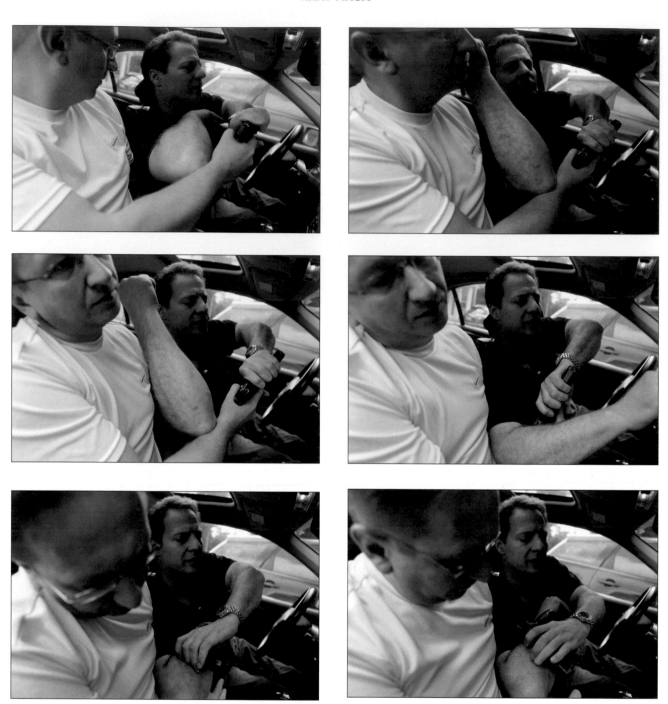

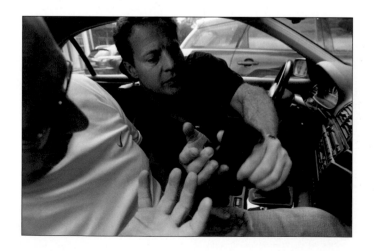

Attacker is in the back seat behind the driver

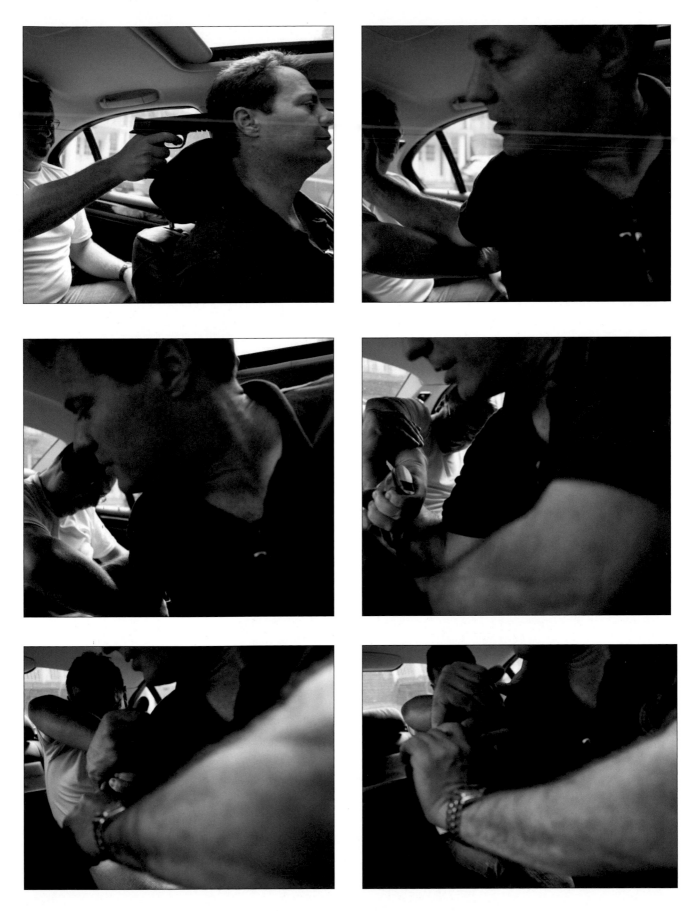

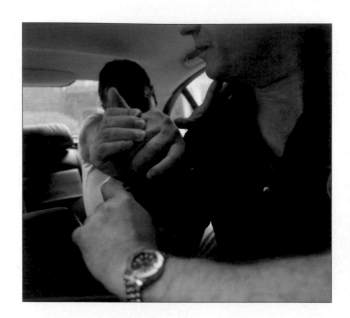
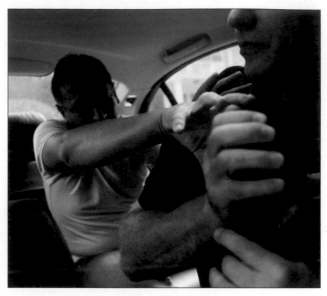

Attacker is in the middle back seat behind the driver

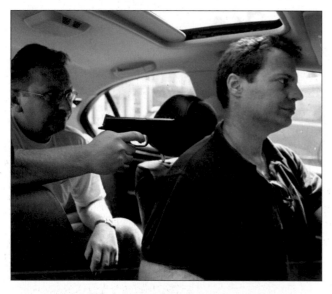
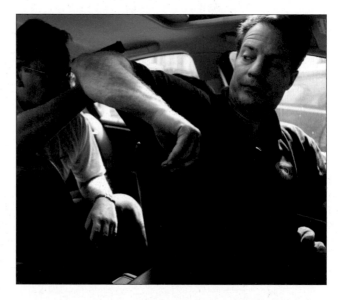

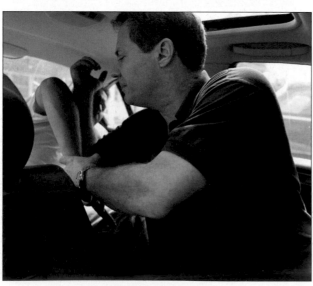
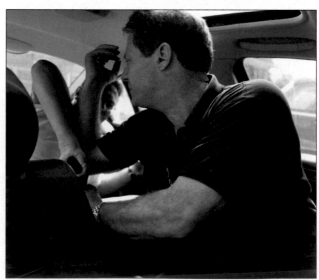

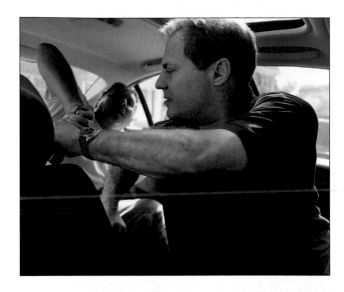

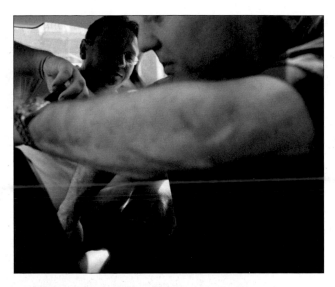

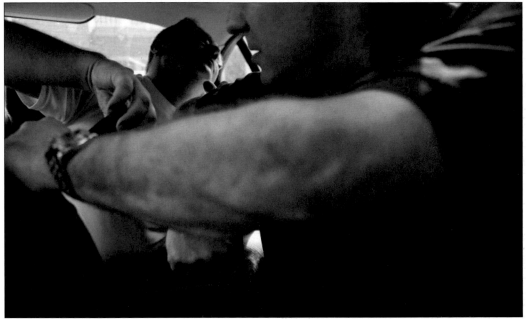

Attacker is in the backseat behind the passenger's seat

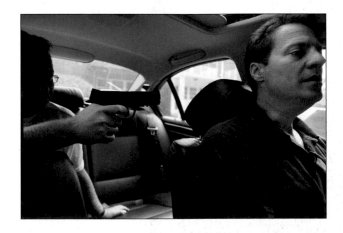

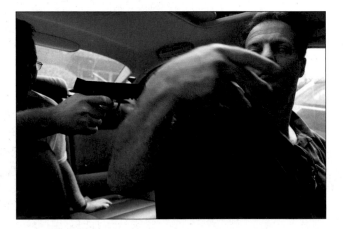

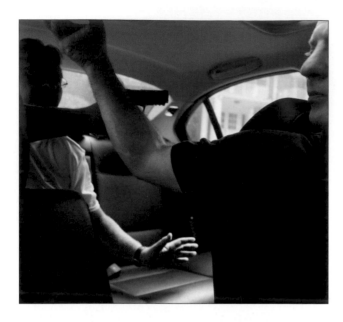

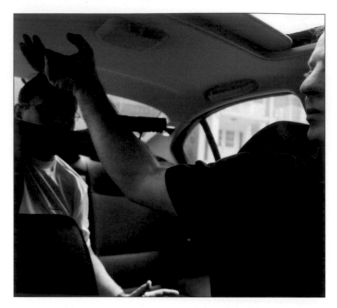

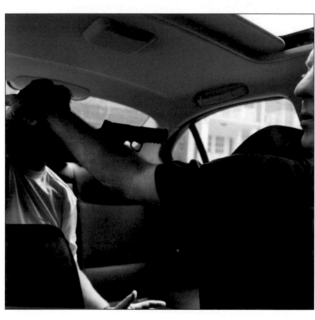

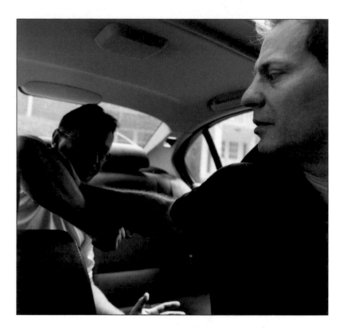

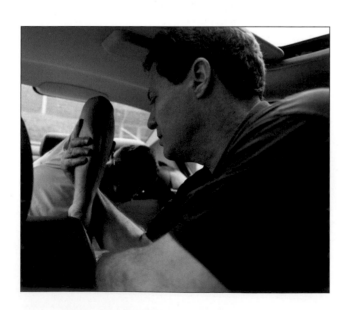

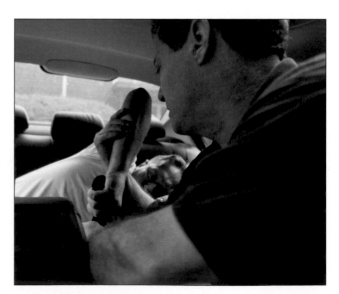

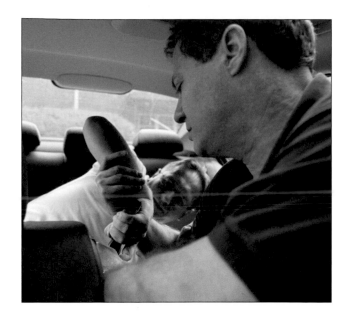

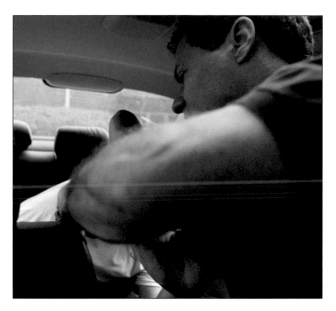

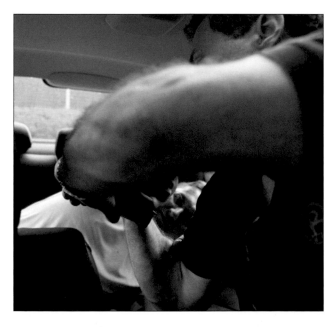

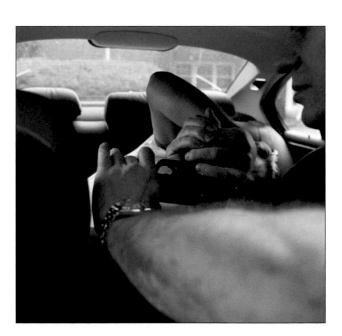

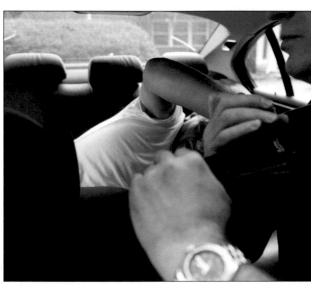

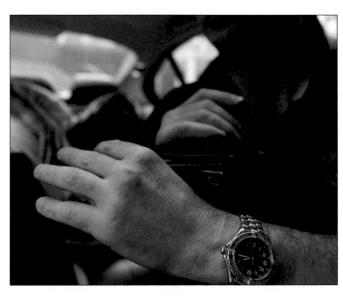

I would recommend using a BB pistol or another type of training device and trying various times in a confined environment, like the inside of a car. Since your movement is limited, you need to stick to the principles and verify that you do not get shot at while your training partner is attempting to increase the challenge and wrestle with you.

Applications for Uniformed Armed Personnel and Civilians

This chapter, while used for Special Forces mostly for hand-to-hand combat scenarios, is also applicable for training civilians to handle kidnapping situations and bar brawls in a civil manner.

Using an Assault Rifle as a Sidearm

These techniques are useful if you get caught in a close combat and you have used up your last bullet or your gun has just stopped functioning. The enemy is right near you, and you can't expect him to patiently watch you try to fix your weapon.

Another scenario: You are stationed to patrol a civilian area, and the crowd is trying to attack you with a knife or get the rifle out of your hands. If an attacker grips one side of your rifle, you can try to use the other tip to create leverage, or to strike him. If he grabs your weapon with both hands, use his pull to kick his groin.

Finally, this lesson will bring your intelligence in using any object to your advantage up to par. Objects such as your briefcase or a barstool can be used as a weapon or a shield. Some of the strikes discussed below are demonstrated in the Club and Chain chapter, using a club instead.

Barrel/bayonet stab or butt strike

1. The soldier stands with his barrel pointed at an enemy soldier.
2. The soldier lunges forward, stabbing his enemy with his barrel (remember to bring your rifle back to your body with the same motion). The stab can be directed at the attacker's throat, abdomen, or heart.
3. The attacker approaches the soldier from his left side.
4. The soldier stabs the attacker with his barrel over his left shoulder.
5. The attacker is approaching the soldier from his right side.
6. The soldier is using the butt of his rifle to hit the attacker over his right shoulder.
7. The soldier notices the attacker coming in from behind him.
8. The soldier strikes the attacker with the butt of his rifle backwards.

Butt strike forward, slash and uppercut

1. The soldier delivers a roundhouse strike with the butt of his rifle.
2. The soldier is delivering a slash strike with the barrel of his weapon directed at the carotid artery (note that the same motion can be used to slash opponent's throat if you have a bayonet.) This move can be used as defense against another soldier who tries to stab you with his barrel. Continue the defensive slash with a straight stab to his throat.
3. The soldier delivers an uppercut strike with the rifle butt pointing upward.

Clip strike forward with a front kick

1. The enemy soldier approaches in a close range, not leaving enough room for the soldier to extend his rifle forward.
2. The soldier strikes his enemy with a magazine strike to his face. This magazine strike has proven to knock people to the ground easily. You can also start with a front kick and as you close the gap, finish with a magazine strike.

Note: Use this technique only if you have no choice, as modern military magazines can be jammed with a direct hit. If the immediate close motion would save your life, heck with the magazine.

Uppercut butt strike to the groin
Evasive rollover with a barrel stab

1. The attacker reaches and grabs the soldier's barrel.
2. The soldier attacks with his rifle butt to the attacker's groin.

Note: Rifle strikes are similar to club strikes. Refer to club strike pictures in this book to get a clearer understanding.

Rollover on the butt of the rifle if you detect a knife attack from behind you.

This you need to practice. It will help you in a quick evasive move from one point to another, if you feel your knees are shaking.

1. The attacker, armed with a knife, approaches the soldier from the back.
2. The soldier notices at the last second and rolls over forward.
3. The soldier gets up and faces the attacker.
4. The soldier stabs the attacker with the barrel (if your safety is not on, you may have shot him instead).

Defense Against a Bayonet Stab

When we teach this topic, we give students two options for a beginning stance. One is common as the soldier stands or walks with his rifle hanging on a sling, parallel to his body. The other is when the soldier runs with his barrel pointed forward.

Defense against a bayonet stab with a rifle butt strike

1. The soldier stands with his weapon parallel to his body and the attacker prepares to stab him with his rifle's bayonet or barrel.
2. The soldier blocks the stab with the middle of his rifle by swiveling it from a horizontal to a vertical level deflection. The soldier moves diagonally away from the attacker's barrel.
3. The soldier executes a counterattack, slashing his barrel at the opponent's carotid artery.
4. The soldier follows with a butt roundhouse strike to the opponent's head.

Defense against a bayonet with the barrel of a rifle

1. The soldier runs with his barrel pointed forward as the attacker confronts him with the same stance.
2. The soldier uses the tip of his barrel to deflect his opponent's barrel with a slashing motion.
3. The soldier follows with a barrel stab to the opponent's throat. This technique is demonstrated in the Club and Chain chapter with a club.

Note: If the attacker is trying to hit you with his rifle from other directions, use your knowledge of club and stick defenses. Soldiers should use their assault rifles as if they're clubs, utilizing the unique shape of the assault rifle.

Defense against an assault rifle threat from the front (or bayonet and rifle butt strike) with bare hands from the left

1. Assuming the attacker is right-handed, he steps forward to stab the defender with the bayonet attached to his rifle. The same technique is used if you are taken as a hostage with an assault rifle pointing at you.
2. The defender, leaning forwards in a fall motion, uses his left palm to deflect the barrel away to his right hip, and pivots clockwise, away from the barrel's direction.
3. The defender then lands on his left foot about forty-five degrees away from the attacker. His hold of the barrel switches from his left hand to his right hand. At the same time, his left hand grabs the rifle around the trigger, reaching with the soft part of the forearm in case the attacker goes for a butt strike.
4. The defender pulls the rifle with both his hands and leans his torso backwards, to help the attacker finish a roundhouse butt swing. This stops the attacker from continuing and gives the defender the advantage of being one step ahead of the game.
5. The defender kicks the attacker's groin while using the weapon for balance.
6. The defender turns to the left, sharply extracting the rifle out of the attacker's hands.

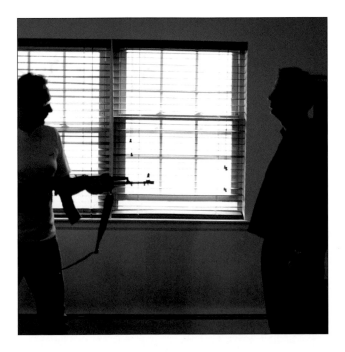
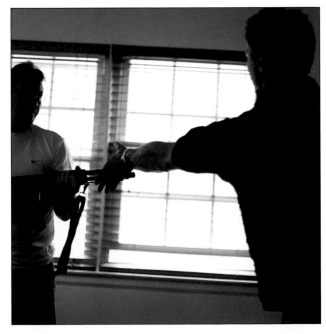

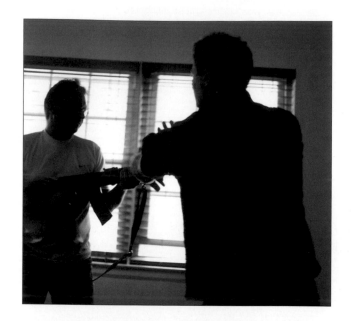

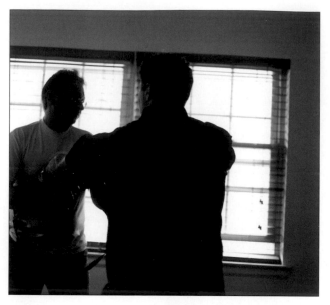

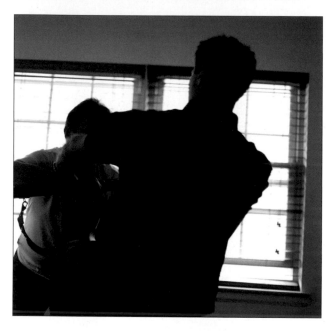

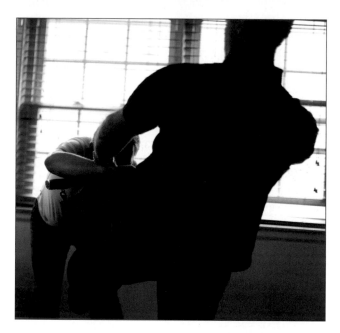

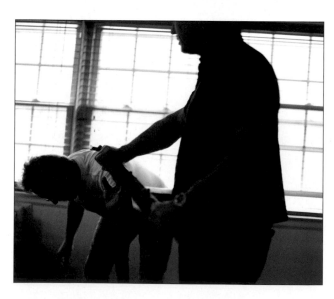

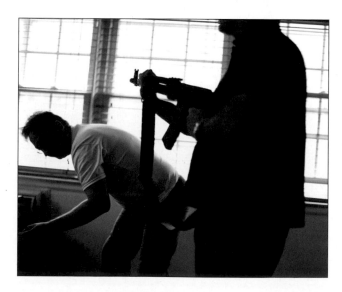

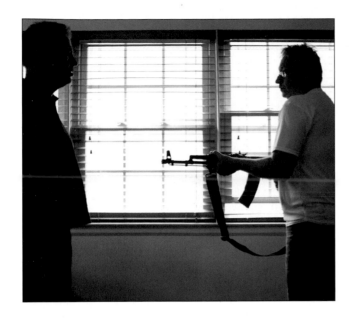

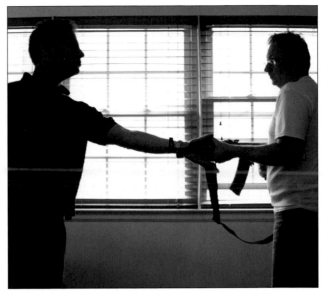

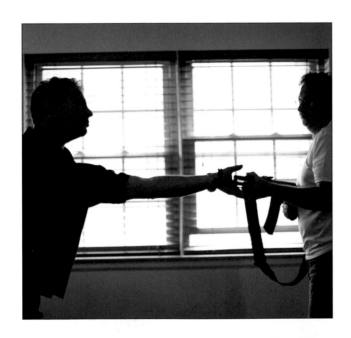

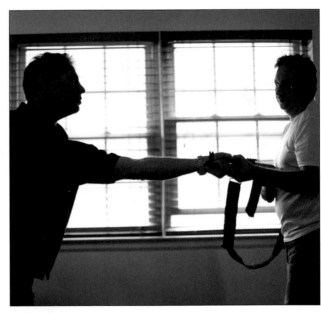

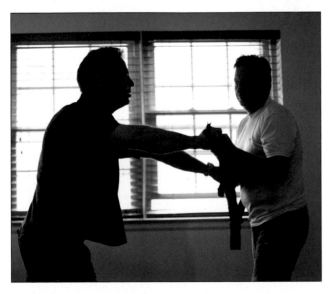

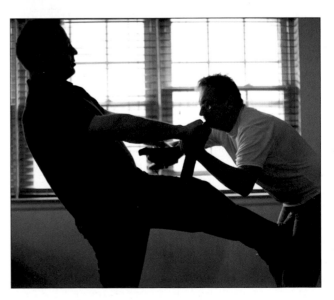

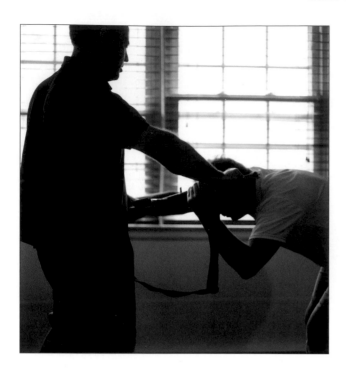
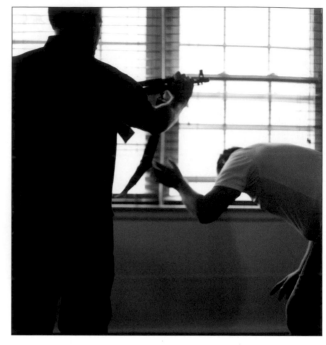

Defense against an assault rifle threat from the front (or from the bayonet) to the right

1. Assuming the attacker is right-handed, he steps forward to stab the defender with the bayonet attached to his rifle or is holding the defender at gunpoint.
2. The defender uses his right palm to point the barrel to his left hip while moving forward and switching the barrel's grip to his left hand.

3. The defender pulls the barrel behind his back and delivers a slightly angled front kick to the attacker's groin.
4. The defender continues to hit the attacker over his head with a hammer strike.
5. The defender grabs the assault rifle with his free hand around the trigger area.
6. The defender extracts the weapon out of the attacker's hands by pivoting sharply to the left.

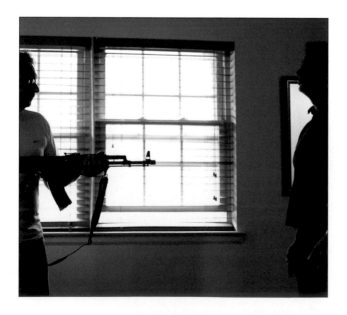
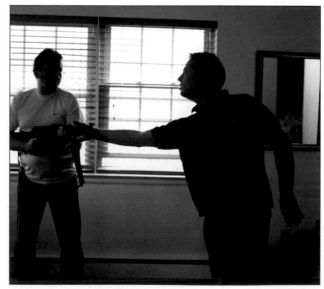

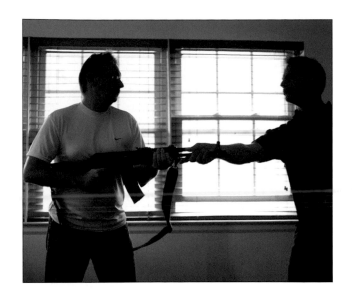

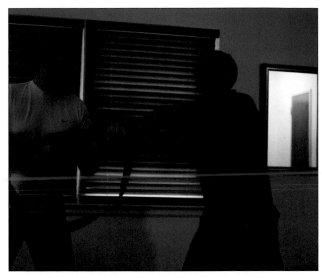

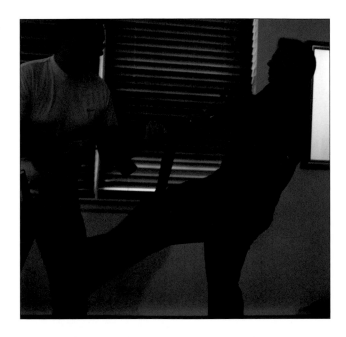

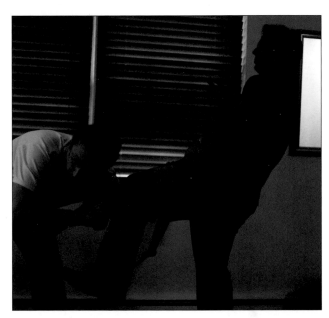

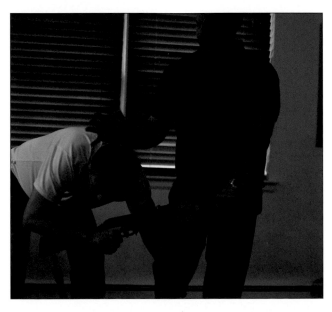

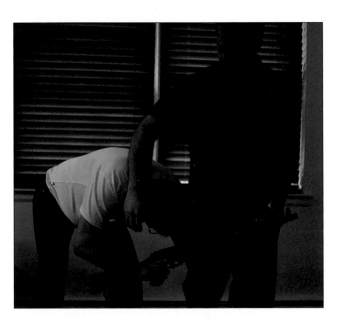

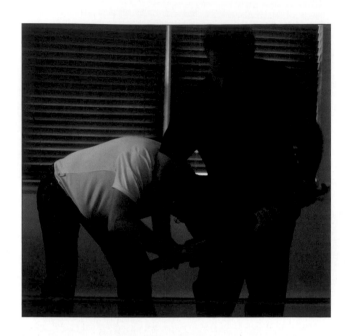

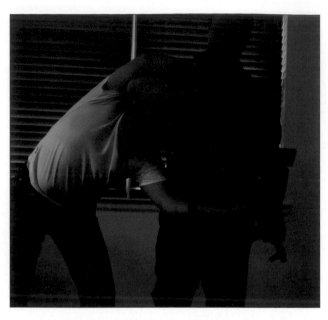

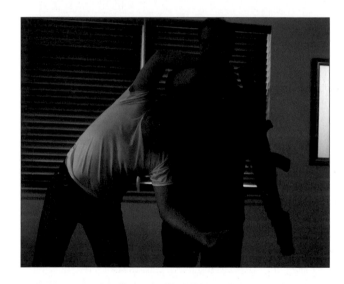

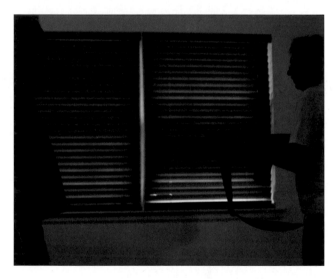

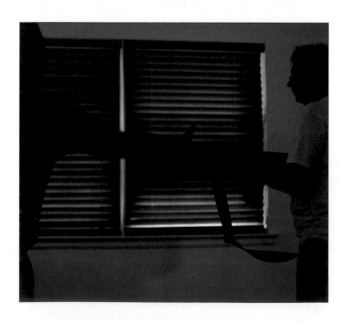

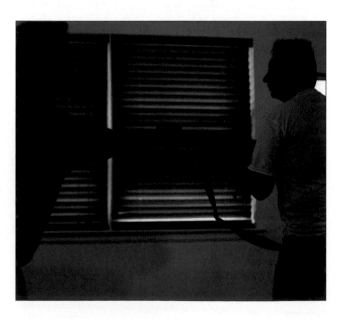

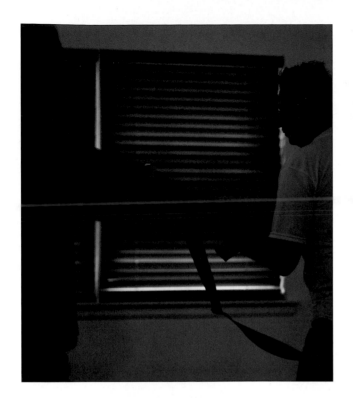
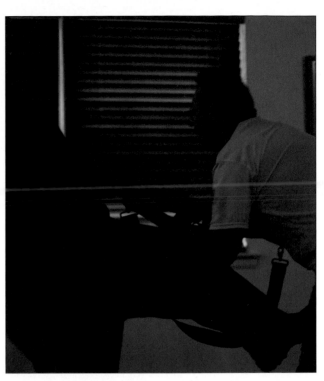
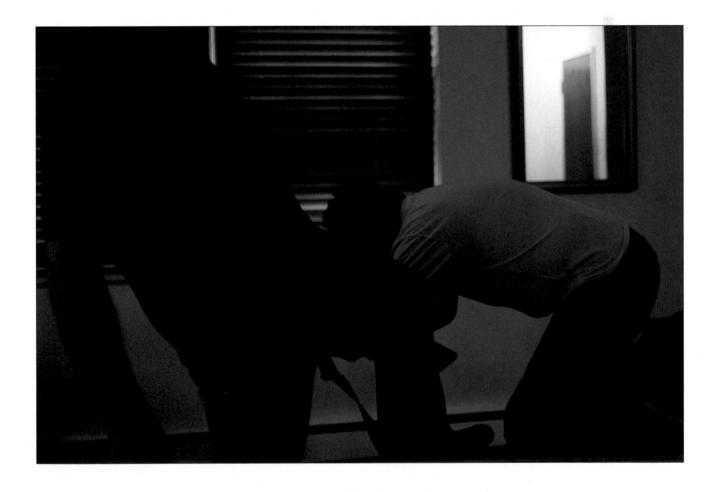

Defense against an assault rifle threat from the back

1. The attacker pushes his assault rifle barrel in the defender's back.
2. The defender pivots, leaning on the barrel, and moving it away from his body. The defender hooks the assault rifle with his left hand.
3. The defender counterattacks with an elbow strike to the opponent's head.
4. The defender moves forward to extract the weapon.

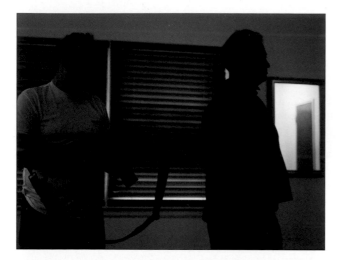 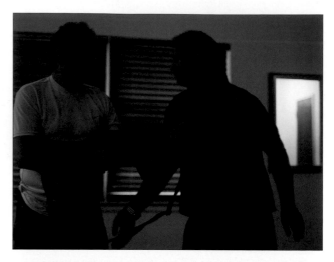

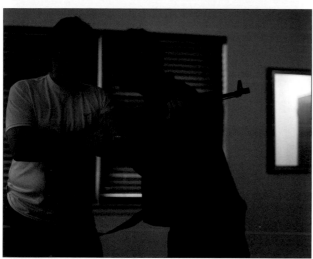 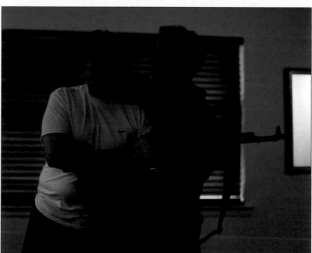

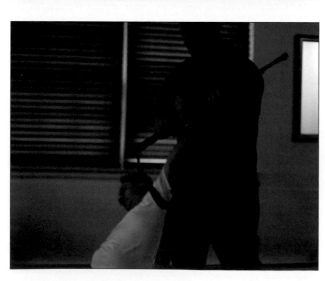 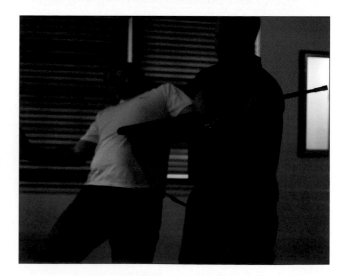

Defense against a Captor Pointing an Assault Rifle at Hostages

Rollover and throw while another group member signals for attention. When you are part of a group that's been taken hostage and one guard is patrolling you with a machine gun, you can wait until the guard is distracted. If you have time to confer with the rest of the hostages, you can stage a distraction through a group member standing away from you.

When the barrel is pointed away from you, you have two seconds to make your move. The plan is to drop your body forward to a rollover as far as you can, and as you rise on your knee, jump forward and create a cradle with your arms for the guard's waist and groin, lifting him up in the air. There is no way he can shoot you if you have reached that far. You then drop him back down to the ground, head first. If he were still holding his gun, it would smash his chest with the fall. You then jump on his back and break his neck. If, however, another guard joins in, you may want to consider grabbing your opponent in a head hold from behind, and roll on your back to make him your shield.

All you need now is a training partner, a stopwatch, and the following photo illustrations, and you are on your way to being proficient in this technique. A toy pellet gun would be even better to boost your confidence. You can select a new training partner, instruct him to play a role guarding the group, and even have some training partners move too much to make him "shoot" them. This will give you a real challenge.

You want to start by warming up and rehearsing the rollover technique learned in the ground-fighting chapter.

1. The attacker is a terrorist or guard, pointing an assault rifle at the group you are with.
2. The attacker is distracted by one of the far group members as the defender dives to the ground.
3. The defender rolls forward.

4. The defender gets up on his knee.
5. The defender jumps forward.
6. The defender grabs the attacker keeping his left arm on the attacker's belt and right arm under his groin from behind. Note that the defender's head is against the attacker's lower back and the defender's legs and back are ready to stand up and lift the attacker's body. Watch your back!
7. The defender lifts the attacker's body.
8. The defender swings the attacker's body down.
9. The defender throws the attacker to the ground.
10. The attacker falls on his assault rifle and the defender is right on his back.

Note: This can be learned in the following steps to achieve an execution time of no more than two seconds:

Step 1: The defenders practice rolling over through two partners without touching on a straight line. Roll over on one hand since it is quicker.

Step 2: A group of soldiers stand as attackers with dummy assault rifles while a group of defenders practice grabbing and holding the attacker's waist and groin.

Step 3: The defenders practice lifting the attackers.

Step 4: The defenders practice jumping from the ground on one knee to lift attackers.

Step 5: The defenders practice their rollover, getting up on one knee and jumping forward to align the defender's forearm with the attacker's belt and swing behind to grab their body for a lift and throw. They should stop at each step and practice until they are fluent.

Step 6: Teach the choke and practice the head hold.

Step 7: Practice fluently, with two training partners at a time, and have the group review the performance. Time the execution and aspire for it to take less than two seconds.

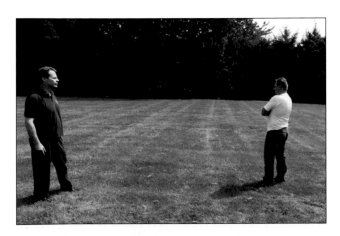
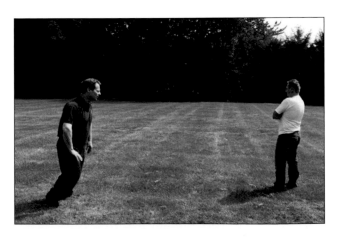

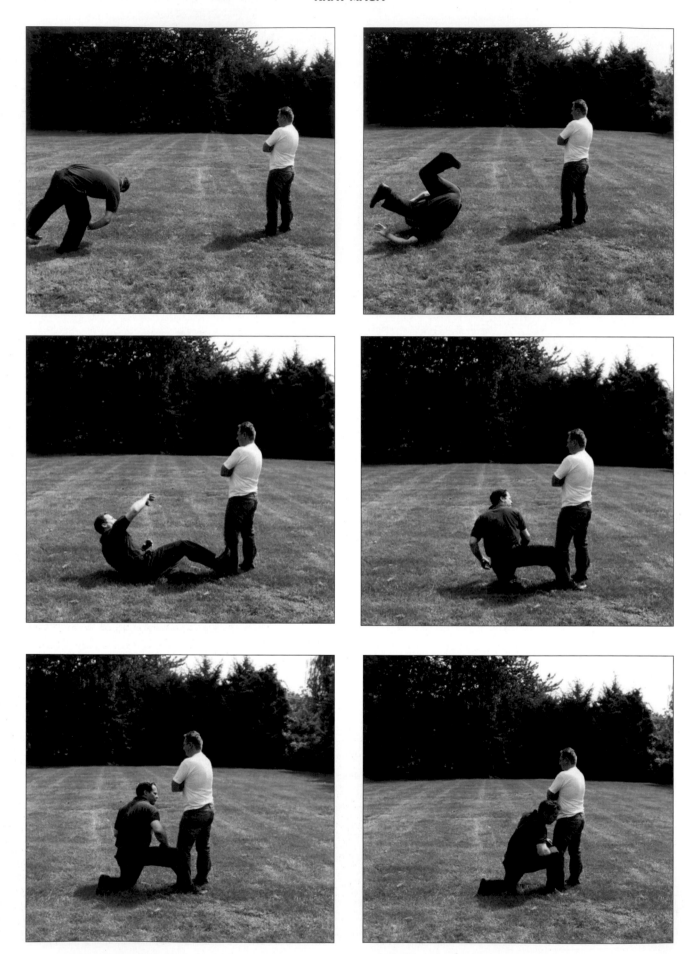

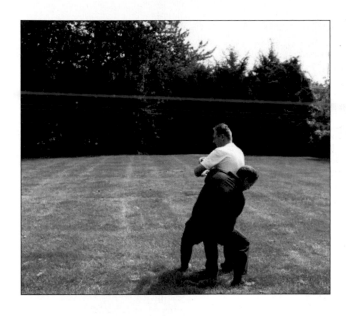

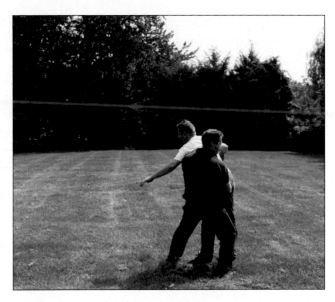

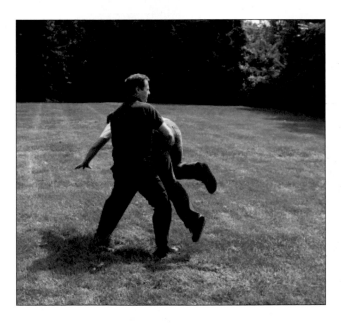

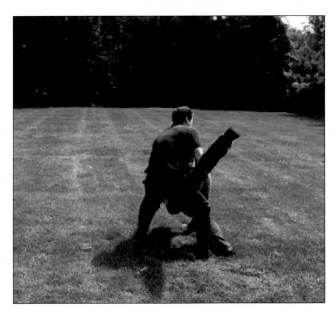

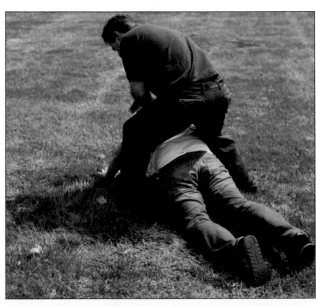

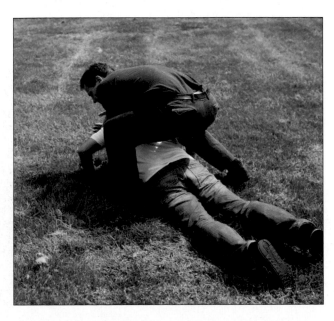

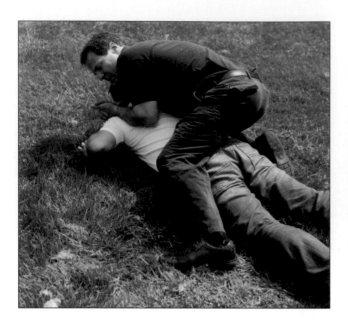 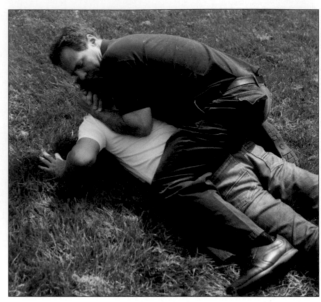

Body Leads

Modern police forces are trained to handcuff and arrest suspects.

However, in the days when European police officers were taught to serve and respect citizens in a nonviolent way, they were trained in these techniques. An officer would hold a violent person down in a painful hold until he calmed down. In the days when police officers carried a nightstick, most criminals were not carrying guns. However, one day it all changed.

The question is, why should we learn to restrain an individual if he would still pose a danger to our lives? Obviously, it is a matter of judgment. You would not want to hold a terrorist who is about to shoot you down into an arm lock, especially if you need to take care of a few more terrorists first; you simply cannot afford the time to give your attention to just one of them while not being able to control the others.

But you can learn the techniques on how to restrain someone so you have a challenge in learning how to get out of these scenarios. Or, you might find yourself in a scenario where your best choice would be to temporarily restrain another individual. A kidnapped civilian may find an opportunity to escape by learning a few extra options.

These holds can be used against violent people until the police arrive. If executed correctly, there is almost no damage to the opponent. At times, a bar fight can end with a drunken attacker unharmed on the floor or being escorted out.

Obviously, you are taking a risk when grabbing a person with your two hands and trying to restrict his movement while inflicting pain on him. He could simply punch you before you are done with our move. However, at times you can sense that your opponent is not the most dangerous guy, and if circumstances allow, you may prefer not harming him. If you are confident that you are not endangering your life, you can quickly grab the attacker and make him understand that you are not to be messed with. At times, if he keeps badmouthing even as you lessen the pain inflicted upon him, you may keep him under control until the police arrives.

When we learned release from body holds and chokes, we did not spend much time on release from wrist holds. If you asked yourself why I did not mention wrist locks more, it is because it is faster to strike at a pressure point for self-defense purposes. So even if an attacker is attempting to grab one of your hands with both of his for an aikido throw, you should move in and strike his face with your other hand. Or you should just not give him your hand.

Body lead number one

Suppose you shake someone's hand and pull his arm toward you.

You then use your other arm to hook his and create leverage on his elbow.

Then, make him feel pain by making him walk with you as you keep him on his toes. If he tries to punch you, all you have to do is pivot his wrist like a motorcycle throttle. He will stop immediately and start to scream instead.

1. The defender uses his right hand to grab the opponent's right inner forearm, pulling it towards him, using his left palm to push away the opponent's chin and stretch his arm.
2. The defender creates a hook with his left hand under the opponent's elbow.
3. The defender leads the attacker away.

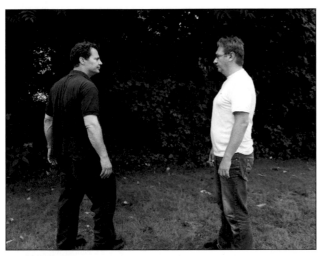

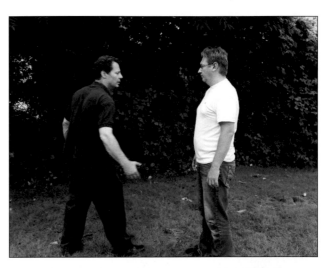

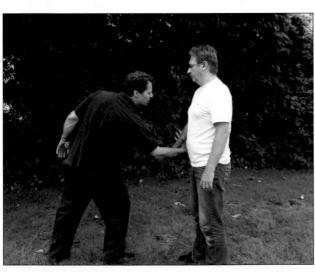

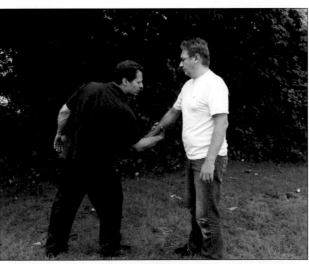

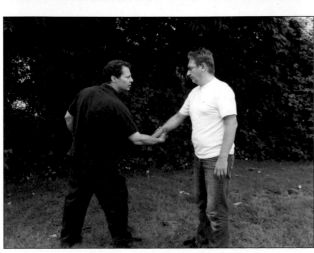

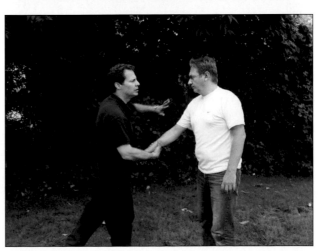

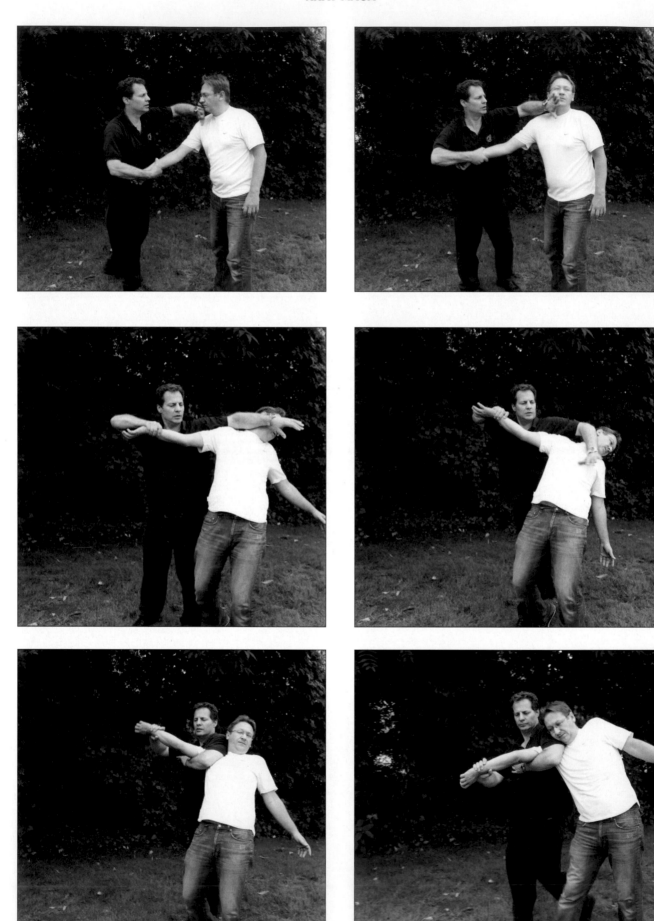

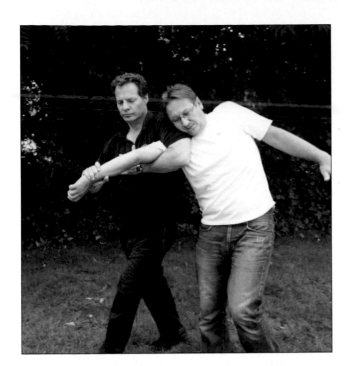

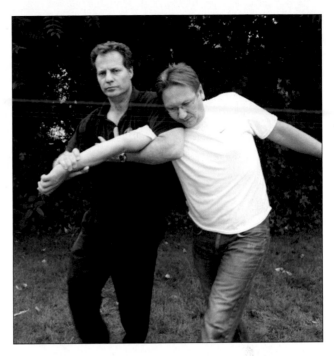

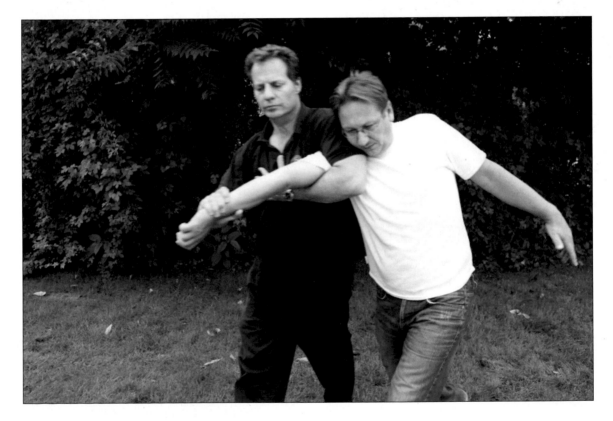

Release from body lead number one

1. The defender inserts one leg between the attacker's legs after he starts to walk.

2. The defender reclaims his arm as he falls to the ground, as the attacker instinctively reaches to use his arms to break the fall.

3. If the attacker falls on his face, you may not need to do anything.

4. If the attacker releases his arms to break the fall, you may need to counterattack according to your judgment.

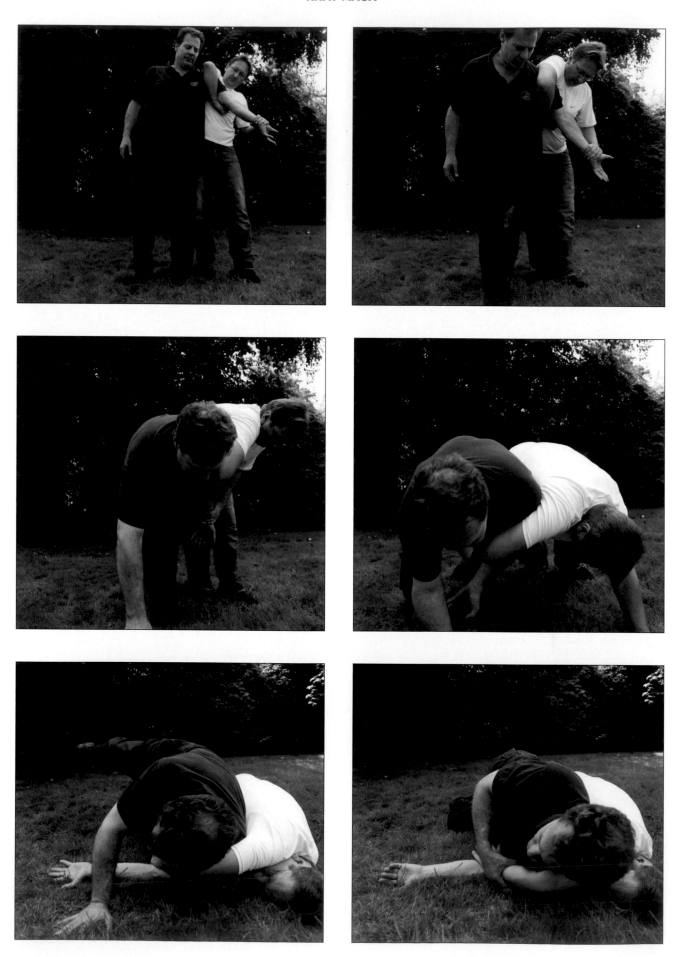

Body lead number two

1. The defender grabs the back of the attacker's hand, lifting his elbow and pointing it up perpendicularly.
2. The defender grabs the attacker's elbow with his free hand.
3. The defender points the elbow at the ground.
4. The defender brings the attacker to the ground.
5. The defender sits, waiting for the police to come, using his legs to hold the opponent's hand.

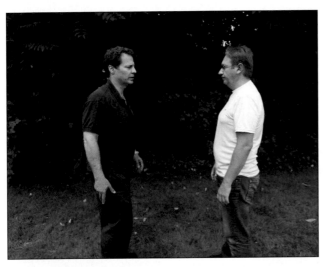

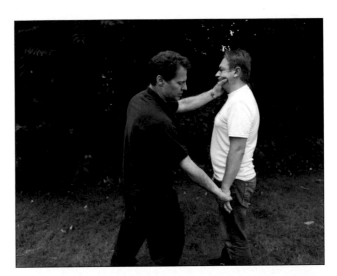

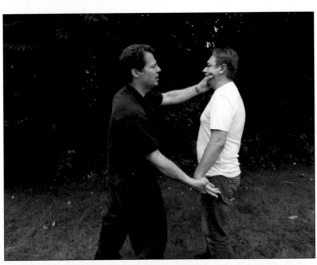

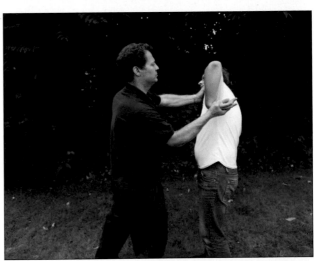

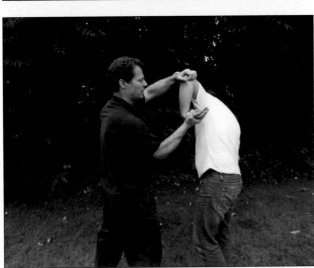

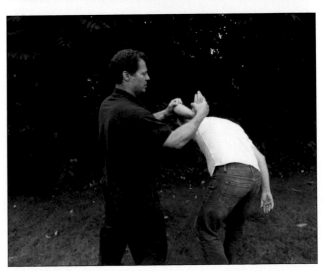

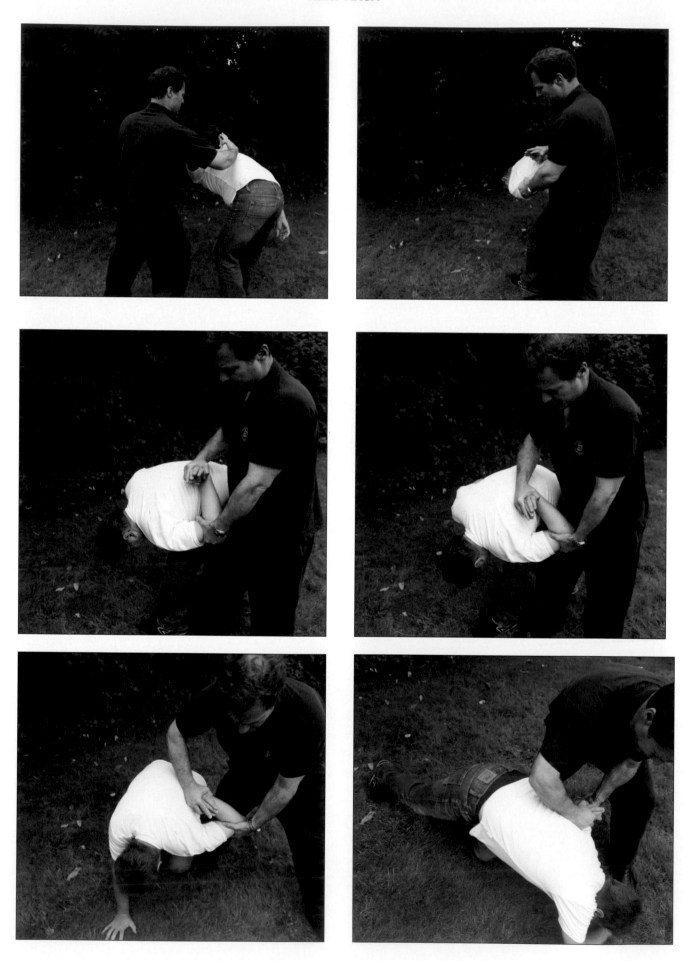

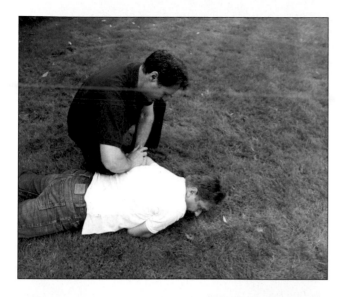

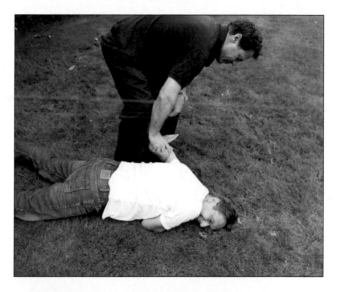

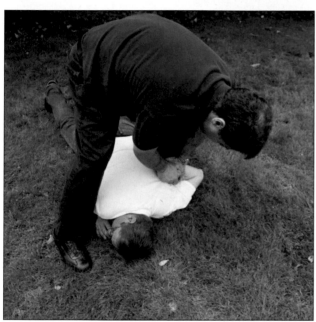

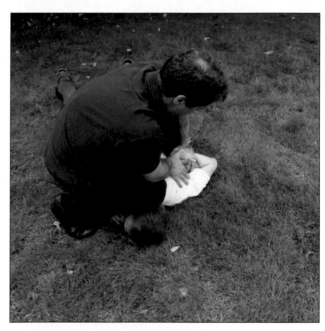

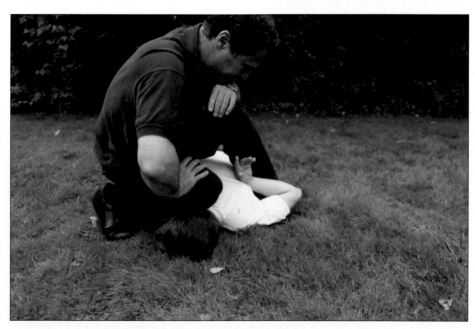

Release from body lead number two

1. The attacker holds the defender's elbow behind his back.
2. The defender drops his torso to the ground to extend his hand upwards. The defender lands on his free hand and continues to bring his body to the ground, extending his captured arm.
3. The defender delivers a scissor kick to the opponent's leg.

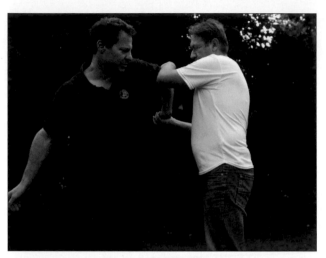

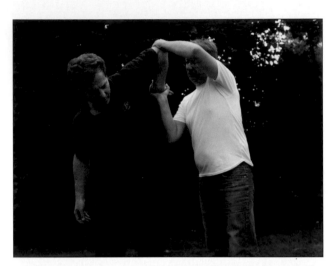

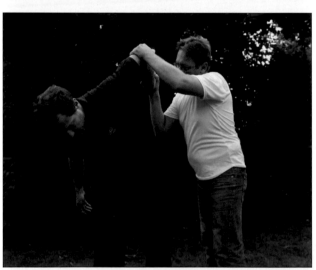

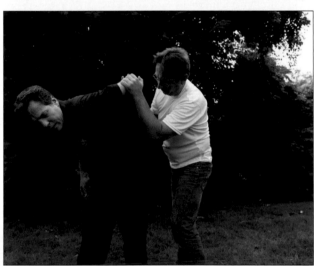

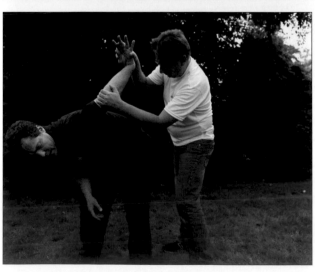

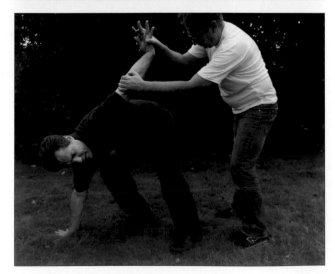

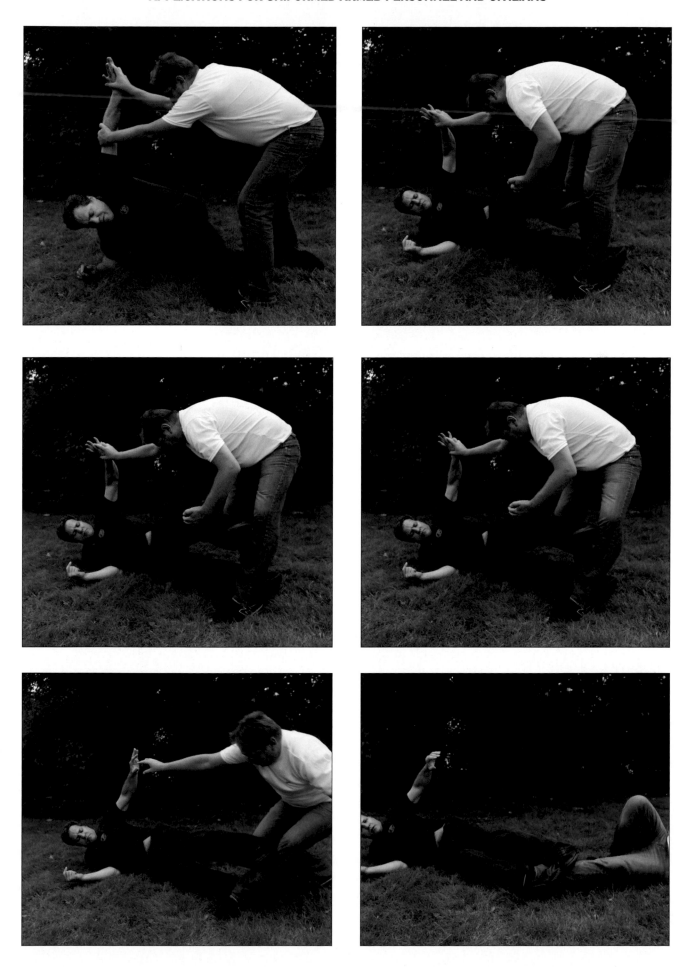

Body lead number three

1. The defender grabs the back of the attacker's hand, squeezing all his fingers and lifting his elbow up perpendicularly. The defender bends the attacker's wrist by twisting the attacker's fingers toward the attacker's elbow.

2. The defender grabs the attacker's elbow with his free hand from the inside.

3. The defender pulls the attacker's elbow toward his chest and switches the hand grabbing the attacker's wrist. The defender uses his free arm to grab the attacker's head and leads him to his destination.

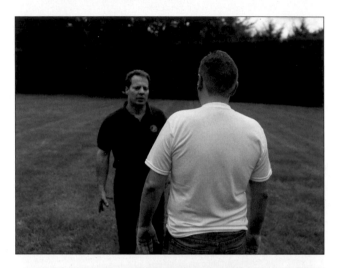
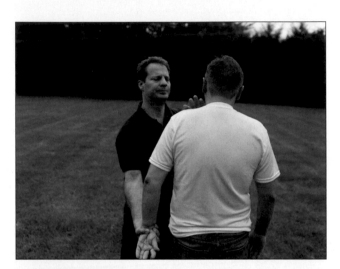

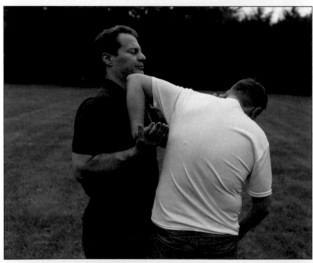
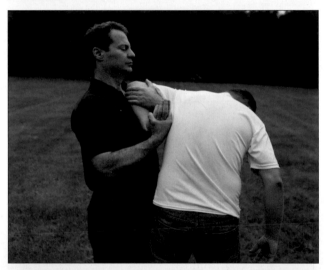

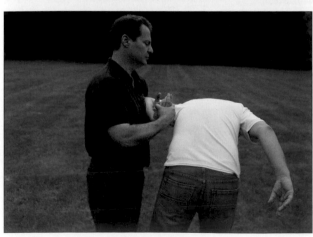
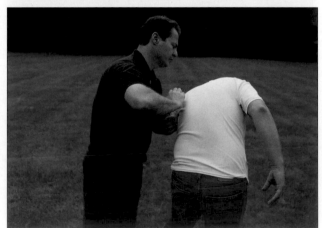

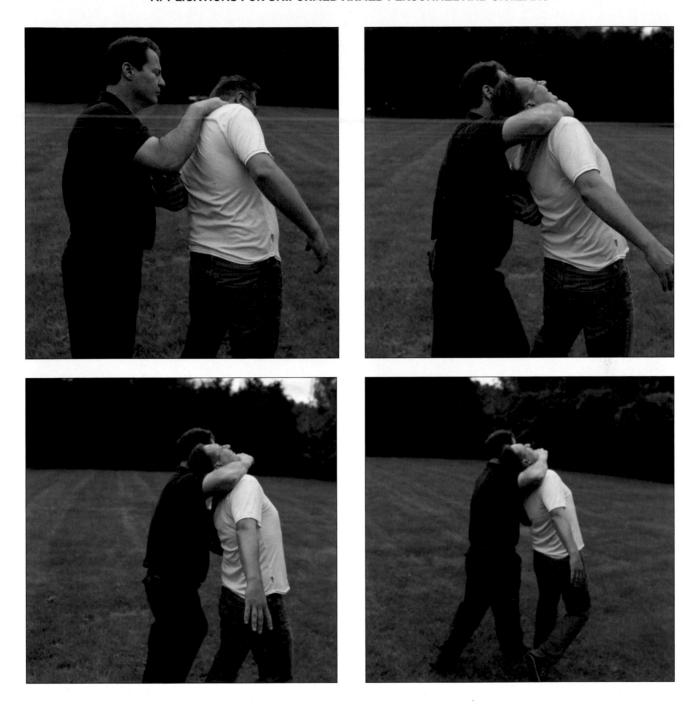

Note: Releasing from this hold is the same as in hold number two if executed in its early stages. Otherwise, you may use your right hand to pull the opponent's wrist down and pull your head out as you drop to the ground, making it more challenging.

Body lead number four

1. The defender grabs the back of the attacker's hand, lifting his elbow up perpendicularly.
2. The defender grabs the attacker's elbow with his free hand.
3. The defender brings the attacker's elbow to his opposite armpit, while pivoting towards his opponent, using both hands to apply pressure on the attacker's wrist.
4. The defender leads the attacker out to his desired destination.

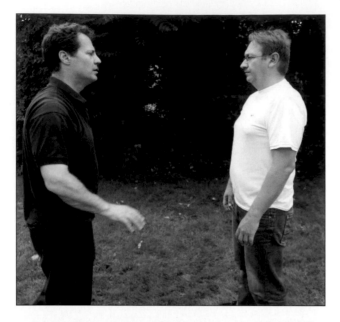
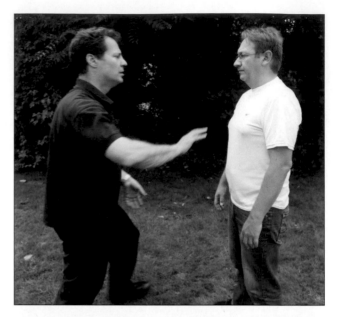
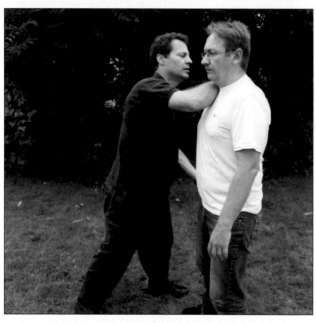
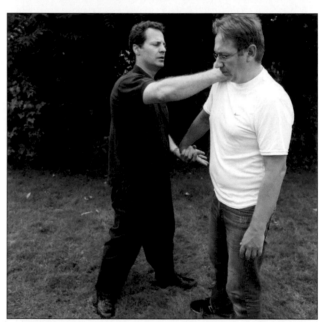
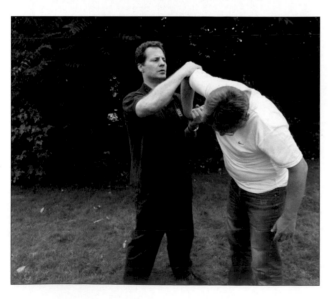
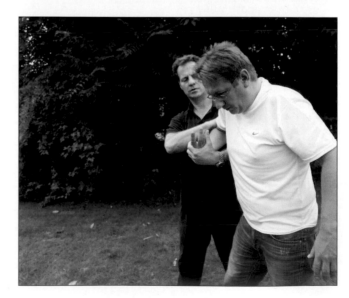

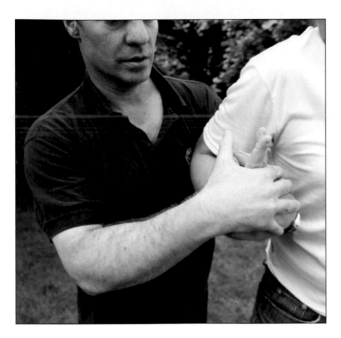

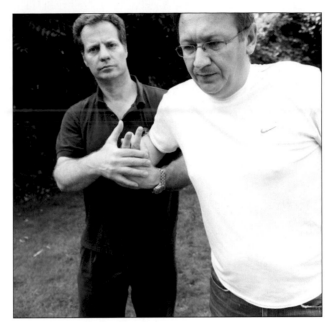

Notes: Releasing from this hold is the same as in hold number two.

You should understand that in wrist manipulations, where you inflict pain to restrain an opponent, the opponent might cry. However, when being left alone, he may come back and attack you. You might have plenty of opportunities for a counterattack or you might have none. When you are fighting for your life, leave the nonsense alone. This isn't like someone twisting your arm in elementary school, which is a situation I am sure you will be able to make it out of. This is not the same. You might feel discouraged trying to get out

of that wrist lock due to the pain in your wrist and fingers, but if you bite your teeth for a quick moment and duck down while extending your elbow, you are free as a bird. Immediately move in to kick the opponent's knee as shown in the aforementioned techniques.

When I demonstrated knife defenses, I explained leverages on the wrists not for the purpose of throwing, but rather to control our opponent's weapon.

You could use wrist manipulations also to control a subdued opponent and use his body as an obstacle against another attacker.

First Aid

Lifting and carrying an unconscious person

Firemen and military soldiers are trained in carrying the wounded in emergency scenarios, but no one ever plans for it to be a one-person job. However, when one person has no choice but to carry an unconscious person out of a dangerous area, the common fireman style will hardly ever work.

The following technique was developed for use in scenarios where you need to quickly evacuate and to carry someone yourself, if the person is unconscious and you cannot wake him up. A human body can be compared to a heavy water mattress whose center of gravity is hard to get a hold of.

Here is the technique for lifting an unconscious person by yourself and evacuating him away.

1. The unconscious person is on the ground.

2. After you determine that you cannot wake him up, position him on his back and lie down next to him with your back to the floor.

3. Grab the hand that is farther from you and put it on your shoulder. Roll with him so that his body ends up on your back while you are lying on the ground facedown.

4. Jiggle your body around so he's positioned exactly on top of you, and get to your knees with a push up.

5. Push yourself and put one foot forward.

6. Stand on your legs with your body leaned forward and pass his hands through his hanging legs, holding his wrists while the back of his legs are seated on your arms. You may need to grab a wrist, and when you stand up, shake your shoulders while keeping your torso parallel to the ground until you grab his other wrist.

7. Stand up straight and you are ready to go.

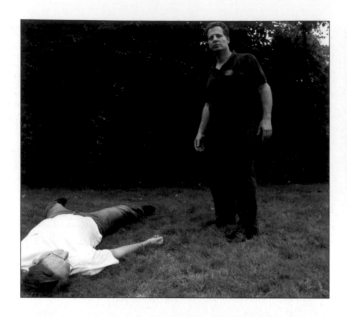

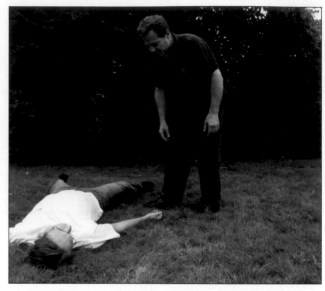

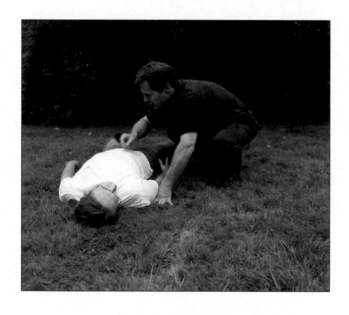

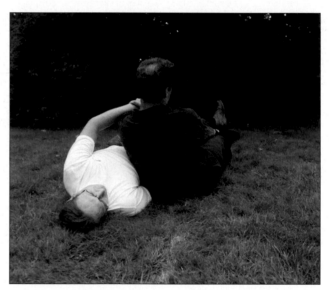

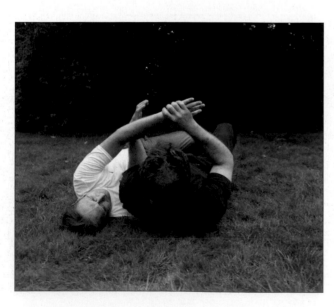

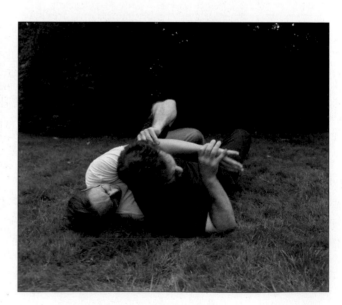

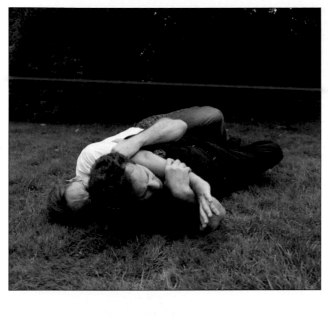

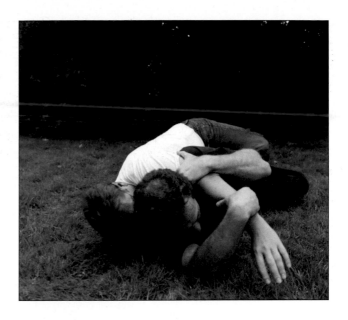

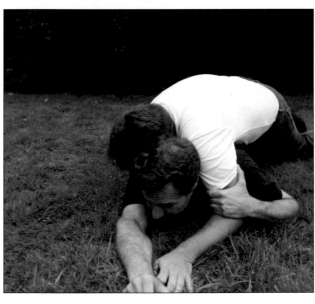

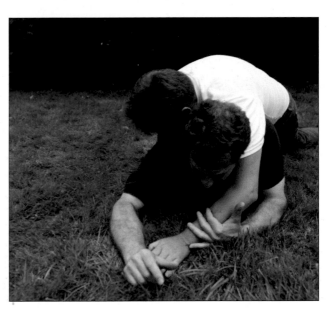

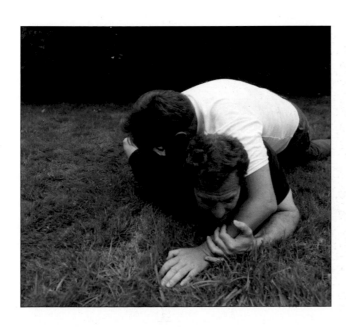

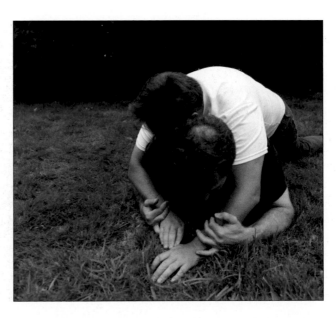

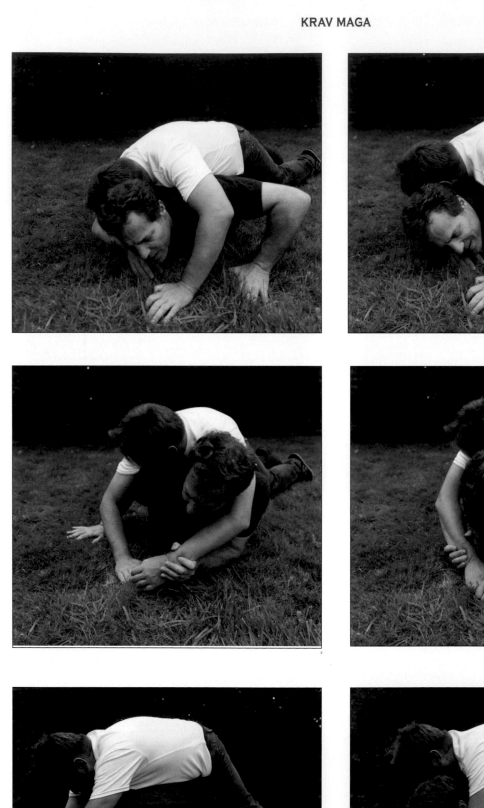
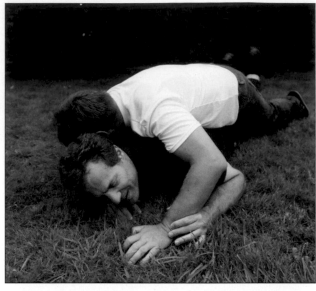
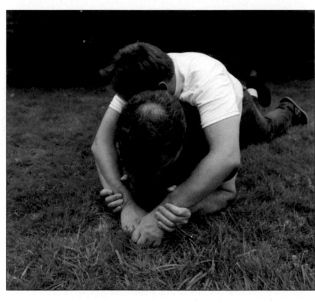
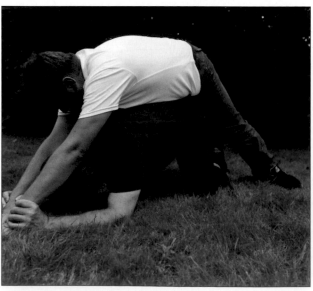
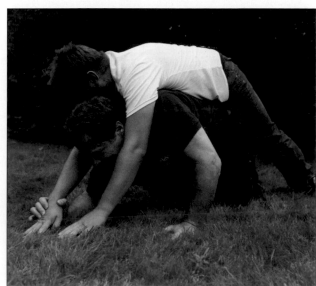

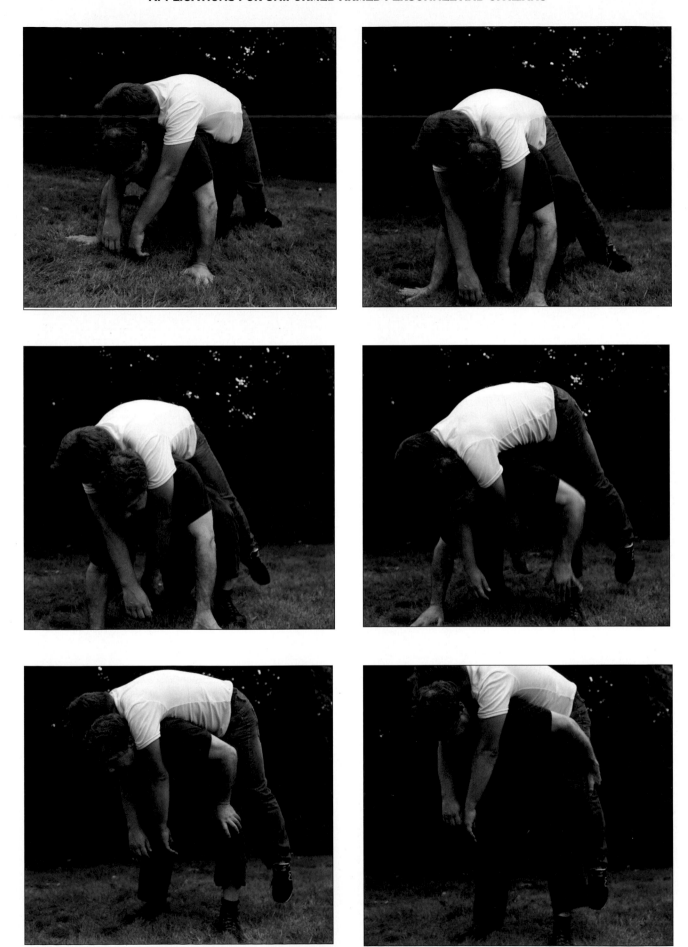

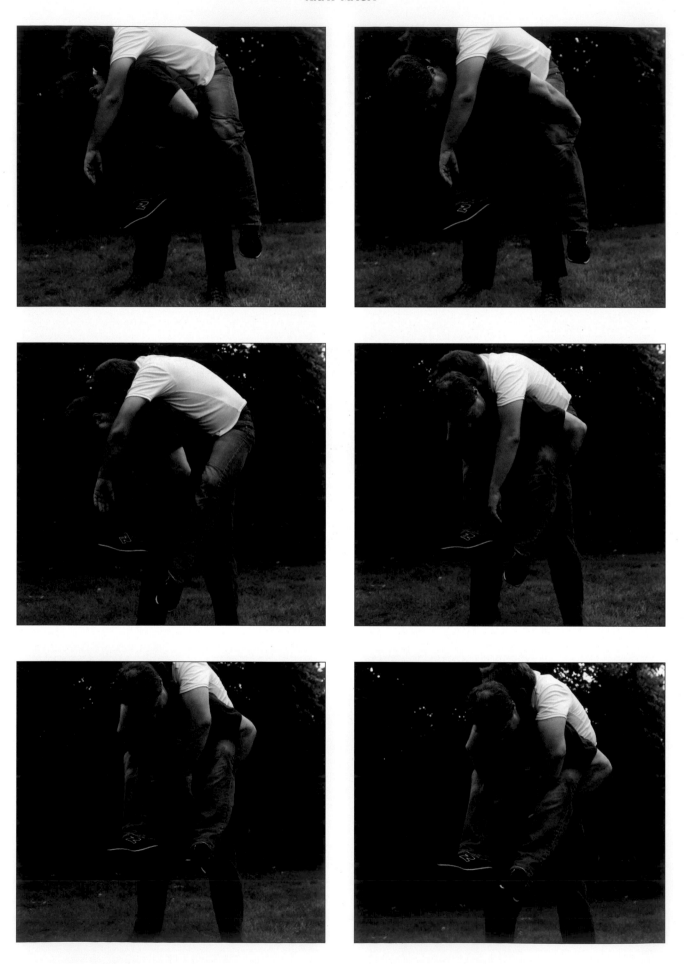

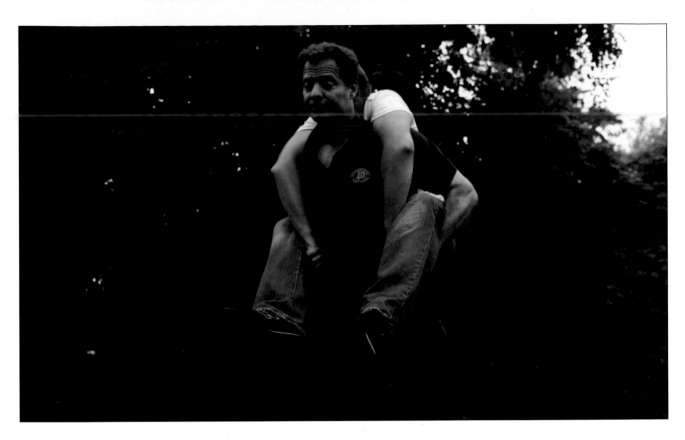

Sentry Removal

Considering some sentries have full gear and sometimes a helmet, you should choose a weapon that will be swift and quiet so as to not alert the compound the sentry is guarding.

Knife through the back ribs to the heart

1. Close the gap between you and your opponent without making any noise.
2. As you extend one hand to cover his mouth, stab with the knife in your other hand, aiming from the kidney diagonally up to the heart. Keep the blade parallel to the ground to facilitate ease of passage between the ribs. For this technique, you would need a long knife of good quality, such as a military modern bayonet.

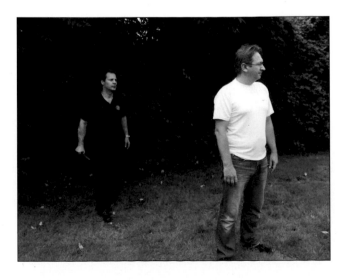
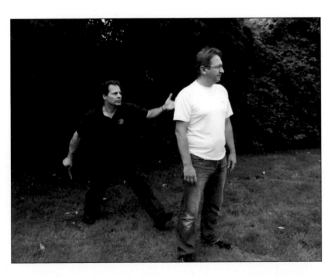

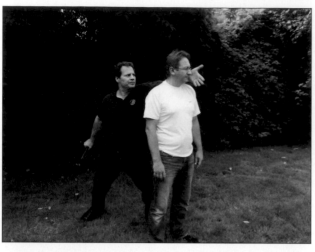 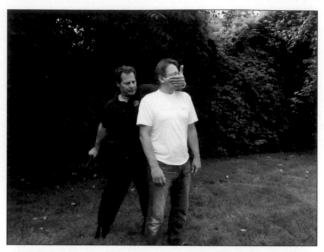

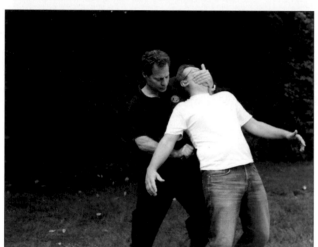 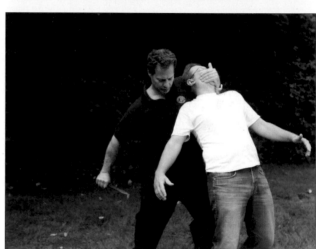

Knife to the clavicle or throat slash

1. Close the gap without making any noise.
2. When you get close enough to your opponent, jump on him and grab his mouth. Use your knees to bend his torso backward toward you.

3. You can either stab him with a top-down knife hold straight in the clavicle and cut his carotid artery, or slash his opposite artery and windpipe if you are holding the knife in an underhand hold.

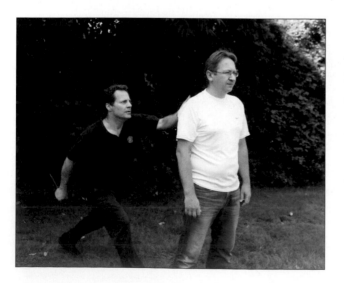 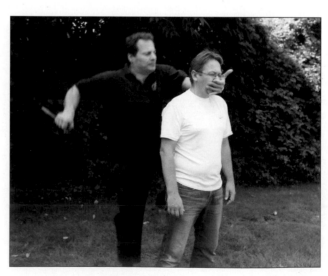

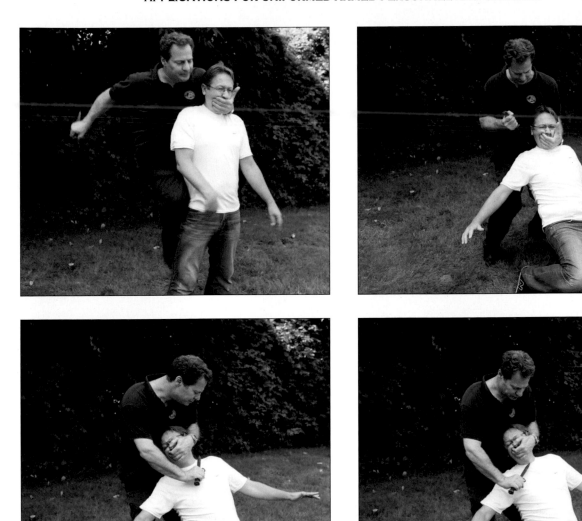

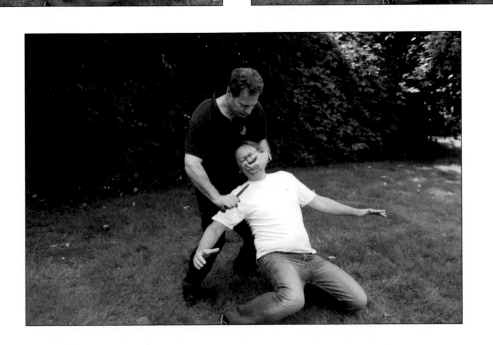

Simple head smash to the ground

You should remember not to try this on a soldier wearing a helmet because you may not eliminate him immediately. However, this technique is very effective to use on anyone else. There is hardly any resistance if an opponent is pulled from the head down, and throwing the head backwards makes it almost impossible to stop.

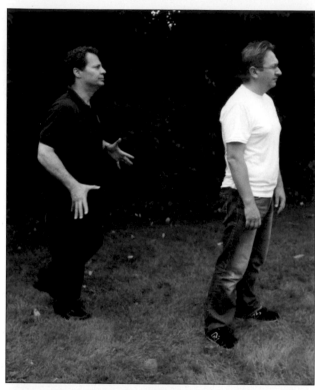

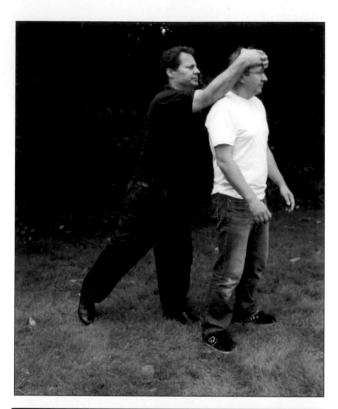

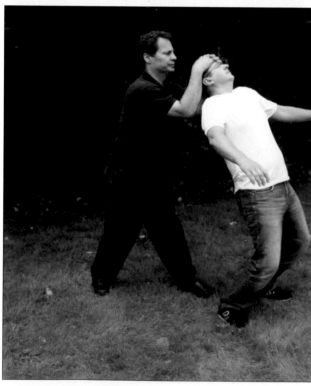

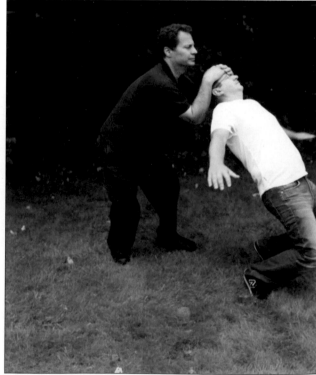

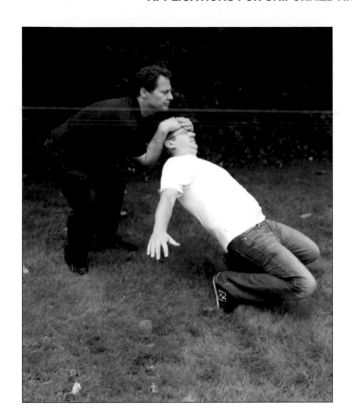 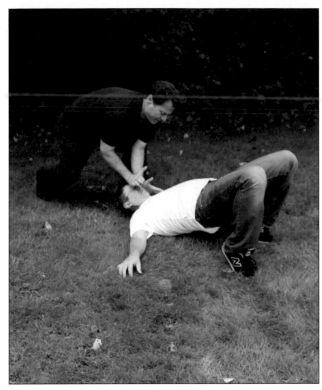

11
OTHER KICKS

Krav Maga has developed kicks from all angles like other martial arts have. It has, in fact, gone one step further and applied better principles, and found the best reason for them. However, any Krav Maga student must know that in self-defense situations, when the only rule is to survive at the attacker's expense, one should resort to basic kicks since they are much faster and have a longer range. Simplicity is the key.

Jump kicks, however, can be used in certain scenarios when chasing an opponent. Pay attention to see if there is less risk in running faster and resorting to closer confrontation. These kicks should be taught after the self-defense chapter has been learned and completed. They can be used as secondary kicks for a continuous attack, when your opponent has moved back after your initial kick, or in tactical defensive moves. While it is a good idea to develop challenging training partners, always ask yourself if there is a reason for using complex techniques in life or death matters.

Generally, a kick should be aimed at the center of the opponent's body, at the groin level. An extended leg parallel to the ground facilitates the maximum reach. If two opponents attempt to kick each other at the same time, the one that aims at the belt area will have more reach than the one that aims for the head. Since a high kick requires kicking in a 135-degree angle upwards, the kicker would need to get closer to the opponent to close the gap.

If you execute a high kick however, your opponent may be able to reach you with a leveled kick to the belt area without getting that close. Therefore primary kicks should be aimed to the belt area from all angles.

Use secondary kicks as a tactical defense move, moving your body away from your attacker's line of attack. If your opponent executes a straight kick at the same time, you will be safely out of the way.

Follow these steps to use a secondary kick for continuous attacks. First, retract your basic front kick to a ninety-degree angle to ease the continuous attack and defense. At this position, if the opponent closes the gap and doesn't execute a complete defense and counterattack, you can continue with a slap kick. Since the opponent is close, and your leg is at ninety degrees, it is quicker to extend your leg than to shift your whole body forward so you can use your fist.

Preferably, all kicks would be executed in a continuous two-stage flow. The first motion would be to close the gap and lift the knee to ninety degrees. The second would be extending of the leg to the opposite direction of your body. Use a perpendicular seesaw motion for the front kick, and corkscrew leg and body motion for side kicks. For a roundhouse kick to the front, use a combination of the seesaw and corkscrew motions together. For roundhouse kicks to the back, use the corkscrew motion to bring the leg close to the opponent's side of the head or body, and then use a horizontal stomping motion. This also makes it a combination of the corkscrew and seesaw motions. In executing a roundhouse kick to the front, we start with a front kick, lifting your knee higher than the waist, pointing to the opposite side of the opponent's cheek. This ensures that when you screw the ball of the foot into the opponent's cheek you will be able to extend the foot way past the opponent's head and knock him out. In this way, a front kick could turn into a slap kick or roundhouse kick to the front, and a side kick could turn into a roundhouse kick to the back.

All kicks can be performed on the spot; however it is more logical to punch from the spot since it is faster to swing your hand than your leg. I would stress the importance of teaching a swift body movement to close the gap with kicks.

Low kicks, such as a side kick to the knee or a back attack kick to the shin are a last-resort, last-second decision for when an opponent is coming in from the back or the side. This is because a normal hand strike range is not possible backward.

When the opponent attacks with a knife, on-the-spot low kicks are valuable counterattacks. In most of these moves, a slight body sneaking and a small step to calibrate the motion are essential. This is really a swift shifting of the body weight and landing on the base leg while kicking with your other leg. The positioning of the landing base leg facilitates a quicker, more comfortable, and more accurate kick.

Attack Kick to the Rear

The back attack kick is a perpendicular swinging upward stomp. The power of this kick is derived from leaning the torso forward and fully extending the leg backwards to where the heel is at the contact point with the target, locking the knee before the contact. After the knee is locked, it utilizes a seesaw motion similar to the front attack kick. The pressure points aimed for could be the opponent's shin, groin, or chin.

1. The defender notices the attacker approaching to his side.
2. The defender closes the gap with his toes pushing his body to the side, leaning toward the opponent.

His rear leg crosses behind the front leg as far as possible, while his hips are pivoted to the point that the buttocks are pointing to the opponent. The defender lands on his base foot with his heel pointed toward the opponent.

3. The defender extends and straightens his kicking leg as he turns back and drops his upper body, facing down to lift his heel upwards and strike anywhere on the opponent's body.
4. The defender retracts his leg to ninety degrees and calculates his next move.

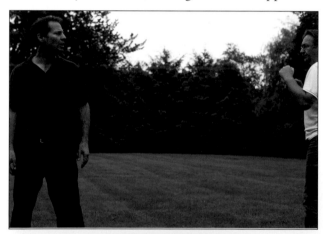

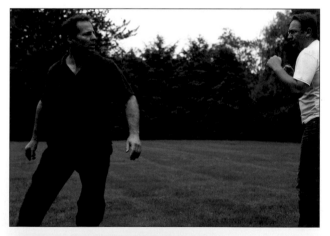

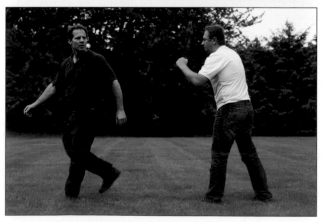

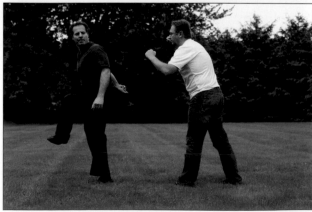

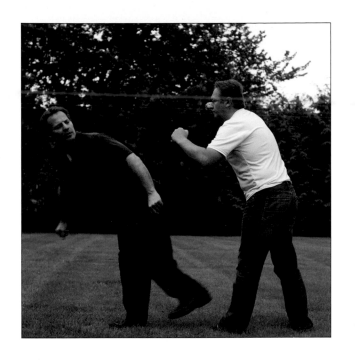

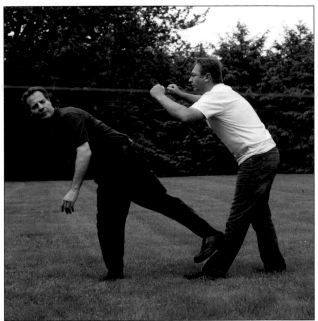

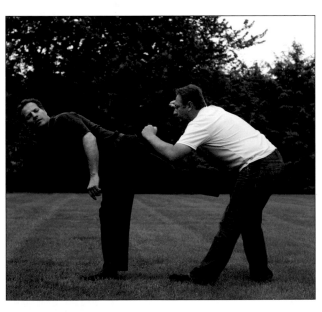

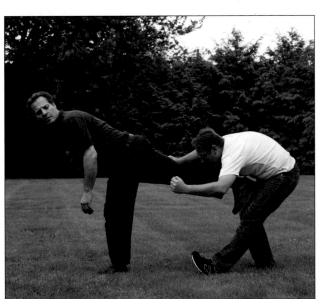

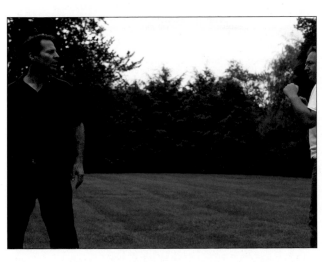

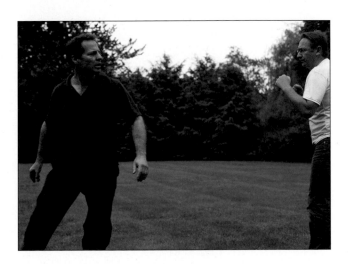

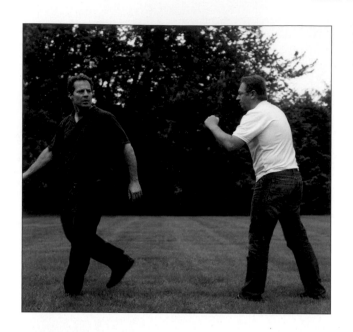
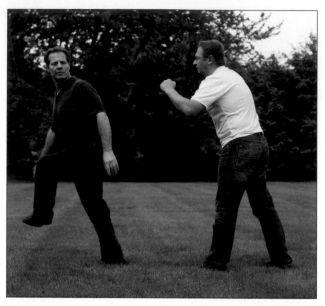
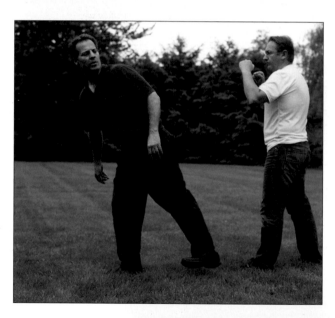
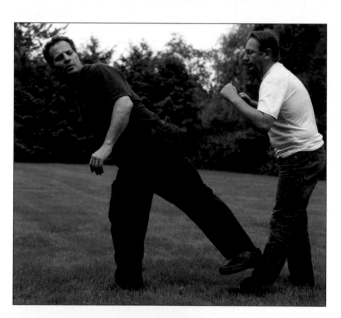
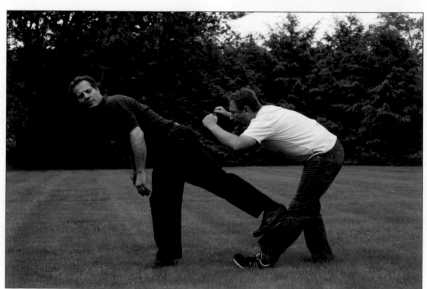

Roundhouse Kicks

Roundhouse kicks require getting closer to the opponent to reach pressure points on the side or front of the opponent's body. Although Krav Maga fighters prefer attacking with simple motions, certain scenarios might hold an advantage in tactical roundhouse kicks.

Roundhouse kick to the side

1. The defender stands with his side to the opponent.
2. The defender advances close to the opponent for a side kick.
3. The opponent is too close and the defender swings his leg in a side kick motion to the side of his opponent's shoulder, continuing with a horizontal stomping motion to the opponent's face or chest.
4. The defender retracts his leg to a ninety-degree angle.

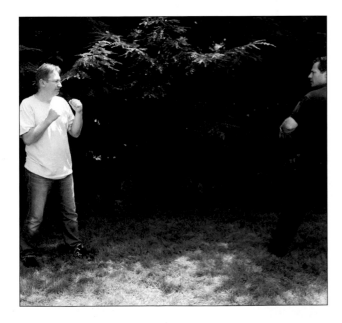

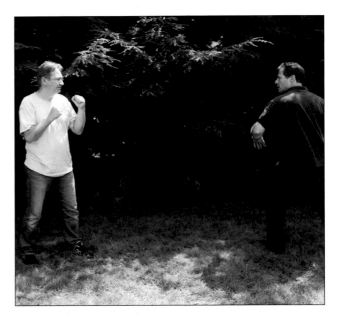

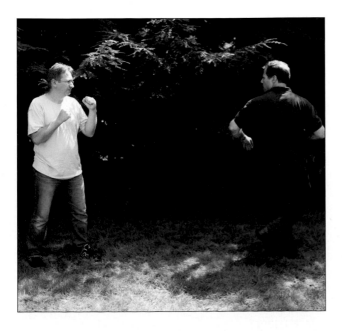

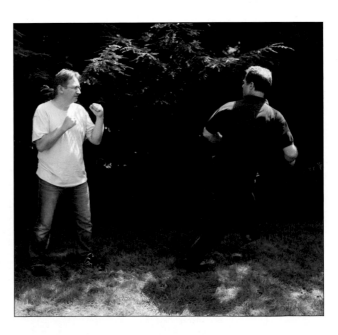

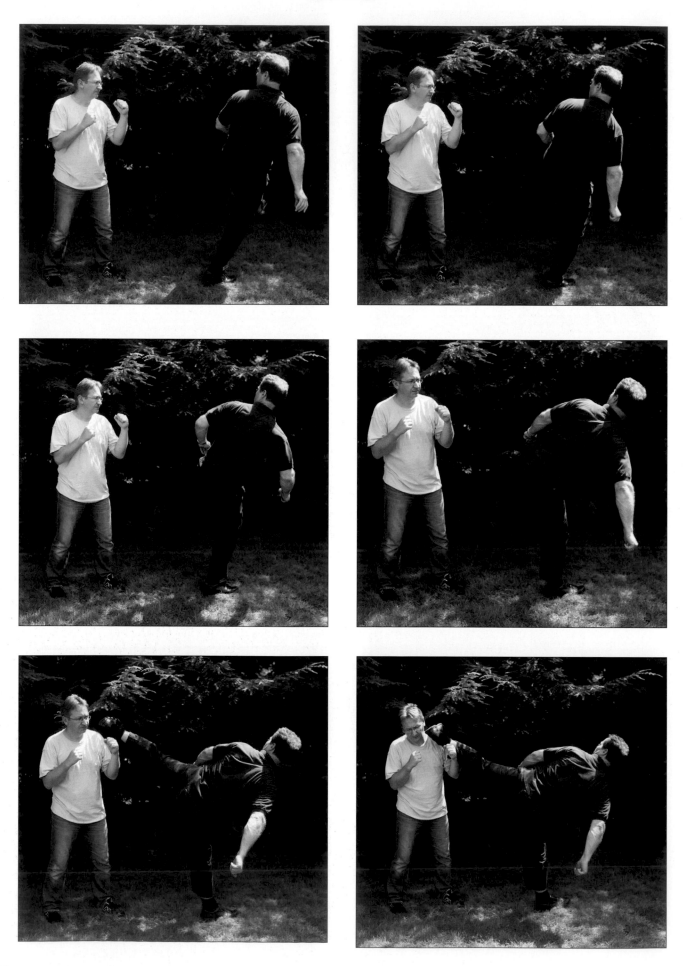

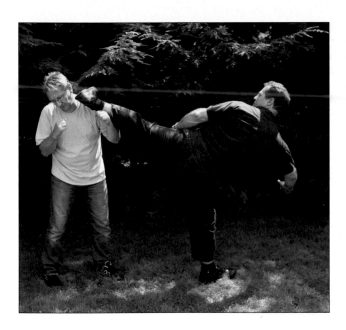 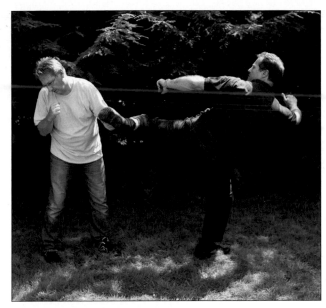

Roundhouse kick to the front

1. The defender stands in front of the opponent.
2. The defender moves in for a high front kick, with his knee pointed to the side of the opponent's chin to help the kick to pass the target.
3. The defender turns his body in a corkscrew motion, the ball of his foot on the opponent's cheek.
4. The defender retracts his leg to ninety degrees and then considers his next move.

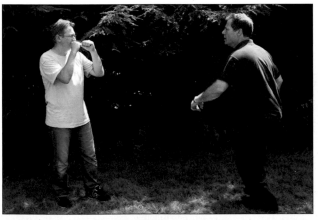 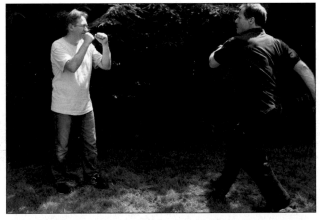

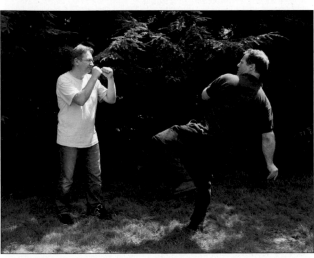 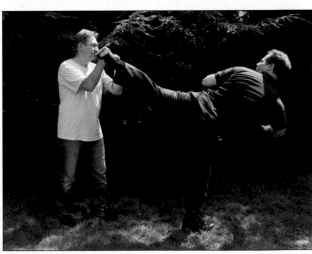

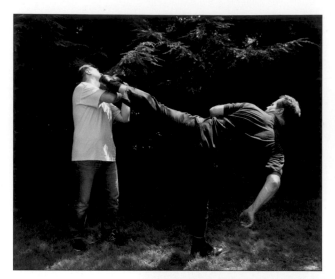
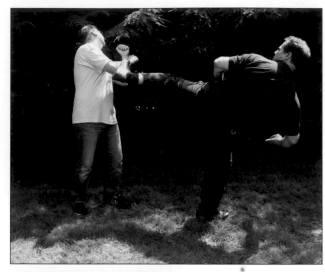
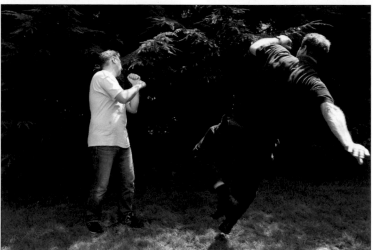

Defensive roundhouse kick to the front with the rear foot

Roundhouse high kicks, although not preferable because of their lesser range, can be used as secondary kicks after the primary front and side kicks. In addition, they can be used in timing tactics where the defender waits for the attacker to attack. As the attacker closes the gap, the defender steps out of the way and executes a roundhouse kick repositioned to keep out of the opponent's line of attack. One of the examples in this book is shown in defense against a straight knife hold with a kick.

1. The attacker is advancing forward.
2. The defender steps to the side with his left (front) foot and executes a roundhouse kick to the attacker's face with his right foot. Although his rear leg should not initially be used, the change in body position takes his rear foot closer to the opponent.

Defensive full turn roundhouse kick to the back

1. The defender crosses his left foot over to his right side.
2. The defender keeps his weight in the center as he pivots, landing with the instep of his base foot facing the opponent.
3. The defender swings his leg for a roundhouse kick.
4. The defender retracts his leg to a ninety degrees.

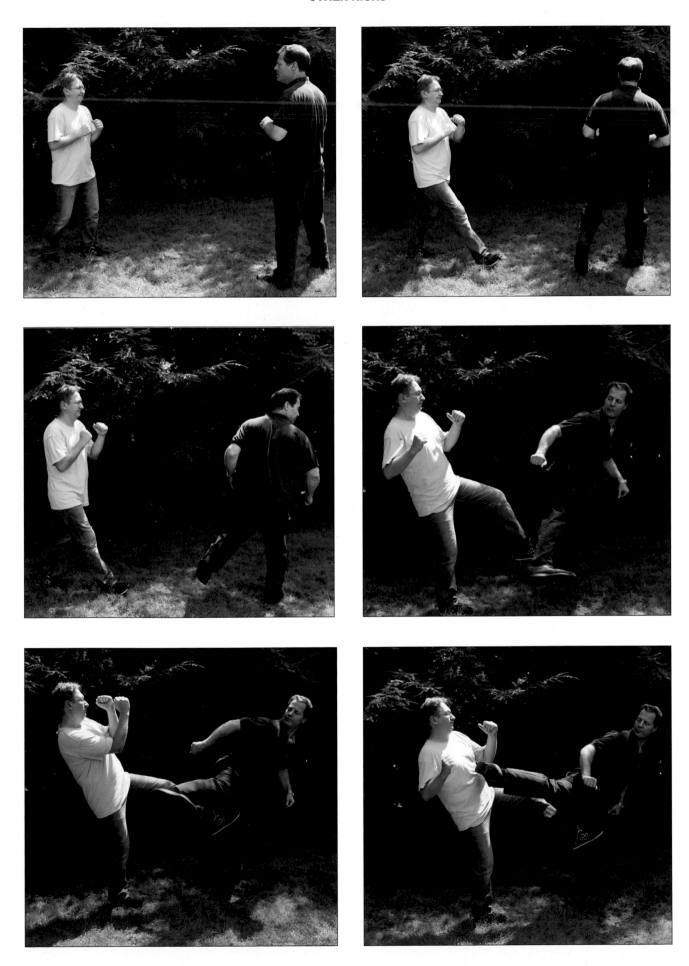

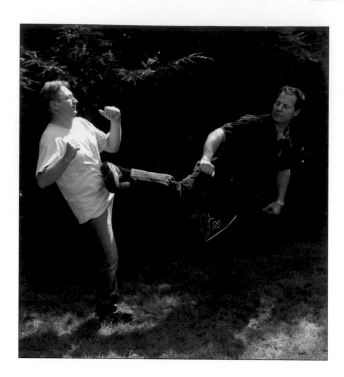 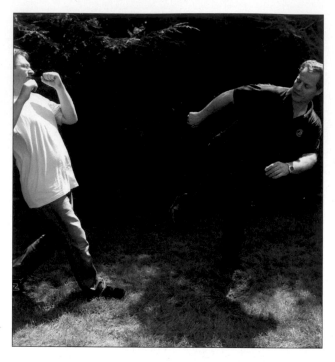

Notes: The problem with this kick is that students tend to find it too difficult to do a full fast turn and land accurately at the right angle. It is really easy if you keep your weight in the center between both your legs as you turn, and as you land on one foot, lift the other simultaneously. You should land with the inside of your foot parallel to your opponent. Then continue with a roundhouse kick to the side. After you have mastered this technique, you should ask your training partner to hold a punching mitt and close the gap slowly at first and then with increasing speed. As he moves closer to you, you should time your evasive step and kick the mitt. Remember, practice makes perfect.

If you are stretched out and ready, your can time your kicks. Let's say you want to kick with your right foot, as your opponent approaches you. You can turn your body to the left, stepping away from the opponent's line of attack. You then execute a kick with your right leg. You can also cross with your left leg over your right leg, moving your body away from your attacker, and give him a full turn roundhouse kick with your right heel. With a little practice, you can pick any side you want to move to when kicking . You can kick the low or high areas. Remember, we are using a low front roundhouse kick like in the defense against a straight knife stab in a prior chapter.

Outside Slap Kick

1. The defender moves forward for a front kick, where his base foot toes are pointed toward his opponent, lunging and crossing the front foot from behind or the front. If from the front, you need to swing the kicking leg across the base leg prior to the slap.

2. The defender extends the side of his leg to the attacker's cheek, slightly pivoting his body to the other direction. The slap kick should pass the opponent's head, moving it with the blow.

3. The defender retracts his leg to ninety degrees, ready for his next move.

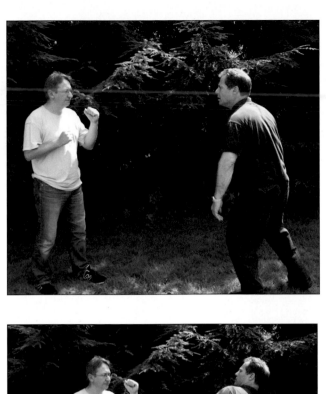
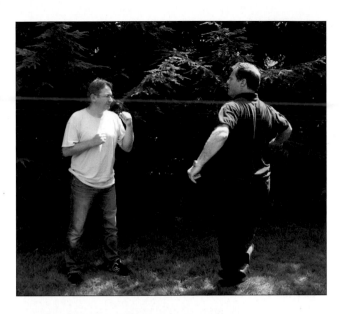
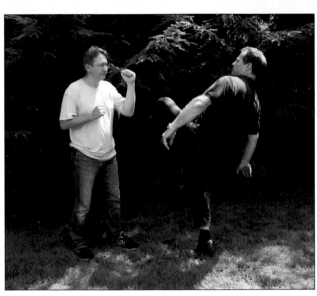
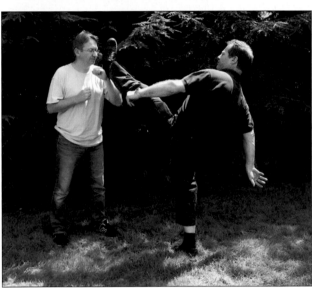
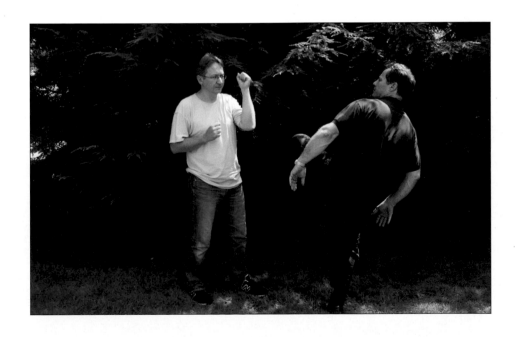

Inside Slap Kick

1. The defender steps forward landing on his base foot at a twenty-degree angle in front of the opponent.
2. The defender slaps the opponent's face with the inner side of his foot, with his body leaning backwards, and to the direction of the slap.

3. The defender retracts his foot to the previous position.

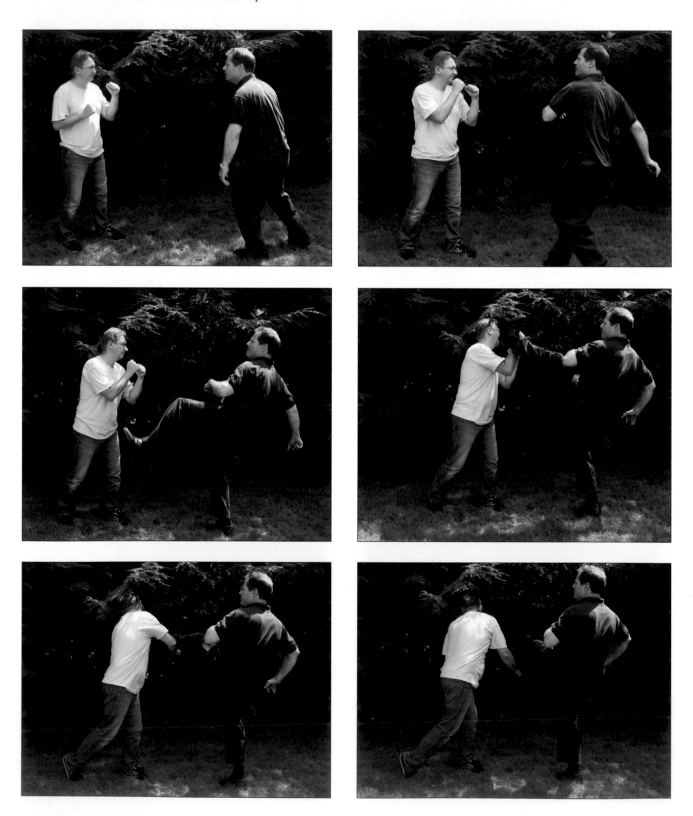

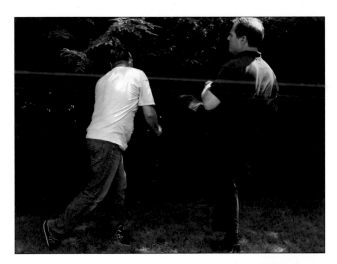

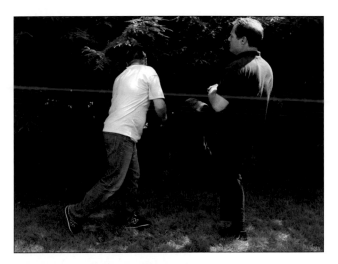

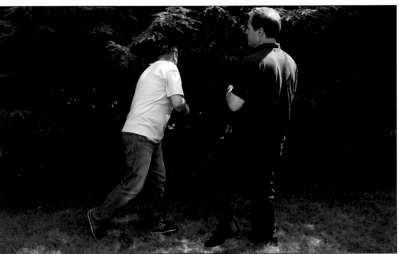

Jumping Kicks

Jumping kicks can be used to chase an opponent standing at a greater distance for a quick attack. If you want to stop an attacker from focusing on another target, you can sprint and reach him quickly with a jump.

Front jumping kick

A front jumping kick can be done by jumping with one leg and kicking with the other, or jumping and kicking with the same leg with the other going in a climbing motion.

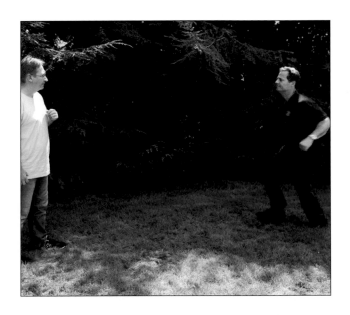

1. The defender runs toward attacker.
2. The defender jumps on his right leg and kicks with his left. The free leg is bent as the knee points backward to the right side, creating balance.
3. Using both legs for balance, land with all your weight in front of your opponent. Do not try to pass his body even if he is lying flat on the ground. You will endanger yourself if you land with your feet on his body, tearing your knee ligaments.

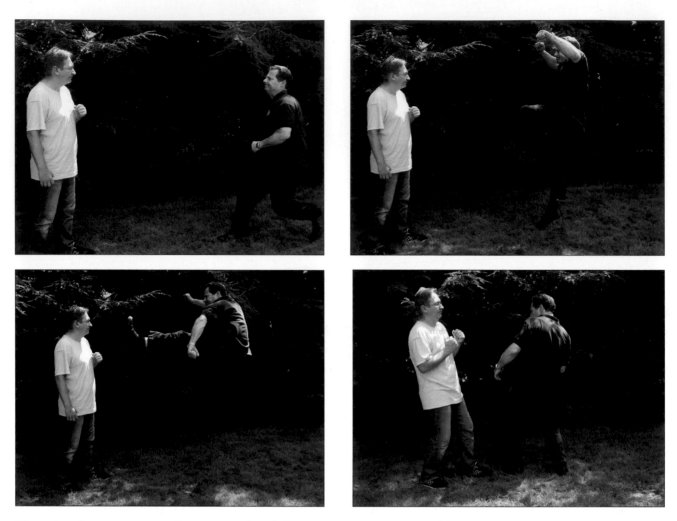

Note: Another variation, as demonstrated in defense against an attacker holding a knife in an under hold position, is where the defender jumps on his right foot and kicks it.

Jumping side kick

1. The defender sprints towards the attacker.
2. The defender jumps on his right leg.
3. The defender pivots to his right, keeping his left side forward.

4. The defender kicks the attacker with his left leg, moving his body in a corkscrew motion.
5. The defender lands on his right leg.

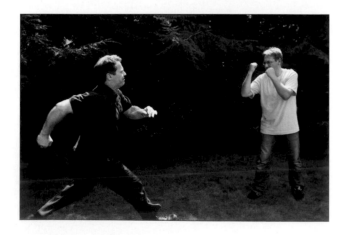
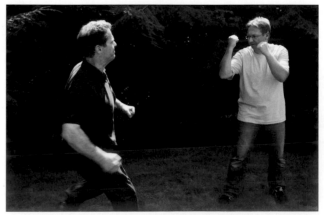

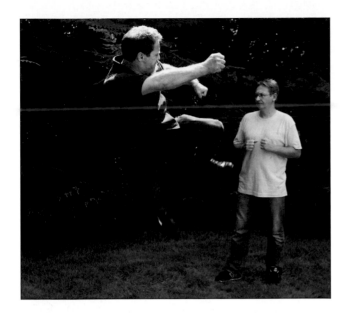

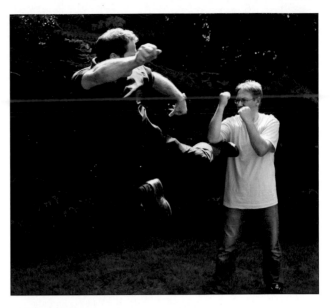

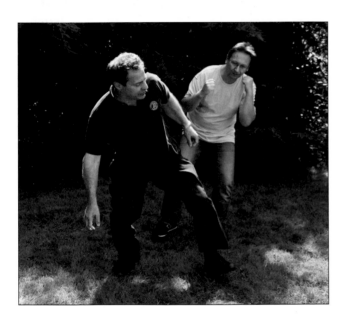

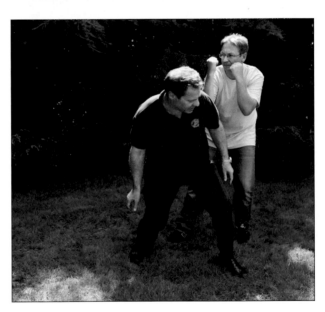

Note: It is possible to switch front to side jumping kicks in the same jump.

The defender jumps to front kick the attacker, but the attacker moves to the side. The defender pivots his body and side kicks the attacker before landing.

Defensive Front Kick

This kick is basically a quick push with the heel of your foot, shifting your body weight forward. You should use the whole bottom of your foot to block an opponent from charging at you. Generally in Krav Maga we classify two types of front kicks: attack and defense. The attack is done with the ball of the foot with upward motion toward the groin or the chin, or a slightly forward motion with the heel to the sternum. The defense is done by locking the knee before the whole foot contacts the target while shifting body weight forward to stop the attacker's momentum.

In the following demo, the training partner is crossing his arms on his chest and moving in. The arm-crossing protects his vital organs and pressure points.

1. The attacker advances toward the defender.
2. The defender lunges forward, landing with his base foot at a forty-five degree angle to the opponent.
3. The defender executes a defensive front kick.
4. The defender retracts his leg if possible, or lands on it if too much weight was shifted in the attempt to stop the attacker.

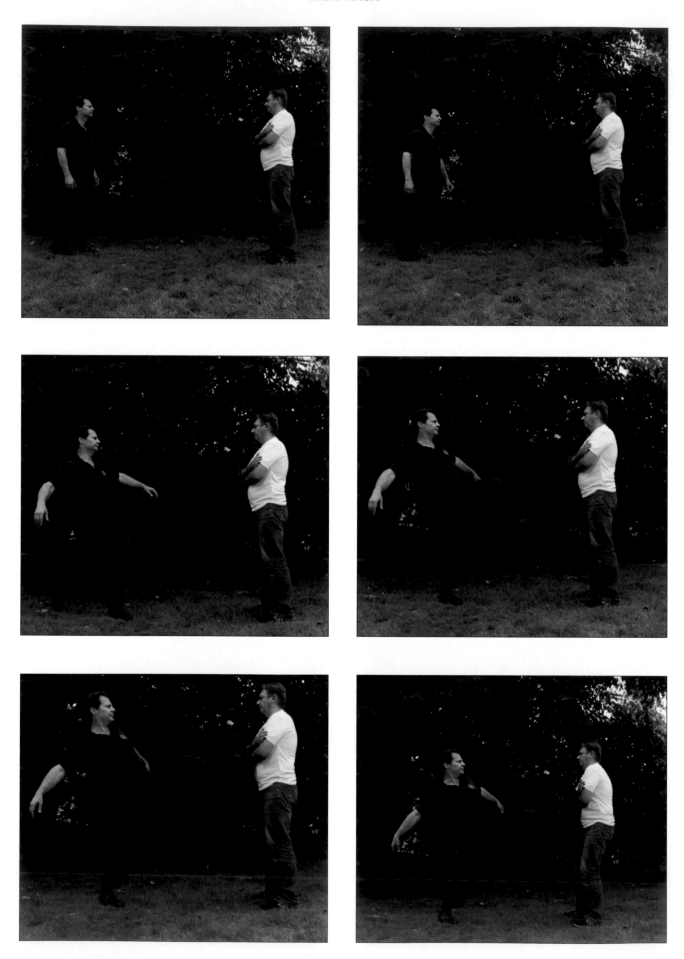

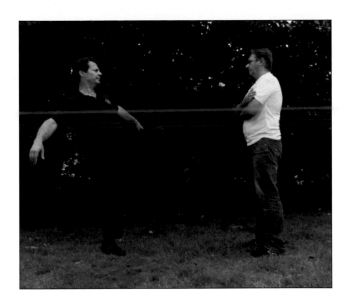

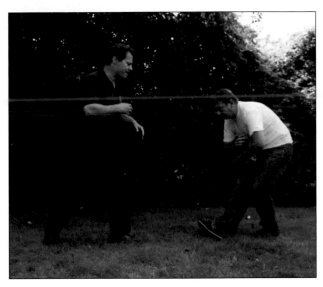

Aggressive Attack with a Defensive Front Kick

This technique is designed to clear an opponent quickly and aggressively out of the way, although it does involve risks.

1. The defender steps forward, kicking to the opponent's chest, keeping both his fists in front of his face and sending them forward. The extension of both arms and fists in front of his face creates a penetrating tool into the opponent's counterattack

as well as creates a distraction. A possible attack from the opponent would be deflected to the sides. This might prompt the opponent to move to either side.

2. After the initial attack, the defender continues to the relevant direction with a horizontal back-hand strike and a knee kick, or another front kick ending according to the situation.

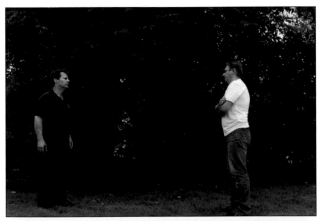

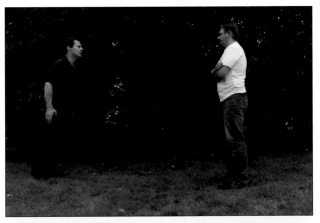

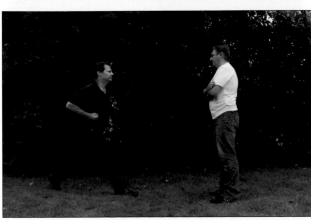

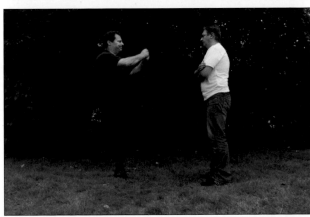

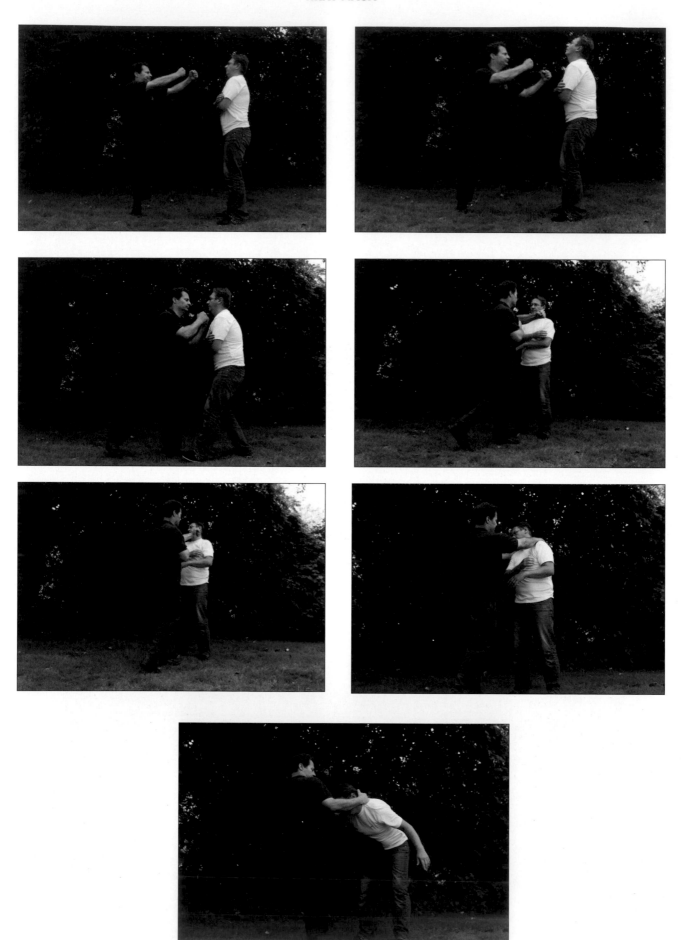

Stomp Kick

This kick is very useful in grappling scenarios from the front and back to the top of the opponent's top foot. See the chapter on close scenarios.

Kick to the Temple When the Attacker Is on the Ground

1. The attacker is on the ground.
2. The defender lifts his leg backwards to ninety degrees.

3. The defender kicks the attacker in his temple.

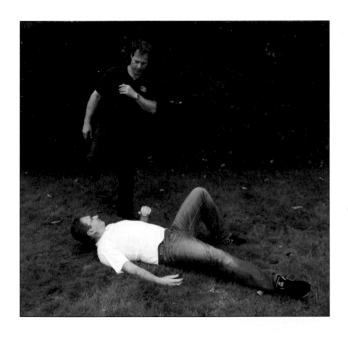
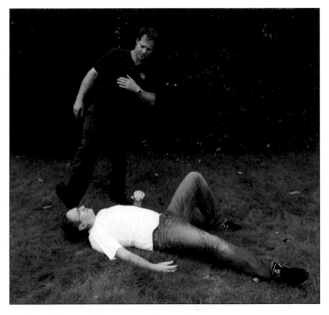

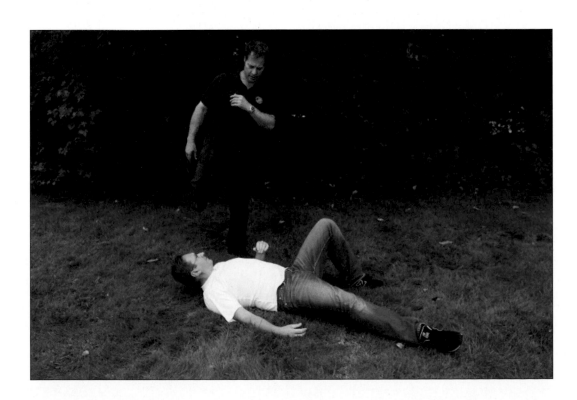

Defensive Kick Backward (Horse Kick)

1. The defensive back kick derives its force from a body leaning forward and then stomping backward, executed in a swing motion.
2. The defender stands with his side to the attacker.
3. The defender advances forward, landing on his base foot, heel pointed toward the opponent. His torso is positioned sidewise to the opponent.

4. The defender swings his leg to position his heel in front of the backside of the body. The defender swings his torso forward and down in a seesaw motion as he kicks backward.
5. The defender retracts his kicking leg to a sidewise position, ready for his next move.

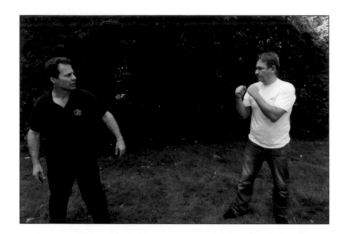 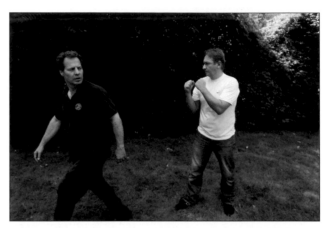

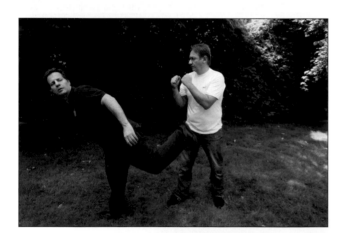 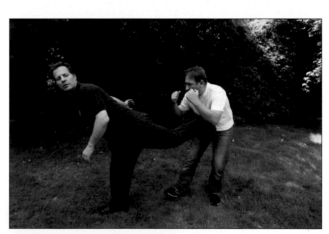

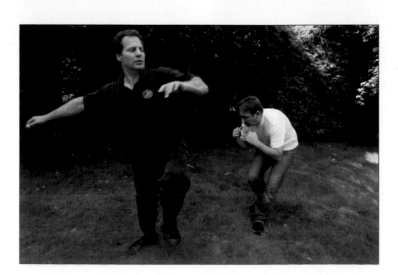

Sheering Kicks

A sheering kick is the Krav Maga refinement of a low kick to the calf, where the objective is to drop the opponent to the ground with one kick. It involves a forty-five degree upward kick contacting either of the opponent's legs. The angle is a key factor in this kick since it counters forces of gravity to create a loss of balance and to lift the opponent. If you kicked the front calf, and the opponent defensively moved away, you would spin backwards and kick the back calf. These kicks lie on the border between science and art. Remember, while they show impressive talent, I would not risk my life using them in a self-defense move.

Sheering kick to front leg followed by a full turn roundhouse kick to the opponent's back leg

1. The attacker stands at a forty-five degree angle.
2. The defender positions his base foot to kick the attacker's front calf upwards at a thirty-degree angle.
3. Attacker lifts his front leg defensively.

4. The defender continues with a spin to the back.
   a. The defender kicks the attacker underneath his rear leg calf with an upwards forty-five degree motion.

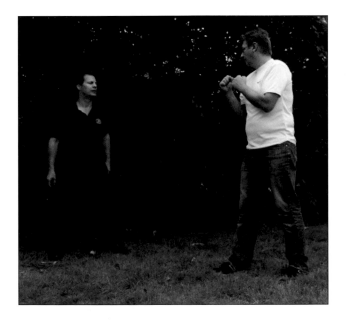

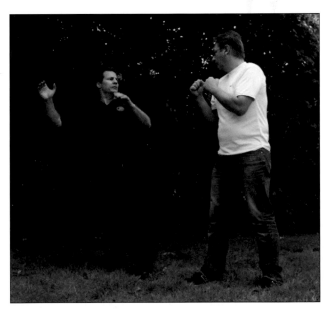

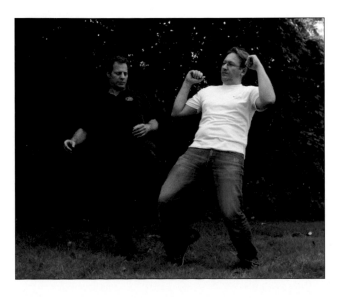

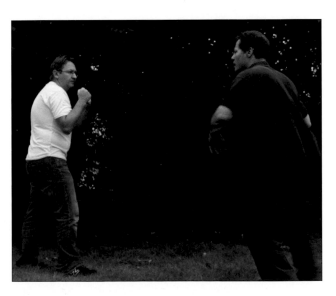

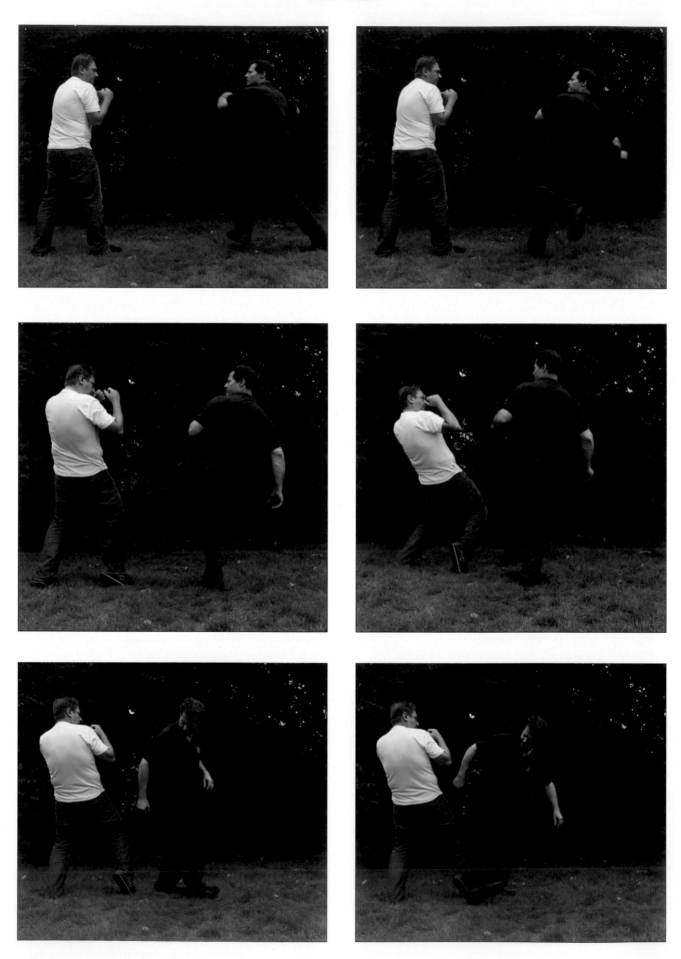

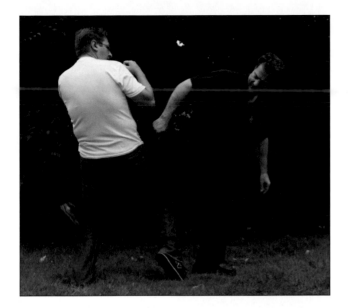
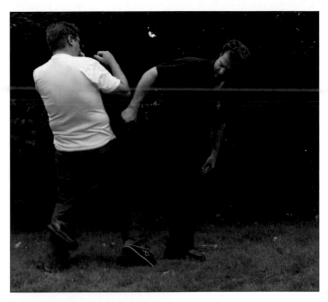

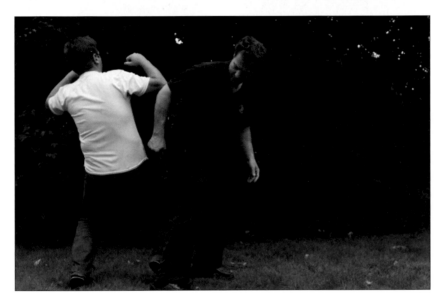

Note: When with a well-rounded training partner, these kicks could be easily blocked with a low defensive kick. I would not recommend them in any sort of fighting. You never know how experienced your opponent is.

Athletically Challenging Drills

In Krav Maga, advanced students are encouraged to try out athletically challenging drills. Some students make them their second nature when sparring. These complex techniques are not followed with detailed photo illustrations, since their components have been previously demonstrated. Some of these combinations are further demonstrated in the following chapter about advanced training methods. The reader is encouraged to look back to the components of each, and combine the parts to make a whole using hints for each combination.

Front kick and full spin roundhouse kick combination

This is a great technique that uses the momentum of the first kick. The retracting leg provides a pull for the spin here. The spinning roundhouse is executed when the first front kick is completed before the kicking leg has landed (see the chapter on advanced training for details).

In and out full turn slap kicks

Another athletically demanding combination is a full turn slap kick involving three different kicks with the body spinning in the same direction. The performer uses the outside of his foot, followed by the inside of his other foot, followed by the outer side of his first foot during a continuous spin.

12
PRINCIPLES OF DEFENSE AGAINST MULTIPLE OPPONENTS

When you are outnumbered, remember, it does not necessarily mean you are out-powered. By moving closer to one of your opponents and getting away from the rest, you can deal with one combatant at a time. You can use the body of one as an obstacle for the rest of the group.

Getting Out of the Center of a Circle

When encircled, throw two punches with one elbow to the three weakest group members.
1. The defender is surrounded by a group. The defender assesses his course of action looking for the weakest link.
2. The defender turns his head over his right shoulder, appearing to look at the attackers behind.

3. The defender pivots his body forward striking one opponent with his right elbow while at the same time he delivers a left punch and his right arm continues to deliver a punch to the middle opponent.
4. The defender takes advantage of the temporary shock for the rest of the group and bursts forward, escaping out of the human ring.

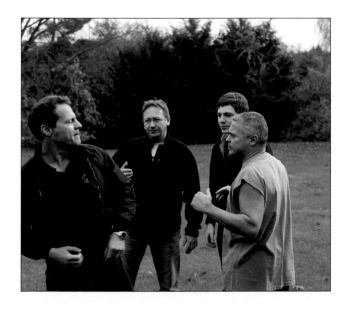

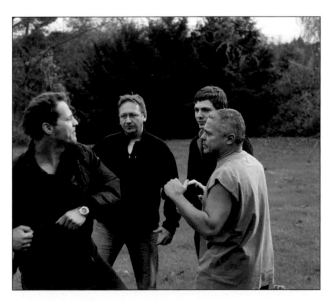

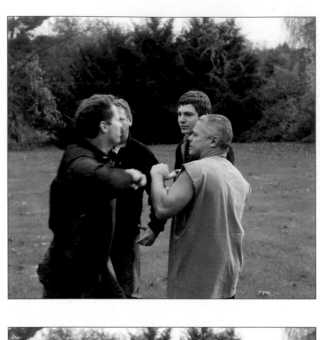
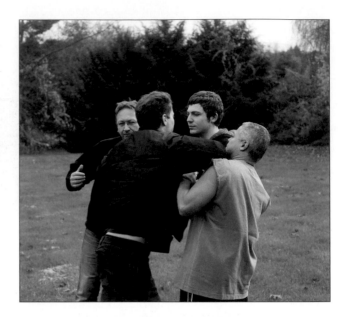
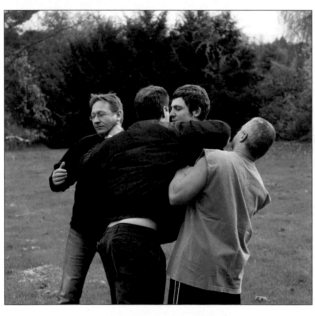
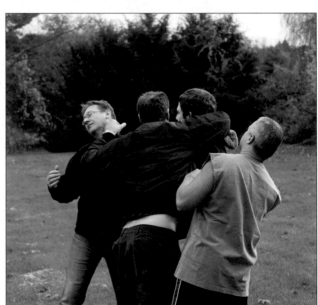
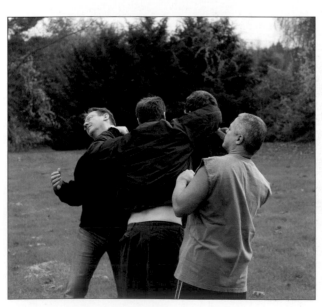
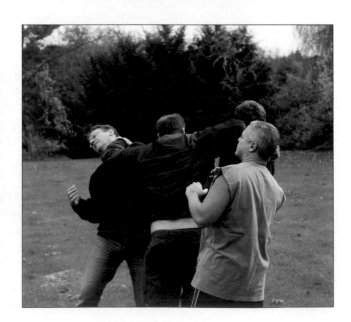

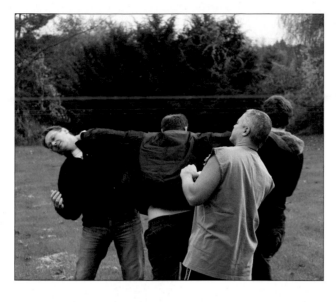

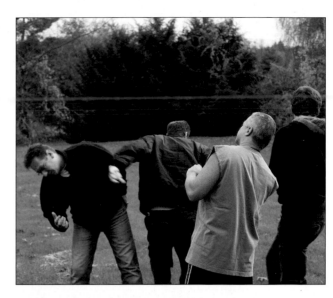

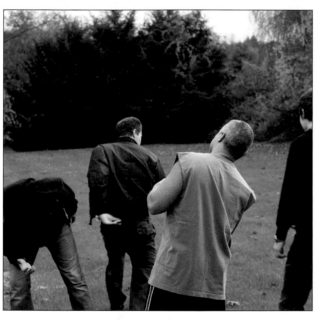

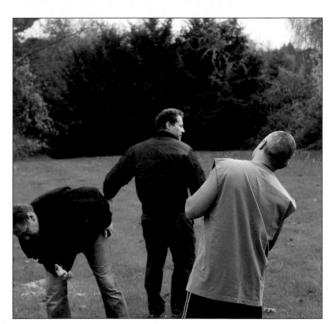

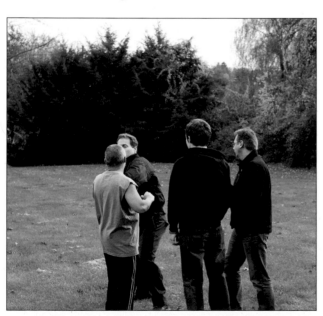

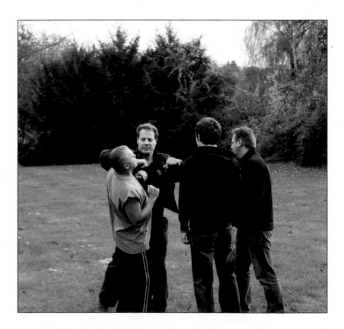

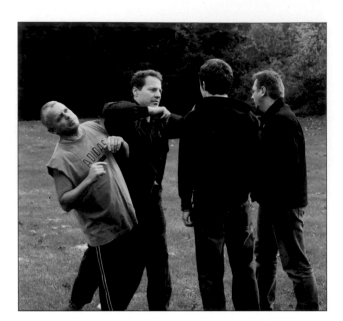
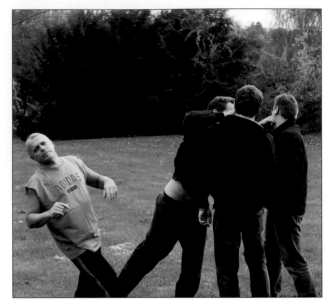

Attack by Two People, One with a Knife and One with a Club

1. If possible, the defender assesses the skill level of the attackers.
2. The defender goes for the attacker with the club first.
3. The defender deals with the club attack.
4. The defender takes possession of the club, throwing the attacker between himself and the next attacker.
5. The defender uses his club to thwart the attacker with a knife.

Note: for the steps and details in these techniques, refer back to the chapters on club defense, knife defense, and handy objects.

If you had no choice but to deal with the attacker with the knife first, you would still need to use your hands for defense against the attacker holding the club,

and you may use the knife for a counterattack if you have to. Remember, if you receive a club blow to your head, your newly acquired knife will not help you.

When attacked by multiple unarmed opponents:

As your opponents close the gap, move closer to one of them and deal with them one at a time according to the principles you have learned in previous chapters. Do not forget to try to assess whether any of them have weapons. Your next move would be to see if you would like to fight for a weapon first to use against the others, or if you would overpower someone else and use him as a shield against the others. You do not have much choice. You will choose whatever's closest to you, or, if time allows, move toward another nearby opponent. If you can assess the group's weapons and their ranges, you basically need to fight the one that can reach you faster.

Favorite Old Aikido Technique

I use this technique for fun and to teach you a few principles.

1. Two attackers hold down the defender's arms.
2. The defender pulls the lighter opponent using the heavier one as an anchor. The defender brings his right arm up while pivoting to the left with his forearm over his head, pulling the opponent's wrist

behind his back, assuming the lightest opponent is on the right.
3. The defender throws the lighter opponent onto the heavier one, hence getting rid of both.

Note: If you only have one training partner, you can grab the door handle and pull your training partner behind your back, letting his body hit the door. Also, remember that if the two opponents grabbing your wrists were standing still, you could have kicked them one after the other in the groin with alternate feet, or kick one in the groin and the other in the knee with the same kicking leg.

Advice for Hijacking Scenarios

If under a terrorist attack, assume you are fighting a group. If in a building, or on an aircraft, you may need to eliminate any enemy you encounter. You definitely do not have time to hold down one opponent. To avoid a recurring attack, make sure the opponent you just took care of is not alive before you go ahead and clear the rest of the area. In this case, it is faster to kill than to restrain.

ADVANCED TRAINING TOPICS
13

Getting Accustomed to Continuous Motion in Krav Maga

You need to be accustomed to continuous attacks. The logic behind these motions is based on the change in distance and the gain in time when reaching a vital pressure point, or when chasing after an opponent moving in different directions. Whatever move you devise, keep it logical, and do not make it too long—unless you want to use Krav Maga as a dance or exercise routine.

In the chapter covering defenses, I analyzed defense moves that utilize all the Krav Maga principles. But what happens if another equally skilled individual is fighting you? It appears that if you are both trained well, the defender always wins, since the Krav Maga defense moves completely neutralize the attack moves.

There are many martial arts experts that teach you not to be aggressive. We arrive at the same conclusions, but only after making sure our lives are no longer in danger anymore and exploring the best techniques.

I will present a few continuous attack scenarios that will demonstrate a few principles and show various connections. Generally, as the range increases, a follow-up kick is executed, and as the range decreases, a follow-up hand strike and then an elbow strike, a knee kick, or close range neck manipulation comes after.

When throwing someone on the floor or smashing an opponent's head against a wall, take into account that he can get up again and attack you. Why would you want to waste your time? Throwing an attacker out the window can be a good choice in certain scenarios.

There is nothing wrong in practicing martial arts on a regular basis. However, as you get accustomed to various options and scenarios, you grow accustomed to bad habits as well. Your second nature may be more suitable for the mat and not for the street. If, however, you completely understand the differences and get sufficient training in both, you might be able to make the switch. But devoting too much time to sports martial arts or fighting sports will make you try them instinctively, passing on more efficient opportunities and exposing yourself to more unnecessary danger and possible death.

Variation Number 1: Front Kick, Front Punch, Side Kick, Back and Hand Strike

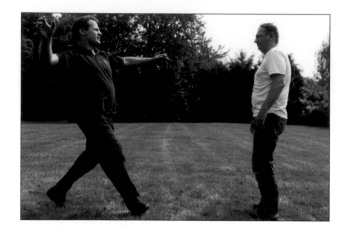 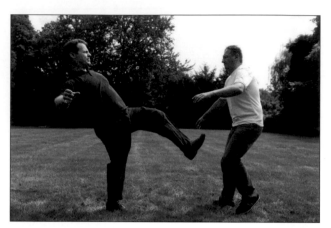

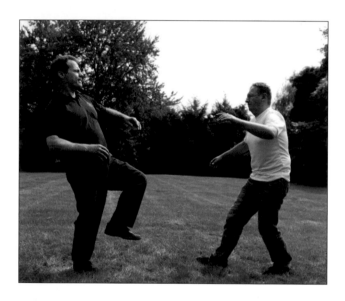 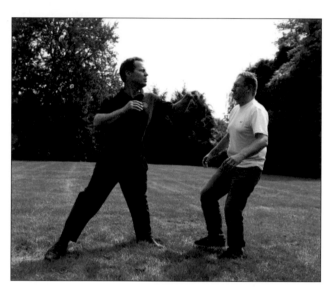

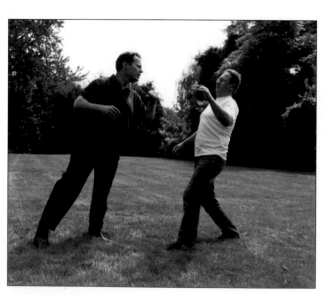 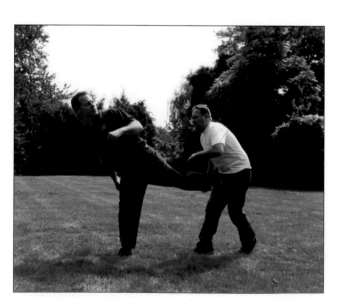

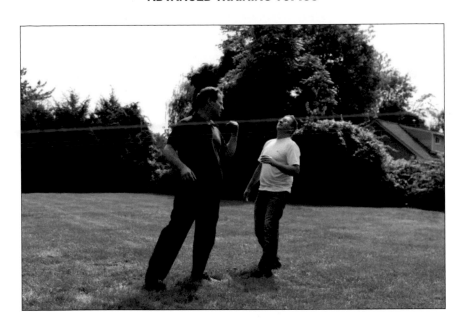

Variation 2: Front Kick, Front Hand Punch, Back Hand Punch, Back Leg Kick

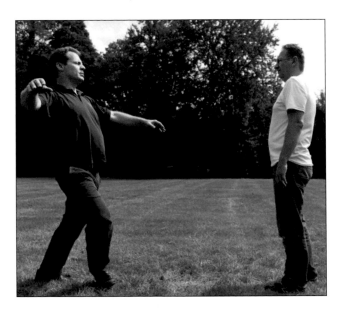 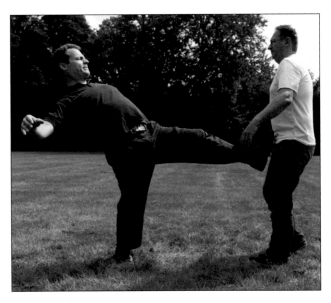

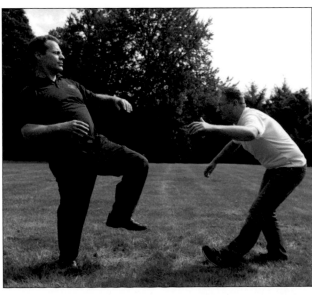 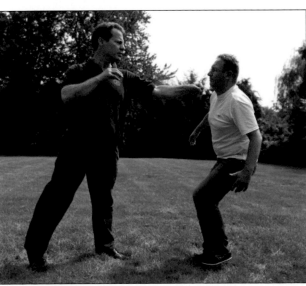

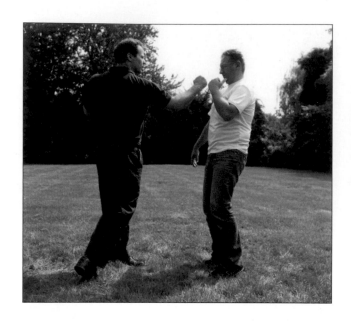
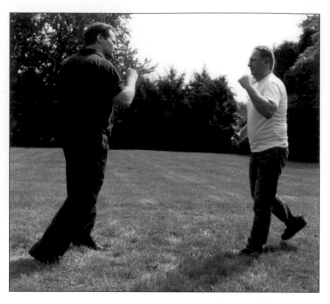
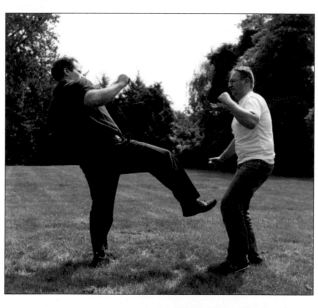
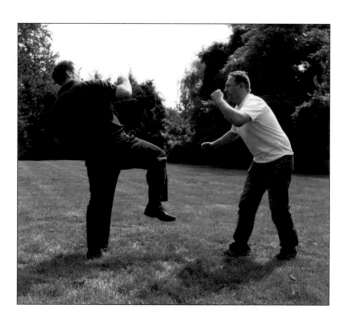
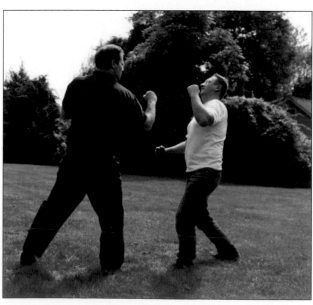
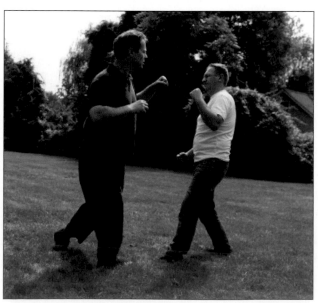

Variation 3: Front Kick and a Switch to a Full Turn Roundhouse Kick

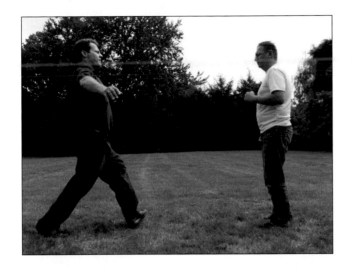
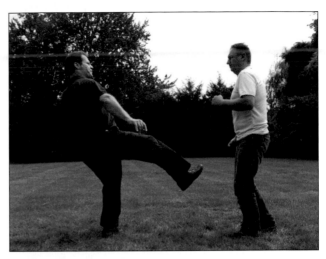

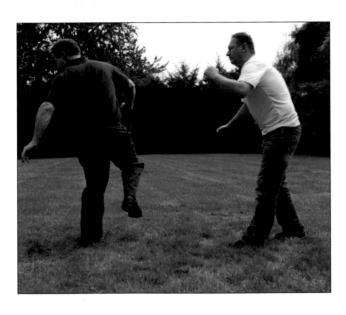
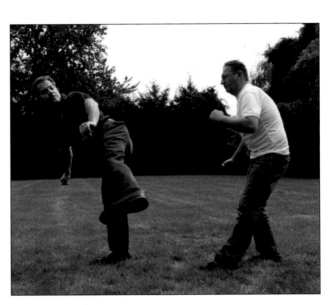

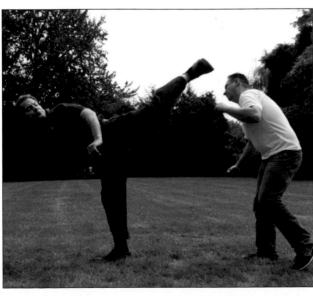
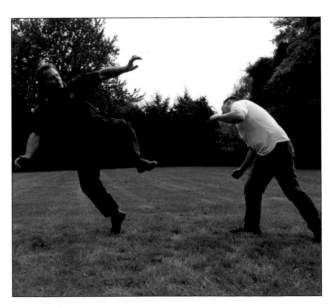

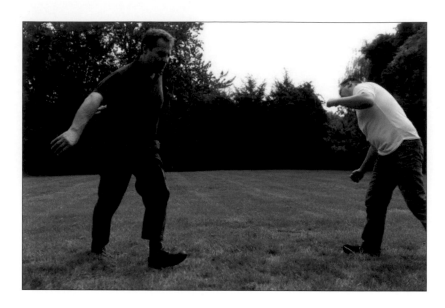

Variation 4: Side Kick and a Backward Switch to Another Side Kick (continue with back hand strike, elbow strikes, and knee kicks)

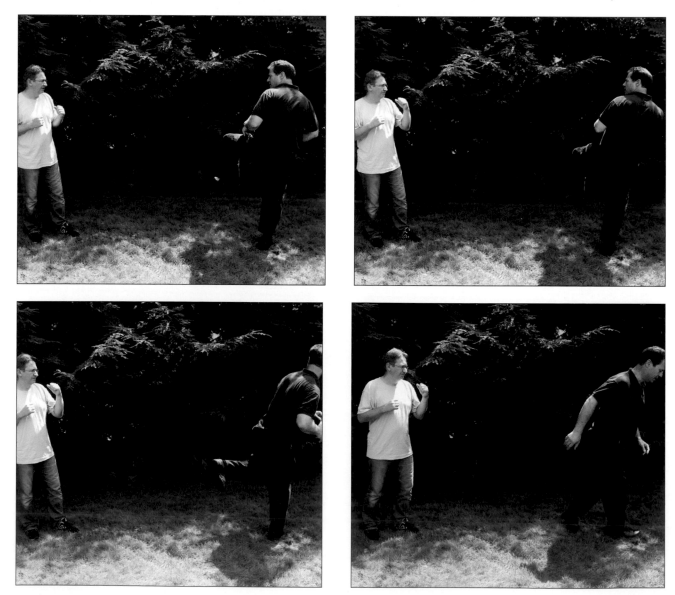

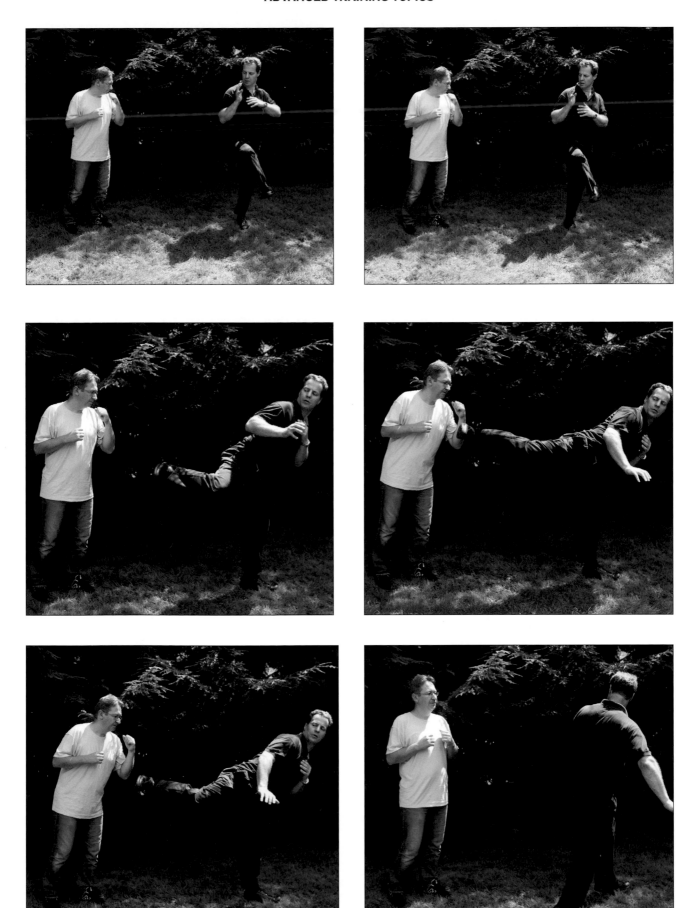

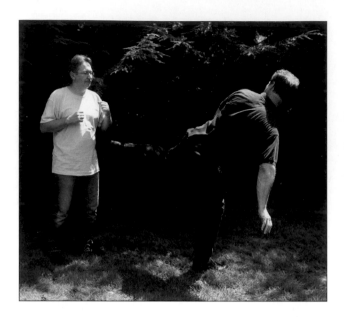 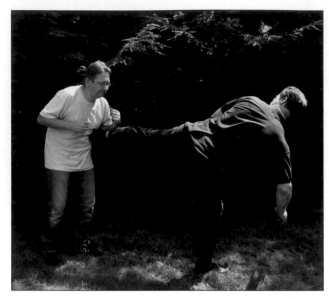

Variation 5

Front kick, then three hand strikes, then two horizontal elbow strikes, then grab the opponent and go for seven knee kicks, and finish with hammer punch (not demonstrated).

General Suggestions for Training

Do not forget to warm up appropriately for your training.

When learning Krav Maga, remember all the steps. They help train the body in following the basic principles of Krav Maga. They promote the breaking down of movement into the correct sequence. Cherish the emphasis points that help you save your life, and do not get bogged down by anything else.

Club or sword fighting can be simulated using any kind of plastic or wood instrument, and proper headgear can be acquired. Krav Maga moves are executed against the first intention of strike. Sparring is always a good way to check fluid response time of students in a surprise attack. Protective gear enables training partners to be less intimidated and try to hit their partners faster and stronger, creating a more realistic environment. However, more often, students tend to evade strikes by moving back and forth without getting accustomed to immediate and efficient solutions. In a way, the stick fighting method could start to resemble sword safety methods in predetermined blow and defense drills. You can create a few drills to demonstrate what happens if you do not succeed, but remember it is all up to the first blow.

Same with sparring using fists, kicks, and grappling. Only a continuous drill in a single motion or a sequence of motions will create an advantage and give you an understanding of fighting concepts and the ability to use judgment in applying them in motion. Remember that having your students wear protective gear while hitting each other with sticks does not promote many fighting benefits, unless the drill is designed to eliminate the immediate danger of getting hit first.

Krav Maga moves are designed to end the initial intentions of the attacker before he begins or finishes his attack. Modern streets are not swamped with samurai swords. If the instructor or student has an interest in sword fighting, he should go to a local fencing club and apply Krav Maga principles and weed out techniques that don't work. Remember that the samurai and aikido schools found in neighborhoods around the world use long-term training and drills using heavy swords in controlled environments to avoid accidental death. French and English fencing schools are much more dangerous and fast paced. You can also go on YouTube and watch various martial arts attacks to enhance your learning and confidence.

Training Techniques

The previous chapters consisted of teaching principles of Krav Maga through techniques that utilize the best motion and reaction time available to the human body. At the end of each chapter, you should practice these techniques in fighting drills as part of the learning process starting in a previously known sequence and continuing on to random sequences to allow real-life judgment and reaction to take place.

When there is more time in the budget, the Krav Maga instructor can include supervised fighting games with more rules that make defense moves harder to execute and more physically challenging. For example, using legs can be practiced between partners with a moderate amount of force. Another fighting drill involves using boxing gloves for practicing defense and counterattacks.

When kicking, a full technique should be used in a realistic way. However, cut the motion short once contact has been achieved. Learn to hit the skin without continuing onto vital organs or bones.

When punching, the same safety feature is applied. If one retrieves his hand without passing the target by too much, the effect can be controlled to cause a mild shock with a few split seconds of disorientation rather than a complete knockout and further damage.

The instructor should give clear instructions to the practitioners, and be sure he trusts them before starting the training. At every slight shock, the instructor should stop the fighting game, recognize the training partner that achieved a tactical advantage, and give the other time to recuperate. Remember that we do not want a full knockout in training, since recovery time can take up to three months.

For close fighting and grappling, drill your students in fighting games that involve controlling their opponents in a short range, preventing them from kicking vital pressure points while controlling their spatial comfort. This should also improve their ability to deliver blows, gouging or tearing down their opponents' soft pressure points. The grappling games will get trainees comfortable in falling, rolling, pushing, and pulling, while searching for a vital pressure point to strike in the close range.

The instructor must stress to students that too much of this training can lead to misconceptions, potentially costing you your life. In reality, ease and speed are utilized by the core Krav Maga self-defense techniques.

Krav Maga grappling drill

Two groups send representatives to the center of the training room.

Two training partners hold a ball and each one tries to take the ball in the opposite direction by taking it back to their group. Instead of a ball, each one tries to take his training partner back to his group. The game forces students to practice changing directions between pushing and pulling before the opponent has the time to redirect his resistance, emphasizing the importance of reaction time.

When to stop a fist fight simulation

It takes a person a few split seconds to recuperate from a slap to the cheek before trying to strike back. When an opponent is disoriented for even a couple split seconds, the Krav Maga trainer will stop the fight. Another option is to let the leading fighter continue with a combination of controlled attacks to keep the opponent disoriented for a few more seconds.

Students should understand that in reality, all it would take is to lift the restraint from the ending part of the striking limb in motion and penetrate their targets about three inches. Keeping realistic range in training is crucial for natural positioning in combat.

Instinctive defenses

Training partners alternate their roles of attacker and defender. The attacker tries to smack his partner on top of the head or shoulder. The defender practices outside defenses. The attacker tries to knee the defender, and the defender blocks this with the outside of his forearm.

The training partner in the attacker role tries to touch the defender on his sternum or forehead. The defender practices inside defenses on the opponent's wrist. The attacker tries to push the defender with both hands. The defender taps the attacker on the wrist, moving both the attacker's hands to the side. If he tries to move them down, the attacker should follow with a headbutt to discourage him from repeating his mistake.

From a close distance, the attacker repeatedly tries to shove his foot into the defender's stomach. The defender, initially with his hands to the sides of his body, blocks with the inner part of his forearm. The defender repositions his arms across his chest, moving to block the kicks by sliding them off with the outside part of his forearms in a continuous line to the back of his hand, keeping his fists closed.

Knockout simulation fighting game

The student leans his forehead onto the back of his hand. His hand is on a long stick perpendicular to the ground. The student turns in circles until he gets dizzy. He then drops the stick to the ground and tries to run to a predetermined corner of the room. From here, he can try to punch a pad or place a ball in a hoop. The purpose of this drill is to simulate a dizzying sensation and attempting to control your body when losing balance. With practice, there is improvement. Remember: Don't get knocked out with a punch when training. If you have a concussion, you can't fight for three months.

Measuring knockout power

While invaluable experience and confidence is gained through full-contact fighting, Krav Maga tries to break down the essential elements of fighting to simplify training, so students can master it in a short amount of time. The focus of training gears your mind and body for maximum benefit.

As a rule of thumb, the more you do something, the more it becomes a habit. When it comes to self-defense training, the Krav Maga training system teaches you in an intense few days what you would take years to learn in other sports and martial arts.

In Krav Maga, the emphasis is on instilling good habits from inception so they don't stab you in the back.

A few gender-related questions may come to mind. Can a female knock out a male with a punch? Can a female break someone's windpipe; KO him with an elbow to the chin? Can she kill him with a kick to his testicles?

Again, while scientifically the genders do have slight differences in their body composition, the differences between any two people (regardless of gender) are equally significant.

So if we distill this question, the questions that come to mind are: What is the minimum force required to knock someone out with a non-projected straight punch from the hip to the face with quick lunging to close the gap?

What is the minimum force required to squeeze someone's testicles until they die? What is the force required for someone to elbow his opponent for a knockout?

An exact answer would give students confidence in their striking force and give them a realistic sense of their options. Of course, you would also need to find a method to test your students' force with some sort of a mechanical computerized device.

Many reality shows claim to measure fighting arts and come up with numbers that are a result of complex mathematical formulas. Measuring force and direction is more complicated than that. Force can be measured by multiplying mass by acceleration. Force is measured in newtons and mass in kilograms or pounds, and acceleration is measured in units of distance per second. While Newtonian theories have been suppressed by the laws of special relativity, in human body speeds, they are still useful in approximate general comparisons.

There are many components that affect punches, like your body weight, your opponent's body weight, distance, how hard the surface you are punching is, how hard the opponent's body is. It appears that many scientists have a hard time measuring the force of a punch or kick in a meaningful way.

If we search for an answer, we see scientists trying to measure it with computers, sensors, spring-operated machines, and even CAT scans. The results of one CAT scan were interpreted by a karate expert who claimed that in a karate punch, the brain is a major contributor to the knockout because there is an increase in brain activity. Perhaps a better interpretation would be that the increased brain activity was just anticipation of the pain that would occur.

Traditionally, many karate styles recognize the need to develop a knockout or killing punch, in an attempt to correlate the ability to break one-inch boards or bricks with the ability to knock someone down.

We all know that the human body has bones that might be even stronger than wood or bricks, and other parts that are weaker. But it certainly is more mobile. Training should put more stress on reaching the target before becoming a target. There are many full-contact karate tournaments, but a very small percentage that end with a knockout, a trip to the hospital, or an accidental death. And yet, we do hear of the occasional street fight that ends in death with just a single punch.

Many boxers and martial artists spend a lot of time honing a technique that maximizes force and overcomes the limitation of gloves and other protection gear to deliver it.

So, to the average person trying to learn pure Krav Maga, there has to be some merit in learning how to punch quickly. If not, perhaps they should spend their life honing the competitive approach to increase force.

When a boxer knocks someone out, it is indeed because he causes his opponent's head to accelerate rapidly. The opponent's head decelerates rapidly because it is attached to his shoulders by a neck.

The brain has inertia and collides with the inside of the skull, causing trauma, dysfunction, and perhaps permanent damage.

The shift of fluid or a burst of blood vessels can cause trauma, internal bleeding, and possibly a coma or even death. In addition, the nerves located at the back of the neck can command the body to fall to the floor instantly. Perhaps this is a primitive mechanism designed to prevent further injury by putting the body to rest and healing its damage from the blows.

Hitting someone's head with a padded fist is still effective in causing loss of consciousness, but may require more force.

However, the unconsciousness is not caused by a blow to the brain. It is caused by the collision of the brain with the inside of the skull. Force won't tell us anything about what happened there. For that, you want to study momentum and its effect on impulsive damage.

Swinging strikes can change the complex calculation of the amount of force exerted on a target. But in a boxing fight, you rarely get a good chance to land a killer punch since the range might be too close or too far, meaning you cannot move your target at enough speed due to deceleration or not enough acceleration in too close of a distance. Or you may have enough speed but not judge the distance right and so may not put in all the force you would otherwise be able to.

With minimum projection, an average person can deliver a linear strike from his waist or shoulders to his opponent's face measured at least one and a half times his/her body weight, equivalent to the force exerted on a scale's spring that is calibrated to measure weight.

The forward lean of the upper body and shoulder twist shifts the body weight in the direction of the blow. The backwards lean of the torso helps to propel the leg upwards and contributes to the force of the kick. The momentum or the motion of mass with speed is the cause of effective blows and kicks.

In pure Krav Maga, when you strike, you basically accelerate your arm to maximum speed and follow by reaching the target at maximum speed. Carry the target about three inches, if possible, maintaining maximum speed while retracting the hand and maintaining a maximum weight shift.

The one and a half times body weight figure does not come from a formula; it is based on years of experience. Simply convert the newtons to pounds or kilograms and compare to your body weight. Be sure you can generate at least a few times more and that you have enough knockout force.

There are very complicated formulas to calculate force. In most scientific experiments done to measure the force of a punch, it appears that they didn't check to see if the results make sense.

You can't measure the maximum possible power to project in a split-second KO opportunity through a scale spring or some sort of boxing machine. Most KO's are done in a split second. The body naturally limits the parameters and gives its best shot for that time frame.

One of the questions to ask when trying to test the force required for a knockout punch is whether the punch was thrown in a non-projected fashion. Boxers do have a distracting fast jab to buy a few split seconds to get more force to a finishing punch. However, in Krav Maga, this is not a training option. If you assume your opponent might stab you with a knife, you do not always have this extra split-second luxury.

The human nerves play a role in sensing impact and commanding the brain to lose consciousness and prevent further injuries.

A single punch can cause death if it impacts the cervical bone and the cartilage cuts into the spinal matter, releasing a small amount of cerebro-spinal fluid and increasing the pressure in the brain. In just a split second, this can cause death. I do not know of any scientific experiments that can measure the force required for that, and what these numbers mean. We can try and find out if the average person without specialized training can be taught to deliver that kind of punch without any major changes to their muscular structure.

At the same time, we would like to find a way to measure athletes in their fighting sports potential.

With trial and error, we can increase the force and change the techniques of punching or kicking. The mechanics of the human body are too complex to mimic and measure accurately.

The force could be deflected through the angle of contact or could be increased with acceleration limited by starting positions that are too close or too far.

So first of all, the pure Krav Maga punch provides the non-projective parameters with optimal lunging capacity. Follow-up circular punches promote full body use of speed and mass.

The estimate of pounds required to knock someone out is given by trial and error. I am 200 pounds. When I was 150 pounds, I had no problem in knocking out a 250-pound man with a single punch to the front of the chin.

Trying to hit one of these boxing machines, I found that without projection or drag I was able to put time and a half my body weight into the split-second contact with no effort. I made sure it would be a lunge from a natural stance with no projection to strike at the same time I closed the gap. So there was no contact with the ground during the punch and I was not able to push it.

In my real knockout experience, I think I've used more force than is required because the man I was up against was taller and flew backward on his back, lifting his feet up.

I was trained in pure Krav Maga to punch my hand about three inches into the target, so it was not a mechanical and crash-like impact since my hand retracted and did not bounce from his chin.

It depends on the nerves of course, but let's concentrate on the minimum force required to KO someone from a front punch to the chin, since this is the most efficient approach, and when we are speaking about efficiency, we try to use the minimal advantage we might have against our opponent, which is the window of opportunity.

The way to measure a knockout force in pure Krav Maga is to have someone who has a fair amount of experience punch three inches into a mitt, and then get a sense of how far and fast it moves. Then he can compare the results of his students when they punch the training mitts, and know how to train them to achieve sufficient force.

Even if not a knockout, the strike should have enough stopping power to control the attacker and find another pressure point. This way, you can overcome even the biggest attackers. Part of the Krav Maga instructor training teaches you to make good judgment calls.

Things to consider when demonstrating Krav Maga techniques

When staging a demo of your techniques, consider the following:

Many Krav Maga instructors use jujitsu since it is more impressive. The human eye likes dramatic stuff. A person slipping on a banana peel is something that will raise a smile on any child's face. It is all about the action. The board-breaking karate punch has nothing to do with efficiency, nor does it consider the fact that your opponent is trained in counterattacks.

Another thing to think about is that an opponent's forehead is stronger than the boards or bricks you are breaking. You could break his nose but might need a few more kicks to finish him, unless you are just hoping for a concussion. If you like judo throws, instead of grabbing his body, why not go for a palm strike to his chin as you do a leg throw? You could also use your inner forearm to strike to the back of his neck if you are executing a hip throw. I hope you realize that if you wait long for the short strikes, you have skipped a better opportunity to finish the fight before he gets too close to you.

You want to eliminate the threat and not bring it closer to your body. Of course the question is how weak or how strong your punch was when he was standing up, and how many seconds you had to keep hitting him before you get sufficient resistance. If your stand-up strike was powerful, he will be flying away from you and towards the floor and you will never be able to get him in a judo throw and finish him on the ground. If your strikes are too weak, you lose your advantage of finishing him quickly and now have got yourself into a grappling game, maybe with a larger opponent. If so, you might not get the chance to hit him again. By demonstrating the artistic play of two bodies in motion, which has nothing to do with the efficient conclusion of a fight, you are selling garbage in the form of self-defense. If your audience buys it, you might be tempted to keep selling them what they are buying and teach them anything but self-defense. The idea of this book is that if you do it most efficiently then it is Krav Maga. Otherwise it is not.

The Secret of Krav Maga

The secret of Krav Maga is not really to master all other martial arts but rather to completely understand their principles, and to use your judgment in what option is best in each scenario, prioritizing the dangers starting with the opponent's capabilities (quick reach, reaction time) from any angle. In the process of training, you master the use of your body as a weapon, and master the most effective way to deliver strikes, defenses, and escapes.

Rhythm in Krav Maga

If you hit hard, you avoid getting hit, unless you miss. Of course, if an opponent hits you hard and you do not know how to avoid it, you could be gone yourself.

Almost any attack hard or soft can cause a distraction, which puts the defender in a temporary state of confusion, unable to see what is going on.

The essence of a good reaction is the ability to identify the original attack and take advantage of the counterattack in the split second when the opponent tries to reach you as you block or evade this attack.

The real problem with feinting the first move is not whether or not the strike or kick was fully executed, but whether the place they were executed facilitated a possible hit. It becomes more of a problem if the point is close to the border of your range.

Let's say you try to identify the opponent's capability from a certain distance and he keeps changing his body position as he gets closer.

You should not have much of a problem moving in and preemptively attacking because he will be in the middle of not knowing where he is.

But let's say your opponent kicks the air, and as you block the air and counter, he deflects your counterattack, and manages to counterattack you—you could be in danger.

The recipe for a good reaction lies in pure Krav Maga techniques and principles. Learning to apply them is a crucial factor in this training system.

Once you have mastered these techniques and principles, you need to go through a few simple drills where the training partner is trying to change his attack or combination in an attempt to break your line of defense. The defender should repeatedly succeed in his defense.

Martial arts and fighting sports have a different concept of self-defense.

The idea in boxing is to throw punches at any angle permissible on the human body. The back is not allowed, perhaps because it is unfair to attack from the back, or perhaps because it is assumed that once an opponent turns his back it is a sign of surrender.

The idea is to hit as much as possible and to get hit the least. This series of training methods promotes fitness and agility that will allow boxers to enter and exit in and out of the hot zone and throw quick jabs and powerful KO's. Most boxers will take some time to feel their opponent's strengths and be cautious not to stay too close until they figure their opponent out.

In Krav Maga students are not trained to fight in a ring. If they tried to use their tactics in the ring, they would be disqualified according to the rules of the sport. If they try to "fair fight" they will find that they do not have enough relevant experience. But Krav Maga students get well-rounded self-defense training that makes them aware of the whole picture quickly.

While boxers can take their time and get closer and farther and try and attack from a different angle, Krav Maga students learn how to use their legs to block and attack at a greater distance, their fists for punching, and elbows for the closer range.

In addition, they learn to use the opponent's momentum to their advantage to escape from grappling attempts and to smash, crush, or tear a soft pressure point.

Not all boxers are career boxers, and not all Krav Maga students are Krav Maga practitioners and take their training to the highest fitness level. The question is, if they did, would boxing training be good and useful to them? One thing for sure, it would definitely help them keep fit and would definitely help them compete in a boxing match. There is always someone who gained a lot of confidence with one knockout punch. I, however, do not believe it is a confidence-boosting factor. As for more training and more competitive fighting experience, I believe you can learn more with a good trainer than on your own. For students who just want to learn self-defense, there is less chance of having enough knockouts to gain complete

confidence, but they might get a nice surprise at what happens when they try to defend themselves.

If however you take boxing drills and use them for Krav Maga training, each boxing drill should be reconsidered and modified to include possible attacks from any distance.

What about the grappling sports like jujitsu, judo, and wrestling? As mentioned before, Krav Maga techniques consider the most efficient approach to any threat, and it is much easier to manipulate a soft pressure point directly than try to restrain the opponent first.

The same would apply to grappling. An experienced grappler would probably be more comfortable at quick maneuvers. Relying on a simpler, less complex and limited approach demands greater fitness.

De-Escalations of Threats

De-escalation comes from the idea that the best method to avoid violence is to try and calm down a possible attacker and avoid a confrontation altogether. Of course, it is an attempt to prevent violence from escalating.

But not being familiar with all the possibilities can increase the chance of injury or death.

Some violence is well thought out, and some tends to escalate. Attackers, angry customers, citizens, and employees take their time and plan their act of violence. Some have a plan and process that increases in intensity during the confrontation.

For the unfortunate victim caught by surprise, trying to de-escalate the situation without knowing all his options might cause the element of surprise to be lost. This means he might be losing his opportunity to defend himself before it is too late.

Most perpetrators often use the element of surprise, picking easy targets that they feel they can manipulate by force and surprise. The defender is often using the element of surprise back to try to cause reversal of fortune.

To make the long argument short, let's say someone verbally or physically crosses the social boundaries to get what he/she wants, disregarding your own physical and audible boundaries.

At the first signs of this, you should counter it with greater resistance and surprise the attacker back without giving him the opportunity to retreat, unless you are certain you have the resources to counter them back!

Depending on the environment, and your resources, you should know what your capabilities are

and be able to judge whether your confrontation could turn into a life-threatening situation.

Be careful you are not misinformed. You get your bearings by what you read and hear and watch in your environment, and from your personal sense of safety.

Of course, when a possible attacker gets close to you and crosses into your personal territory, he might inflict harm upon you before anyone else might be able to help.

In terms of hand-to-hand combat, this means that once someone shows their intention or ability to immediately hurt, you need to neutralize him. As long as you are aware of your body's fighting capabilities, you can apply your solutions. The worst thing that can happen is you losing the element of surprise.

Your opponent has lost his when he shows you signs of violence. If you are a small female, and a man is trying to hurt you, instead of kicking him in the groin and then plucking his windpipe or testicles, if you chose to threaten him by calling the cops, you are losing the element of surprise.

While you talk to him he can finish what he started, or pause, listen to you, and make up his mind and then finish what he started and surprise you again. In fact you should have kicked him before he got closer and was able to reach you.

You could have called the cops if your door was locked, and he could not hear you and was not breaking your door down while you stood behind it with no place to hide.

The de-escalation process does not necessarily mean the use of one technique or another. You want to increase the quantity of strikes using less power to achieve nerve control and decrease in injury.

Perhaps your only resort to de-escalate the violence is to instantly kill your opponent to prevent harm to your body. Once your opponent gains advantages in the element of surprise, he can escalate it to higher levels.

The key is responding in the constraint of reaction time. If you run out of time and distance between you and your opponent, you will not be able to identify his next move and respond to it properly.

Your mind might still be analyzing and thinking about how to respond in the split second during which he might make you unconscious and then choke you to death or cut you to pieces. Remember, you need time to process what you see and to use your body as a weapon. Body language, eye contact, a facial expression of confidence, and a forceful use of voice might deter an attacker, or give him sufficient warning to reconsider. But never say what you will do to him, since you want to keep the element of surprise. If he gets threateningly close, immediately reach for his throat saying "do not stand that close to me," and prepare to get him out of commission.

In conclusion, I hope you have learned a lot from this book and have a good idea of what is good to do and what is not, and what kind of training you are looking for. My hope is that you will understand what Krav Maga is, or what gave it its great reputation. Perhaps the name today is used generically by all sort of folks, but at one point in history it meant something unique. My idea in writing the book was to give you a unique path to find out how to defend yourself as needed. I felt that if I did not put it in writing, the accumulated knowledge and the systematic hand-to-hand combat training system of Krav Maga would have been lost.

This book's purpose was to show you efficient ways of hand-to-hand fighting, and how it can be done quickly and methodically. Generally, if a weaker person goes for a weaker pressure point, he can get good results. You still, however, need to go through the whole process. While every step of the process can increase your awareness, you need to complete your training. Remember that in a short few days, you will learn much more self-defense than in five years of other martial arts. However, you need to make sure you spend enough time in putting your theoretical and partial knowledge together to achieve a level of fluidity. Krav Maga was able to bring your mind into use and draw the whole picture of intensive hand-to-hand combat. Since many people learn a lot more than they expect in an intensive Krav Maga course, they might think they know it all. Well, you need to get sufficient training to have enough techniques selected, and know the agreed-upon attacks and defenses that are the most efficient. But you need to drill yourself with training partners in fluid response to various attacks and defenses, using all the principles together. Finally, you need to try to confuse your training partner and try to surprise him by attacking using variations of parts of the principles. Remember that in training, the student and instructor should not rush to a challenge. No one should want to get hurt, nor should they want to hurt their training partners. After all, why would you want to train with someone you want to hurt? If you do hurt someone you want to train with, you will not have anyone to train with and others will not want to train with you. Once you understand and are able to execute the techniques, you need to get to a point where you forget them in action. Your mind, body, and soul need to freely feel what is about to happen and stop it before you even start to think. This is the ultimate state of Krav Maga.